GW00888565

PATRIC

HOLFC...

with David Miller PhD and Dr James Braly

how to
QUIT
without feeling
S**T

PIATKUS

PIATKUS

First published in Great Britain in 2008 by Piatkus Books

Copyright © 2008 by Patrick Holford, David Miller and James Braly

Reprinted 2008 four times, 2009

The moral right of the authors has been asserted

All rights reserved
No part of this publication may be reproduced, stored in a retrieval system,
or transmitted in any form or by any means, without the prior permission in
writing of the publisher, nor be otherwise circulated in any form of binding or
cover other than that in which it is published and without a similar condition
including this condition being imposed on the subsequent purchaser

A CIP catalogue record for this book
is available from the British Library

ISBN 978-0-7499-4022-5 (HB)
ISBN 978-0-7499-0994-9 (TPB)

Edited by Jan Cutler
Illustrations by Rodney Paull
Designed and typeset in Plantin Light by Paul Saunders
Printed and bound in Great Britain by CPI Mackays, Chatham, ME5 8TD

Papers used by Piatkus are natural, renewable and recyclable
products sourced from well-managed forests and certified in
accordance with the rules of the Forest Stewardship Council.

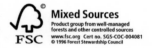

Mixed Sources
Product group from well-managed
forests and other controlled sources
www.fsc.org Cert no. SGS-COC-004081
© 1996 Forest Stewardship Council
FSC

Piatkus
An imprint of
Little, Brown Book Group
100 Victoria Embankment
London EC4Y 0DY

An Hachette UK Company
www.hachette.co.uk

www.piatkus.co.uk

Dedication

This book is dedicated to all the people who have tried, and failed, to break free from addiction. We hope this book will give you the missing piece you have been looking for.

The advice and insights offered in this book, although based on the authors' extensive experience, are not intended to be a substitute for the advice of your doctor or other suitably qualified person.

Neither the publishers nor the authors accept any responsibility for any legal or medical liability or other consequences which may arise directly or indirectly as a consequence of the use or misuse of the information (nutritional or otherwise) contained in this book.

You are advised to seek medical and/or nutritional advice from a suitably qualified practitioner about the treatment of your specific condition and/or before changing or ceasing any recommended or prescribed medication or nutritional or other treatment programme. You are also advised to seek medical and/or nutritional advice from a suitably qualified practitioner before taking any medication or nutritional supplement(s) or adopting any other treatment programme.

About the Authors

Patrick Holford BSc, DipION, FBANT is a leading spokesman on nutrition in the media, specialising in the field of mental health. He is author of 30 books, translated into over 20 languages and selling over a million copies worldwide, including the *Optimum Nutrition Bible* and *Optimum Nutrition for the Mind.*

Patrick Holford started his academic career in the field of psychology. In 1984 he founded the Institute for Optimum Nutrition (ION), an independent educational charity, and was involved in groundbreaking research showing that multivitamins can increase children's IQ scores – research that was published in the *Lancet* and the subject of a *Horizon* documentary in the 1980s. He was one of the first promoters of the importance of zinc, antioxidants, essential fats, low-GL diets and homocysteine-lowering B vitamins such as folic acid.

He is director of the Food for the Brain Foundation and director of the Brain Bio Centre, the Foundation's treatment centre for people with ADHD and autism, depression, dementia and schizophrenia, and those recovering from addiction, where a nutritional approach is used. He is an honorary fellow of the British Association of Nutritional Therapy. He teaches, researches and pioneers nutritional approaches to mental-health problems.

Patrick's work in addiction Patrick has had a major interest in addiction since the 1970s when he graduated in psychology. In his holidays he worked in treatment centres, ranging from halfway houses in the East End of London (whose residents would sometimes resort to hairspray to get their fix) to residential treatment centres for professionals at the other end of the social scale. He also worked in a treatment centre for heroin addicts.

He later specialised in mental illness, from depression to schizophrenia, and became convinced that nutrition was the vital missing key, since the brain not only depends on, but is literally built from, nutrients commonly lacking in our Westernised diets. He studied the approaches of the late Dr Linus Pauling, a twice Nobel prizewinner, and became the student of Dr Abram Hoffer, who pioneered nutrition-based approaches to addiction back in the 1960s, with amazing success.

David Miller PhD has worked in the addiction field for 30 years. He was associate professor of addiction studies at Graceland University in Missouri, where he was on the faculty for eight years. Before that he taught addiction studies at Park University in Missouri for 11 years.

David's work in addiction Over the last 30 years David has practised addiction counselling in private practice, in an intensive outpatient treatment programme, in a detoxification programme, in a family intervention practice and in a food addiction programme. He has also acted as consultant to numerous treatment centres.

The focus of his work and research has been on finding effective treatment methods to aid those for whom traditional treatment has not worked. His research has led him to the conclusion that many of these people are not without motivation but are attempting to cope with physical problems that interfere with their ability to stay clean or sober. He has developed strategies for increasing sobriety skills and has pioneered nutritional approaches for preventing relapse that address the physiology of addiction.

David has been in recovery from alcoholism himself since 1974. Since that time, he has had a desire to pass on what he learned the hard way to those people for whom staying sober is most difficult. His own recovery was extremely difficult for several years. He struggled with hypersensitivity, mood swings, irritability and anger outbursts, even while working as an addiction professional. After several years he found relief from the most disturbing symptoms by taking amino acid supplements recommended by a colleague. This put him on a search for more effective ways to relieve abstinence symptoms. He worked with different types of addiction, including food addiction in people with type 2 diabetes, most of whom struggled with abstinence symptoms that lasted over a long period of time. He pursued and utilised various methods of reducing those symptoms, the most successful being the nutritional strategies we offer you in this book. Several years ago David met Dr James Braly, who has researched, improved and refined nutritional therapy. Dr Braly, David and his wife Merlene have worked as a team committed to furthering this work. Merlene, an expert in addiction and a skilled writer and communicator, also contributed greatly to the writing of this book.

Dr James Braly has specialised in alternative and nutritional treatments for numerous chronic conditions, including addiction, for 30 years and is currently researching nutritional approaches for addiction. Dr Braly has authored many books including *Dr Braly's Food Allergy and Nutrition*

Revolution, *Dangerous Grains*, *The H Factor* and *Hidden Food Allergies*. He has helped establish nutritional treatments in many medical clinics and treatment centres in the US.

James's work in addiction Working with David and Merlene Miller, James Braly has pioneered and developed a highly effective nutritional therapy for addiction. He conducted the first semi-quantitative study of efficacy and safety of intravenous and oral nutritional therapy for recovering alcoholics. He introduced and popularised testing for and treating hidden (IgG) food allergies, the concept of leaky gut syndrome and the importance of lowering homocysteine – factors that affect many people recovering from serious addictions.

During his clinical years in the 1980s, James often made use of high-dose supplements and vitamin and mineral therapy to help addicted clients through severe withdrawal symptoms while coming off coffee, sweets and other addictive foods. Years later he was approached by the Millers to research and develop an intravenous nutrient formula and protocol of diet and supplements that could rapidly reverse sobriety symptoms in recovering alcoholics and drug-dependent clients. For several years he has focused exclusively on helping those with some of the worst addictions, who have struggled to become and stay drug-free or sober.

It is the combined expertise of the authors that makes this book unique. Patrick Holford provides the benefit of his extensive study and experience with optimum nutrition; David Miller has many years of direct experience working, with Merlene, in the field of addiction; James Braly applies his knowledge of nutrition and medicine to the problem of addiction. What they have created together is an easily understandable and highly effective new approach that will enable you to free yourself from your dependence on substances that keep you from being healthy and happy.

ACKNOWLEDGEMENTS

First of all we would like to thank the amazing Merlene Miller, who took all our material and painstakingly pieced it together in a clear way. We think of her as the 'fourth' author, and deeply thank her for her weeks of devotion to this project.

We would also like to thank Dr Hyla Cass, co-author with Patrick of *Natural Highs*, for her permission to use certain sections of the text and figures in this book. Our thanks goes to Oscar Ichazo for his permission to use the material on the Doors of Compensation in Chapter 5. Also, thank you to Jane Nodder for her permission to use material on eating disorders (this appears in the appendices, which are on our website www.how2quit.co.uk).

We are grateful for the work of Kenneth Blum, whose research into the addictive brain has been invaluable to us and has laid the foundation for our approach to healing the addicted brain. We are also deeply grateful to the other pioneers in nutritional medicine such as Julia Ross, author of *Diet Cure* and *Mood Cure*, Joan Matthew Larson, whose book *Twelve Weeks to Sobriety* has helped thousands of people, and Dr Abram Hoffer, the first pioneer of a nutritional approach, who guided us in our work. Dr Joseph Hibbeln's path-breaking research on essential fatty acids and brain cell membranes helped guide us in this very important area of research. We are also indebted to Dr William Hitt for his pioneering work in intravenous nutritional treatment for addiction. We would also like to thank the many scientists and addiction experts who checked and advised us regarding various sections of the book, especially Dr Joanne Lusher from London Metropolitan University.

Also thanks to Gaby, Patrick's wife, for her support and feedback during the months of early mornings and late nights researching and writing this book. David would like to thank his family for their continuing support. We would also like to thank Jan Sloan, Jane Heywood and Bev Youngman for their help in manuscript preparation, as well as Ruth and Monique for help with research, and all the team at Piatkus/Little, Brown, especially Gill Bailey, Jillian Stewart and Jan Cutler for their support, encouragement and sharp editing.

CONTENTS

INTRODUCTION

The vast majority of people have some level of desire, craving, dependency or addiction to one or more substances. Presumably, since you are reading this book, this includes you or someone you care about. Which substances are affecting your life? They may be the addictive substances that are more culturally acceptable within limits (alcohol, caffeine and cigarettes), or the others that are not (heroin and cocaine), or they may have been prescribed (sleeping pills, antidepressants and stimulant drugs).

You may be mildly dependent on these substances: getting on with life, and perhaps experiencing some benefits as well as some downsides. Or you may have tried to quit because you wanted to be healthier, but the discomfort this caused prompted you to start using the substance again. Or you may be – or you may know – one of those people whose lives have been ruined by addiction to the point where they are desperate to quit and may have attempted to free themselves many times but have been unable to do so.

Perhaps you have successfully quit an addictive substance, expecting to feel so much better, only to find, months or even years on, that you still feel lousy. Whichever of these situations apply to you, the chances are that you have experienced some level of what we call 'abstinence symptoms'. These are symptoms that emerge when the addictive substance is removed, and they include cravings; hypersensitivity to stress, noise or pain; feeling 'empty' or incomplete; not feeling 'normal'; feeling anxious or shaky; having problems with memory or sleep; experiencing fatigue, mood swings, restlessness and impulsiveness or depression – in short: pain and misery.

It is these symptoms that often cause you to return to the addictive substance, whether it is sugar, nicotine, caffeine, alcohol or cocaine – so, sadly, most attempts to quit fail. But now you can change that.

We have a revolutionary approach that has been tried and perfected over the past 25 years in the US and is now being revealed to UK readers for the first time. What's more, it's completely natural – you can now beat your addiction, without using any additional drugs, and feel great in around 12 weeks (although some dependencies need to be tapered off gradually and will take longer than this period); for mild addictions you can even look forward to feeling better within four weeks.

Our method has been proven to work time and time again. It can relieve you of your addictions, giving you a new lease of life and freedom from the grip of an unhealthy, and often dangerous, dependence that has probably dominated your everyday existence. What's more, instead of having cravings and abstinence symptoms you'll feel great. The case of Nancy, below, is typical of those we regularly hear from who we have helped to free themselves of addiction.

Case study **NANCY**

'For ten years I was hooked on prescribed antidepressants, tranquillisers and stimulants, plus marijuana. I am 15 months "clean". I definitely feel that I would not have been able to come

*off drugs successfully had I not gone through your programme.
I truly believe that your approach to treating addiction disease
is the best out there. I'm extremely grateful.'*

So what makes our natural method so different and so success-ful? Firstly, let's look at the case of Ben. When he tried to quit his addiction to opiate painkillers he suffered so badly with absti-nence symptoms that he tried all kinds of other unhealthy ways to make himself feel better and eventually made himself very ill indeed. He had tried so hard to get off the drugs and the other substances he was taking – it certainly wasn't because he was lacking in any willpower – but it wasn't until he tried the nutri-tional approach that we offer you in our How to Quit programme that he was able to kick all the bad habits and live life to the full again.

Case study BEN

Ben is a doctor who struggled with addiction to opiate medica-tion for years. When he could no longer hide his addiction, he was told to get treatment or he would not be allowed to practise. He went into a treatment programme and made a commitment to stay off the drugs, promising himself he would never jeopar-dise his career again. He loved practising medicine and could not imagine his life without his chosen profession, but he was soon experiencing high stress levels, hypersensitivity to everything around him and severe cravings. He found that he could reduce the severity of these symptoms with sweets.

Soon he was addicted to sugar, although he didn't realise it. As he gained more and more weight and developed diabetes, he made a valiant effort to eliminate sweets from his diet, but when he did, the old symptoms and cravings returned. He not only craved sweets but also the opiate drugs he had quit. Soon he found himself using them again and having the same problems they had caused him in the past. He was caught again and his medical registration was suspended pending two years without drugs.

Although he had more treatment and started going to a 12-step support group, nothing relieved his symptoms, especially his craving for sweets. However, he thought it was better to eat sweets than to go back to the addiction that could cost him his medical registration forever. He resumed a junk diet and began smoking – anything to keep him from using opiates again. Then, a new disaster struck: he had a heart attack! Hardly surprisingly, he was told that he must change the way he ate and had to give up smoking.

Now, not only was his profession in jeopardy but also his life. At this point someone told him about a place that used a nutritional approach to treat addiction. However, he was worried about what they expected him to give up and was ready to abandon the plan before he even got started.

Then he met David Miller, who encouraged him to give it a try. David shared his own story about the relief he got from not only eating healthily but also from taking amino acid supplements. 'David saved my life,' Ben says. 'I would never have given nutritional therapy a chance without the hope he gave me.' Ben immediately began the amino acid supplements along with other nutrients. He found that his craving for drugs and sweets – and even nicotine – was so much less that he was able to stick with his new nutritional plan. His other abstinence symptoms disappeared within days, and he began to feel better than he had ever felt in his life.

He has now been abstinent from drugs and sugar for several years and, despite some ups and downs in the recovery of his health, enjoys a quality of life he never thought possible.

Like Ben, you can use our programme in order to beat your addiction naturally.

Conventional addiction treatment, *alone*, whether it's giving up smoking or alcohol, does not have a high rate of success.

Generally speaking most addiction treatments report a 20 per cent success rate after a year. After five years this figure is possibly lower than 5 per cent.

With the optimum nutrition approach we are recommending – our How to Quit programme – your chances of making it are much higher. For example, for those with serious alcohol or drug addiction the success rate in treatment centres incorporating our approach is about 80 per cent clean or sober after one year. For minor addictions your chances of success could be higher still. The reason our approach is so successful is that we focus on the area that is the most affected in any addiction: the brain.

All chemical addictions are rooted in the brain. Why? Because it's the brain's chemistry that becomes unbalanced when we become addicted. When we first inhale that cigarette, or drink that first alcoholic drink we create a change in our brain and, depending on the substance and often our own biological make-up, this can cause us to crave more and to feel s**t when we stop.

The reason you get hooked into needing, craving or wanting these substances (or you quit them and still feel bad many weeks, months or even years later), is because your brain becomes, and remains, programmed for addiction. The addictive substance literally mimics and effectively replaces your brain's own natural feel-good chemicals. The more you use the substance the more deficient you become, and the more 'abstinence' symptoms you develop. Just quitting doesn't reset your brain.

To restore balance in the brain you need to supply it with the right building blocks from which your brain makes its own natural chemicals – the ones that your drug of choice has been mimicking. These building blocks are nutrients: the chemicals that are part of our brain's evolutionary design. Your brain is literally made from, and dependent on, nutrients from food. We have found that certain combinations of safe nutrients, including amino acids, vitamins, minerals and essential fats, work better than drugs, and they do so without side effects, which means that you can look forward to relief from the misery of quitting without resorting to another drug that will create yet another side effect for you to get over. What's more, many people start using addictive substances because they feel tired, anxious, stressed, depressed or just generally not good. Our How to Quit programme doesn't just reset your brain out of addiction – it makes you feel so good you don't 'need' stimulants or relaxants.

In this book we bring to you the hottest new discovery in the science of addiction: nutritional treatment that is tailor-made for you and your addiction. It is based on personalised nutritional supplement recommendations to rapidly relieve your abstinence symptoms, backed up with a brain-friendly diet to bring you optimum nourishment and healing. The treatment is safe to use at home and we explain everything you need to know about how and when to take the nutrients that are best for your particular addiction. It doesn't contradict, in fact it complements, any other successful approach to treating addiction. It is, literally, the missing piece – ensuring you feel great, not s**t, months after quitting.

Our How to Quit programme is tried and tested, and based on the evidence of the hundreds of people who have benefited from following it. The success of this approach hinges on the reduction in abstinence symptoms within days of following our recommendations. Here are two examples from people who have tried our approach:

Case study KATHY

'Thanks to you I've quit 30 cups of coffee and 15 cigarettes a day. I feel so much better; my energy levels are improved. I sleep like a baby. I don't miss coffee at all and I'm not smoking. And I've lost three stone [19kg/42lb] in three months.'

Case study AMANDA

'I quit heroin ten years ago but still felt "edgy", stressed and occasionally shaky, and I needed cigarettes, caffeine and sugar to function. Now I "need" nothing – my energy is great, my mood even, and I no longer feel edgy or shaky.'

Our approach is based on decades of research at leading universities and medical centres that has clearly established that addiction is something that happens in the brain. Even if you might start using a substance for a psychological reason, perhaps the bust-up of a relationship, the consequence of continued use of a potentially addictive substance is a change in your brain chemistry. This is such a fantastic and important discovery that, needless to say, the drug companies are scrambling to produce drugs based on it. But, based on past track records, these new drugs usually have serious side effects – even if you're initially told they are safe. This has certainly proved true with the so-called 'safe' SSRI antidepressants and the apparently 'non-addictive' non-benzodiazepine sleeping pills. The bottom line is that you can't cheat nature without paying a price. By working with your brain's natural design, and its need for specific nutrients, you can reclaim your health and well-being without needing drugs or alcohol, stimulants or relaxants.

A big difference between man-made drugs and natural nutrients is that these nutrients can't be patented, and without a patent there are no big profits to be made from this discovery. So, it's up to you to read books like this, to learn about what really makes you feel the way you do, and to take control of restoring your own well-being. But because there are a variety of nutrients, each with its own specific properties, you need to discover which ones are suitable for your particular symptoms. This is the purpose of our book: we will guide you through the information you need so that you can find out for yourself which nutrients will help you to feel good, so that you can break free from the cravings and feeling of 'need' for particular substances. What you will end up with is your own tailor-made How to Quit programme.

In most cases, people following our How to Quit programme cut the number and severity of their abstinence symptoms by a third up to a half within one week, and by a half up to three-quarters within four weeks.

We deal with all the main chemical addictions and dependencies, whether prescribed (antidepressants, tranquillisers, sleeping pills, methadone), illicit (crack, cocaine, amphetamines, heroin, cannabis, ecstasy) or legal (caffeine, cigarettes, sugar, chocolate or alcohol). What we don't cover is behavioural addictions such as gambling or eating disorders, because these bring up other issues that are beyond the scope of this book. (Although we do discuss them briefly in the appendices, which can be found on our website www.how2quit.co.uk)

What our approach does not include or endorse is prescription-drug therapy – that is, swapping one addictive drug with another.

We bring you many years' experience of the role of nutritional therapies in conquering addiction: Patrick Holford has worked with addiction since the 1970s – both in treatment centres and in the study of the role of nutrients in addiction; Dr David Miller has worked with addictions for 30 years in addiction counselling, detoxification programmes and as a consultant to treatment centres; Dr James Braly has researched, pioneered and developed a highly effective therapy for addiction using supplements and IV vitamin and mineral therapy since the 1980s. David and his wife Merlene (who has also contributed to this book) have worked with James, providing opportunities for him to apply his nutritional therapies with clients in recovery.

This book brings together Patrick's years of work in nutrition with the amazing results that David, James and Merlene were reporting from the addiction clinics that have taken on their approach. We give you a detailed description of the treatment with an easy-to-follow Action Plan for ending your addiction – a programme that is backed up by the testimonies of the many people who have beaten their addictions by following it.

So, the question to ask yourself is: do you or anyone close to you need this book? If the answer is yes to any of the following questions, this book will provide the solution you need. Are you taking mind-altering prescription medication? Can you stop smoking without feeling s★★t? Can you stop eating sugar without craving it? Do you regularly drink coffee or other caffeinated drinks to give you a boost? Can you stop drinking alcohol or using an illegal substance without experiencing any of the abstinence symptoms described above?

Perhaps you have picked up this book because someone you love has a substance problem that is affecting their health, relationships or even creating difficulties with the law. This book will help you understand why it is often not possible just to quit despite a hundred-and-one obvious reasons to do so. The more you understand about what anybody with an addiction is going through and what can be done about it, the better able you will be to give them hope and help.

Our How to Quit programme is safe and, in most cases, you can do it yourself or use it alongside other activities or programmes that you are following to support your commitment to quit. It doesn't replace any other invaluable methods – such as counselling or Alcoholics Anonymous (AA) – it just makes quitting any substance many times easier. In fact the late Bill Wilson, who founded AA, became convinced that nutritional therapy was the missing piece of the puzzle when he first encountered the nutritional approach through meeting Dr Abram Hoffer back in the 1960s. (Dr Hoffer pioneered the treatment of addiction with high doses of vitamin B_3 and vitamin C, which are two of the nutrients we'll be telling you about.)

Indeed, we encourage you to use our programme with whichever other approach you may wish to use, as this will increase your chances of success. We also recommend that you include other vital tools such as a supportive community, sleep therapy and exercise, and we have explained all these in the book.

Beating your addiction naturally with our How to Quit programme has many benefits for your health beyond breaking free from addiction: it will give you improved motivation, mood and energy, and the ability to deal with stress. We think it's the missing piece in breaking the hold your dependency exerts, and it explains why so many people fail despite all the will in the world and the great support they may be receiving.

> **C**an you imagine how different it would be if you felt naturally fantastic? Would quitting be so difficult then?

Please be aware that some drugs are harder to quit than others. Benzodiazepines are notoriously difficult, as are cigarettes. If you do have a serious addiction and have tried to quit and failed many times, as well as following the advice in this book we recommend you have some professional support, and we'll let you know how to get it. There are treatment centres using this kind of approach, mainly in the US, although our mission is to get this approach integrated into treatment centres around the world.

One of the early pioneers is The Health Recovery Center in Minneapolis, Minnesota, which treats alcoholics; a three-year follow-up study shows a 74 per cent success rate, which is leagues ahead of other treatment centres. We think even this impressive success rate can be improved by applying the latest discoveries we bring you in this book.

The estimated cost in Britain of problems associated with alcohol alone is £20 billion a year. Class 'A' illegal drug use is estimated to cost a further £10 billion a year. Smoking is the single biggest preventable cause of premature death. Despite all the will in the world, people – perhaps you – struggle to quit because when they do they feel s**t. We bring you a safe, natural and practical way to unaddict your brain and put you back in charge of your life, without the need for chemical crutches.

This book is intended to help those suffering from addiction problems, but if you are a counsellor or health professional dealing with addiction you will also find information here that is hugely relevant to your work and that might transform the way you approach addiction and how you help your clients. As you will see in the book, intravenous nutrient therapy has been used in US treatment centres for many years with astonishing results and we hope that many treatment centres in the UK will add this vital and missing piece to their treatment. We also hope this book will stimulate research to prove what we have seen work time and time again for those with substance dependencies.

How to use this book

This book is divided into four parts, which give you all the background details you need to know about addiction and how it affects the brain as well as how to beat it naturally:

Part 1 explains how your brain becomes addicted. As you read through you will probably find that this part rings a lot of bells. As one person said, 'I have learned more about why I feel the way I do in the last three hours reading this than I have in 30 years in and out of addiction treatment.'

Part 2 describes the 12 critical components for 'unaddicting' your brain, so that you neither crave substances nor feel lousy after quitting, and how to put them into action.

Part 3 looks specifically at each of the major chemical addictions, from caffeine to prescription drugs, giving you a more personalised strategy for quitting or ending craving for that particular substance.

Part 4 puts it all together into your personal and doable How to Quit Action Plan, complete with brain-friendly recipes and addiction prescriptions.

As David Miller said, 'Meeting Patrick Holford and seeing the effectiveness of his nutritional approach completed the components of a balanced and successful way to treat addiction. I have never been as optimistic as I am today. I can honestly say that the suffering addict can now, more than ever, find relief and get a much better start on the road to recovery.'

We hope this book will inspire you.

Wishing you the best of health,

Patrick, David and James

PART 1

HOW YOUR BRAIN BECOMES ADDICTED

Some people feel great, full of energy, getting a buzz from life without 'needing' anything to pick them up or chill them out. The occasional drink, cup of coffee, or whatever, is no big deal, but they don't feel they have to have it to feel good. These people don't wake up in the morning feeling the 'need' for anything. If this isn't you, the first question to ask yourself is, 'Why not?'

Before you can discover how to get out of the addiction/ dependency trap you need to understand how your brain becomes addicted. This information will not only explain exactly how and why you feel the way you do but it will also give you a new awareness of why it is important for you to quit using the substance that you think you 'need' and why it is possible to do this without feeling s**t. That's the purpose of this section of the book.

1.

ARE YOU READY TO QUIT?

Whatever it is that you 'need' in order to feel good, there's something that doesn't feel right about having to consume a certain substance to feel OK. You've probably also found that the original kick you got from the substance you use isn't nearly as good as it used to be. It just doesn't fill that need any more. You might even have noticed that the substance doesn't actually make you feel good at all – just less bad. The 'joy' of the substance has become partly or wholly the fact that it brings relief, however temporary. You might also have found that your relationship with your substance actually causes you problems or gets in the way of your ability to function in the world in one way or another.

What's your addiction?

Take a look at the list of substances opposite. Ask yourself honestly which of these you consume on a regular basis, either weekly, daily or several times a day (tick the box). Or, if you are reading this because you are concerned about a friend, find out as best you can about what he or she consumes.

	Weekly	Daily	Several times a day
Caffeine	☐	☐	☐
Sugar	☐	☐	☐
Alcohol	☐	☐	☐
Nicotine	☐	☐	☐
Marijuana	☐	☐	☐
Sleeping pills	☐	☐	☐
Tranquillisers	☐	☐	☐
Antidepressants	☐	☐	☐
Painkillers	☐	☐	☐
Stimulants (such as Ritalin)	☐	☐	☐
Cocaine or other stimulant drugs	☐	☐	☐
Heroin	☐	☐	☐
Ecstasy (MDMA)	☐	☐	☐
Other	☐	☐	☐

Now, take the first substance you ticked and ask yourself this simple question: *How would you feel if you quit this substance completely for the next fortnight?*

If you wouldn't be able to quit we could say that you are addicted. Another definition of addiction is that you continue to use the substance despite it having harmful consequences – on yourself, your work or your relationships. If you could quit but you know you'd feel rough, we would say that you are *dependent*.

Now look at the list on page 16 and tick the appropriate column so that you have a record of your relationship with these potentially addictive substances. If, on the other hand, you have already quit one or all of these substances and still feel rough, with low energy, mood swings and a feeling of emptiness, tick the box labelled 'still suffering'. What you tick is your baseline.

	Dependent	Addicted	Still suffering
Caffeine	☐	☐	☐
Sugar	☐	☐	☐
Alcohol	☐	☐	☐
Nicotine	☐	☐	☐
Marijuana	☐	☐	☐
Sleeping pills	☐	☐	☐
Tranquillisers	☐	☐	☐
Antidepressants	☐	☐	☐
Painkillers	☐	☐	☐
Stimulants (such as Ritalin)	☐	☐	☐
Cocaine or other stimulant drugs	☐	☐	☐
Heroin	☐	☐	☐
Ecstasy	☐	☐	☐
Other	☐	☐	☐

Take a photocopy of this page and have a look at it again when you've completed our How to Quit Action Plan (as detailed in Part 4). We hope that there will be no more ticks in these boxes, if that's what you want. The advice in this book will also help you recover your *joie de vivre* – a lack of which leads many towards using mind-altering substances in the first place.

Of course, we are not proposing that all of these substances must be avoided by everybody all the time. For most, the occasional coffee, sugary food or alcoholic drink is perfectly OK. Assuming you are not a recovering alcoholic, and if you can occasionally partake without triggering a need to do it over and over or gradually increase the amount you consume, good. If not, then an appropriate goal for you would be to abstain completely from the substance that is a problem for you.

A culture of addiction?

In Britain alone it is estimated that there are over 10 million smokers, and the same number of ex-smokers, whereas six and a half million people drink harmful levels of alcohol. In terms of serious consequences a person dies every month from 'E' pills and amphetamines; a person dies every day from heroin or methadone, every 20 minutes from alcohol and every four minutes from the consequences of smoking.

Not only is the use of these potentially addictive substances going up and up, especially in the Westernised countries, but so too is the amount we spend on them daily. Some of us spend as much on these substances as we do on food. Why?

The answer, most of the time, is that we think or hold on to the belief that they make us feel better – happier, less stressed, more energised, more 'connected', more relaxed or in less pain. The trouble is, the more you have, the more you need (that's the first criterion of addiction: you become tolerant to its effects), and the more you need the worse you feel when you don't have it (that's the second criterion: withdrawal symptoms). Both tolerance and withdrawal happen because these substances change the way your brain's chemistry works until you end up programmed for craving and addiction.

Why haven't you quit?

The chances are you've tried to give up the substance or cut down many times. In the beginning you thought you could just do it with willpower but, despite having the motivation and will, after a few days or weeks, you were back where you started. Why?

Why, despite all your good intentions, did you start using the substance again when you'd decided to stop completely? It probably doesn't even make sense to you that if your feel-good substance is no longer giving you the same pleasure it used to, or if it is creating some kind of problems in your life, you choose to keep using it or keep going back to it.

The answer is simple, and one of the main messages of this book:

> **W**hen you quit, you experience what we call 'abstinence symptoms', which may be more difficult for you to tolerate than the problems that result from continuing or going back to your substance of choice.

The other important message of this book is that there is a way out – it is possible to quit and not feel s★★t.

Someone may have told you that you might feel lousy for a few days, but then you would feel better. But that didn't happen for you. And then, did your desire for the substance overpower your desire to quit? Do you feel a failure because you can't do something you know you should? Despite your desire to quit, is there a niggling voice in your head that says you'll never succeed? You'll soon discover, as you continue to read, that what happens to you when you use a mood-altering substance and what happens when you don't is a result of changes in your brain. The very nature of addictive substances, and the way they reprogramme the instinctive and emotional part of the brain, is a far stronger influence on your behaviour than your rational mind. Unless you reprogramme your brain's chemistry away from dependency, quitting becomes difficult, if not impossible – and at the very least, certainly uncomfortable. Strong, instinctive and largely unconscious forces – sometimes as strong as the survival instinct itself – are at work to keep you consuming your feel-good substance. But once you understand the dynamics, and how to change them, it gives you power to control these seemingly irresistible cravings.

You are not alone

If you struggle to feel good, or less bad, without a smoke, something sweet, something to drink, or some other substance, you are not alone. Addiction or dependence affects most of us at one level or another. The use of addictive substances, whether caffeine in tea and coffee, or alcohol and cigarettes, is part of everyday life for most of us. Most people are somewhere along the continuum from mildly dependent to seriously addicted.

Many of us use a combination of substances to change how we feel: sugar, alcohol, nicotine, caffeine or prescription drugs (to name the legal ones). We harshly judge the use of illegal drugs, such as cannabis, cocaine, amphetamines, heroin and Ecstasy, but your brain doesn't care whether a substance is legal or not. All of these substances contribute to scrambling your brain's chemistry.

The addiction epidemic

In Britain, despite all the campaigns, taxes and over 100,000 smoking-related deaths each year, one quarter of all adults smoke.[1] We drink an average of 16 units of alcohol a week – that's 4.5 litres (8 pints) of beer.[2] A third of 16 to 24 year olds smoke and their average alcohol intake is 18 units a week – more than two bottles of wine. Collectively we drink 70 million cups of coffee every day – the equivalent of two each for adults.[3] One-quarter of our water intake is from caffeinated tea.[4] In one survey of over 5,000 people, the average caffeine intake per day was 241mg (a regular coffee or strong tea is about 100mg).[5] Most of us are having at least three stimulant drinks a day. And some of us are drinking a few cups more to make up for those who don't drink any.

An estimated 7.5 million people in the UK have used cannabis, and up to 2 million do so on a regular basis.[6] One in ten of the UK population use one or more illicit drugs.[7] In the UK the number using cocaine has doubled in the last five years to over 1 million people.[8]

In America 22 million people are classified with substance abuse or dependence problems.[9] Seven million children in the US take stimulant drugs (usually for attention or hyperactivity problems) – that's roughly one in five.[10] In Britain 359,000 prescriptions were written out for just two (Ritalin and Concerta) in 2004.[11] In the UK there's an estimated 1.7 million tranquilliser addicts (that's benzodiazepines alone) and 31 million anti-depressant prescriptions written annually. The number of people addicted to them is unknown. Over 180,000 people seek addiction treatment each year.[12]

ESTIMATED NUMBER OF PEOPLE DEPENDENT/ADDICTED
(per cent of UK population)

Nicotine	15 million	(25%)
Caffeine	12 million	(20%)
Alcohol	4.6 million	(8%)
Tranquillisers	1.5 million	(2.5%)
Heroin	150,000	(0.25%)
Cocaine	20,000	(0.03%)

(Sources: Ash, Drug Scope, Alcohol Concern, Department of Health, NHS)

But am *I* addicted?

Addiction to any substance is a serious problem. Perhaps you think because you do not consume illegal drugs or are not an alcoholic that you are not addicted or that your heavy use of nicotine, caffeine or sugar is not a problem. The proof is in the pudding: if you've tried to kick the habit but ended up feeling so bad you start using the substance again, then you're probably addicted. The longer you're addicted the more your brain's chemistry changes, the less effective the substance becomes and the stronger your desire grows to keep using it. It's a vicious circle.

Abstinence symptoms: why quitting is so hard

As we have said, there are symptoms of addiction that occur while you are using a substance, but even more distressing for most people are those that occur when they *stop* using the substance. We have already explained a little about these symptoms and that we refer to them as abstinence symptoms. These can vary from mild to extremely severe, and they are the reason that most people fail to stick with their attempts to quit.

Acute withdrawal: symptoms when you first stop

The first symptoms that occur when you quit a substance are related to acute withdrawal, and in most cases are the opposite of the effects of the substance. For example, if you are using a substance that stimulates you, when you stop you will feel a lack of energy: lethargy, drowsiness, fatigue. If, on the other hand, you have been using a substance that relaxes you, when you stop you will probably feel a high level of agitation, anxiety and jitteriness. Some substances, like nicotine, do both, and quitting brings on a mixture of withdrawal effects. (If you have a severe addiction to a drug with relaxing effects – such as alcohol, a painkiller or an anti-anxiety drug – it may not be safe to stop taking it suddenly and we would strongly recommend that you get medical support.)

Most of the acute withdrawal symptoms will subside within three to ten days. And most people can make it through those, expecting that then the worst is over and they are in the clear. However, what happens next is that other symptoms will begin to emerge, lasting weeks, months or even years if you don't know what to do to reduce or eliminate them. Some of these may actually become worse over time. The most common ones are listed in our Scale of Abstinence Symptoms Severity on page 26. But before you look at it we will describe in some detail a few of the symptoms that tend to be the most baffling and distressing over time. In Part 2 we'll show you how to quit without experiencing these symptoms.

Hypersensitivity: when everything is too much

One of the most common abstinence symptoms is hypersensitivity to *everything*. Put simply, you have heightened sensitivity to external and internal stimuli: noise, light, touch, pain and stress. People who experience this most intensely are unable to filter out background noises and happenings, and this causes them to feel bombarded by all that is going on around them. If you are troubled by this, you feel constantly overwhelmed by everything going on around you and by all your internal thoughts and feelings. What would usually be considered *mild* stress becomes *major* stress. Sounds that others do not notice become major distractions for you. Pain is more intense, and simply being touched can even sometimes feel like being mauled. People who are the most troubled by this feel overwhelmed by a world that comes at them full force.

In most cases this particular symptom is partly genetic. Alcoholics, children of alcoholics and those with attention deficit hyperactivity disorder (ADHD) have been found to 'magnify perceptual input' (magnify everything their senses experience) and this has been associated with craving for a mood-altering substance.[13] It commonly exists prior to using an addictive substance and probably contributes to the risk that someone will use mood-altering substances at an early age. For some, certain substances, including alcohol, make this symptom disappear. So it would be expected that people plagued by it from childhood would use a substance that offers relief and that they would experience it again when they quit.

You find it difficult to concentrate

Although the inability to concentrate can result from any number of brain disturbances when you quit a substance, it can also be, and often is, related to hypersensitivity. When the buzzing of a fly demands as much attention as the person talking to you, it is difficult to stay focused on what that person is saying. It's not rudeness and it's not intentional. It is just very difficult to maintain a focus when everything around you is calling to you at the same time. It can be frustrating and embarrassing to realise that someone is talking to you but you haven't taken it in.

Your memory becomes poor

Problems with memory result from the inability to concentrate. If you didn't take in what someone said to you or were distracted when it occurred, you won't remember it. Or the memory will be sketchy. You can't recall what was never really recorded in your brain in the first place. Memory problems can also be related to fuzzy thinking, which often occurs when neurotransmitters in the brain are not communicating properly (we explain how neurotransmitters work in Chapter 2). It is hard to remember what you haven't grasped in the first place.

Your mood changes

You may experience anxiety, depression or both as a result of quitting. A certain amount of psychological stress is expected when change is going on. Change is stressful, and it is normal to have some fear connected with quitting your feel-good substance. But stress is exacerbated to the point of anxiety by hypersensitivity and the inability to concentrate and remember.

Maybe what you feel is not what you would really call depression, but is just a general feeling of discomfort or unpleasantness, an inability to feel pleasure. You feel that the colour has gone out of life. Sometimes these feelings come and go and take the form of mood swings. One day you feel good and then soon feel very 'down'. The tendency is to believe when you're feeling good that you are always going to feel good; it's then disheartening when you are again overcome by the inability to feel pleasure.

You crave substances to change your mood

Intense cravings, or what some refer to as 'drug hunger', is a powerful compulsion to alter one's mood with a substance. The abstinent person experiencing cravings knows what will bring relief. Hypersensitivity has been linked to a strong craving for alcohol, drugs and sweets. And alcohol, drugs and sweets normalise it. Feeling incomplete or inadequate or unfulfilled is common with abstinence from any substance that you have used to satisfy you. You experience a feeling of emptiness and a yearning for something, anything, to fill up the emptiness.

You have trouble sleeping

Many people experience sleep problems when they quit addictive substances. A common problem for abstinent alcoholics in early recovery, for example, is unusual or disturbing dreams. This is probably because alcohol suppresses REM sleep. This is the stage of sleep when we dream. And when we miss REM sleep our body tries to make up for it when we do begin to get dream sleep. The same is true with cannabis. This results in a rebound effect and we dream more than normal.

People who quit using other substances have other problems, such as having trouble getting to sleep and/or staying asleep. If this happens to you, you will probably feel sleepy in the daytime or feel tired all the time. Some people experience a difference in their sleep patterns, sleeping for long periods of time or sleeping at different times of the day.

The most serious sleep problems are associated with withdrawal from sleeping pills or benzodiazepines (like Valium and especially Xanex or Klonopin).

CAUTION It is dangerous to come off these drugs suddenly; you should taper off gradually. If you withdraw too rapidly, you may go for long periods without sleeping at all or worse, slip into a coma and die. For this reason we strongly recommend that you seek experienced medical help when tapering off any benzodiazepine.

Record your symptoms to monitor your recovery

Take a look at the Scale of Abstinence Symptoms Severity on the following pages. These are the most common symptoms that people experience when they quit and their brain chemistry is still in dependency mode. Even if you quit something months or even years ago your brain may still be out of balance and you may continue to experience some of these symptoms. Of course, not everyone who quits suffers from all these symptoms. What symptoms you have and how severe they are depends partly on what drug you have used and partly on your own biochemistry. Although we talk about these as 'abstinence' symptoms, sometimes it's these kinds of symptoms that lead you to use a substance in the first place to provide relief. Your brain chemistry can literally be out of balance from birth.

Here are some guidelines for getting and evaluating your abstinence severity score:

1. Use the scale to find your score when you have quit, because if you are still using your feel-good substance, your score will not give you the correct picture. This is because the substance is changing how you feel. The question is how you feel when you are *not* using it. So, use the checklist to determine your score after you have not used your substance(s) for at least one day.

2. If you are going through a medical detox for alcohol or other drug withdrawal, find your score when you are through the acute withdrawal phase.

3. Circle the number that best indicates the severity of each symptom you are experiencing *today* while you are no longer using your mood-altering substance.

SCALE OF ABSTINENCE SYMPTOMS SEVERITY

Circle the number that best indicates the severity of each symptom you are experiencing today (zero indicates the absence of the symptom, 10 represents an extreme, intolerable intensity level). Answer each question as honestly as possible.

	Low level High level
Craving or drug hunger	0 1 2 3 4 5 6 7 8 9 10
Craving for sweets/sugar/bread	0 1 2 3 4 5 6 7 8 9 10
Craving for salt	0 1 2 3 4 5 6 7 8 9 10
Loss of appetite	0 1 2 3 4 5 6 7 8 9 10
Overeating/always hungry	0 1 2 3 4 5 6 7 8 9 10

	Low level									**High level**	
Bloating or sleepiness after eating	0	1	2	3	4	5	6	7	8	9	10
Sense of emptiness/incompleteness	0	1	2	3	4	5	6	7	8	9	10
Anxiety	0	1	2	3	4	5	6	7	8	9	10
Internal shakiness	0	1	2	3	4	5	6	7	8	9	10
Restlessness	0	1	2	3	4	5	6	7	8	9	10
Impulsiveness/acting before thinking	0	1	2	3	4	5	6	7	8	9	10
Difficulty concentrating/focusing	0	1	2	3	4	5	6	7	8	9	10
Fuzzy thinking/head cloudy/ brain fog	0	1	2	3	4	5	6	7	8	9	10
Memory problems/memory loss	0	1	2	3	4	5	6	7	8	9	10
Depression	0	1	2	3	4	5	6	7	8	9	10
Mood swings	0	1	2	3	4	5	6	7	8	9	10
Negative self-talk	0	1	2	3	4	5	6	7	8	9	10
Irritability/impatience with people	0	1	2	3	4	5	6	7	8	9	10
Daytime sleepiness/drowsiness/ dozing off	0	1	2	3	4	5	6	7	8	9	10
Problems getting to or staying asleep	0	1	2	3	4	5	6	7	8	9	10

continues ▶

	Low level	High level
Fatigue/lack of energy/worn out	0 1 2 3 4 5 6 7 8 9 10	
Hypersensitivity to stress	0 1 2 3 4 5 6 7 8 9 10	
Hypersensitivity to sound or noise	0 1 2 3 4 5 6 7 8 9 10	
Hypersensitivity to pain	0 1 2 3 4 5 6 7 8 9 10	
Dry mouth/dry eyes/dry skin	0 1 2 3 4 5 6 7 8 9 10	
Aches/muscle or joint pain/headaches	0 1 2 3 4 5 6 7 8 9 10	

Add up your total score: ☐

When did you first experience the symptoms?

Although we call these 'abstinence symptoms', you may have had some of them *before* you got hooked. Perhaps the substance you became addicted to was the one that worked best to relieve those symptoms. In other words, the symptoms can be the reason you began using the substance in the first place, or they can be the consequence of substance overuse. Which way is it for you? If it is that the symptoms existed before and you used a feel-good substance to relieve them, then they will return even more intensely when you stop using that substance, depending on the degree of damage to your nervous system caused by the substance.

Whether the symptoms are cause or effect, if you have quite a few of these symptoms when you attempt to clean up your act, it's time to do something about it. If you are still unsure whether or not you are ready, ask yourself this:

> **W**ould you be ready to quit if you knew you didn't have to go through the discomfort you experienced when you tried to quit in the past?

See how your symptoms improve

Most people who follow our programme cut their abstinence symptom score by at least a third within one week, and by a half to three-quarters within four weeks simply by tuning up their brain chemistry with our How to Quit programme. And that's the big secret to quitting successfully: creating a level of health and a state of mind free from craving and discomfort.

Are you still unsure if you are really addicted?

Many people tell us that they consume substances on a regular basis, get great joy or satisfaction from doing so, and therefore can't be addicted or dependent. Well, that would depend upon your definition of addiction. As we have been pointing out, addiction is not just about what happens when you use a substance, but what happens when you don't. When we talk about addiction or dependency in this book we are talking about a condition in which there is a compulsion to keep using a substance despite negative consequences, as well as withdrawal symptoms when regular use ceases.

Of course, you can have negative consequences with or without compulsive use and withdrawal symptoms. The substances we are focusing on are harmful in a number of ways even if we are not addicted to them. Many people who are not addicted drink more than they should and may sometimes drink irresponsibly. Caffeine and sugar in excess are not good for us whether or not we are addicted. The big question is whether or not you can easily give them up when it becomes apparent that it is wise to do so.

Case study SARAH AND KENNY

Let's take two people who enjoy sweets and eat them on a regular basis. They both begin to gain weight and to have some health problems. They both decide to lose weight. Sarah, who is not addicted, is able to reduce or perhaps eliminate sweets from her diet. She loses weight and enjoys the accomplishment of controlling the amount of sugar she consumes. Kenny stops eating sweets only briefly before going back again and again to the same pattern of eating. He gradually increases the amount he eats and ultimately develops diabetes. Despite his weight and physical problems he is unable to control his sugar intake. He is addicted to sugar.

Most people feel tired and stressed as a consequence of too much sugar, caffeine, alcohol or cigarettes. Yet the addicted brain says 'have a coffee/have a drink/have something sweet/have a cigarette – it will make you feel good.' If you recognise that these substances are harming you and you can make the choice to stop using them without craving and discomfort – or if you are able to limit them to occasional use (not likely in the case of cigarettes) – you are probably not addicted. But if you continue to consume the substance despite ongoing negative consequences, and if you feel lousy when you quit, you are addicted and need to do something about it.

You *can* let go

If you are ready to quit, we have a How to Quit programme to help you. In most cases this takes 12 weeks to complete – defined as being free from abstinence symptoms. We will show you how to free yourself from the hold your substance of choice has on you. If you are not sure whether you are ready to give it up, come along with us. Find out what can happen if you choose to quit. We will show you that it really is possible to quit without feeling s**t, with this amazingly successful, scientifically based programme.

SUMMARY

▶ If you are dependent on a substance – caffeine, sugar, nicotine, alcohol, or prescription or illicit drugs – you are not alone. Most of us have some type of dependency.

▶ You may have given up using the substance you are dependent on but suffer from a variety of symptoms we call abstinence symptoms – listed in the Scale of Abstinence Symptoms Severity.

▶ You may have had some of your symptoms before you started using an addictive substance and then found that the substance relieved them.

▶ Whether the symptoms are a cause or a result of using the substance, if you have a number of them, or if the ones you have are very severe, you can do something about them.

▶ The How to Quit programme we describe in Part 4 will help free you from the discomfort of abstinence and prevent you returning to addictive use.

2.

HOW YOUR BRAIN MAKES
YOU FEEL GOOD

As we explained in the Introduction, beating addiction naturally is all about 'resetting' your brain away from addiction. In the last few years scientists have made enormous strides in understanding what the biological roots of addiction are and how addictive substances hijack our brain's chemistry until we literally feel our survival is dependent on them.

Most of the scientific research into helping with addictions is being used to find ways of developing a suitable, and profitable, drug fix for what is often a drug problem. However, this kind of approach creates yet more abstinence problems. Some people move from alcohol to sleeping pills, from cocaine to antidepressants, or from heroin to methadone, but each of these prescribed drugs has its problems, including the problem of addiction.

This chapter explains how, when your brain is functioning as nature intends, it provides you with good feelings. We describe how our How to Quit programme works naturally with the brain's inherent design, rather than using more drugs to give us 'quick fixes' (with yet more abstinence problems). The most important point to understand is that your cravings are created by your body and brain to get you to do the things that temporarily restore balance. When you get the relief provided by the substance, and feel good, this is your brain rewarding you. We are going to show you how you can make your brain reward you, that is make you feel good, without the need for addictive substances. What makes our How to Quit programme so different is that it uses this new understanding of the chemistry underlying addiction to help your brain and body to heal itself *naturally*. This is achieved by providing the very nutrients that our brains need to make its own feel-good chemicals – the ones addictive substances mimic.

The amazing brain

Your brain is incredible – a mere 1.3kg (3lb) in weight, and mainly composed of fat, it has the capacity to hold trillions of memories. It allows you to experience the delights of eating, the beauty of music, the ecstasy of love, the thrills of sex, and, for some of us, the bliss of inner peace.

It's also the abode of fear, anxiety, depression and craving. Understanding how this phenomenon works will show you why coffee, cigarettes, alcohol and other drugs produce the effects that they do. The key to the pleasant, even euphoric, effects of mood-altering substances is how they mimic the action of special chemicals in the brain called neurotransmitters. This is described in Chapter 3, but first we'll explain how the brain makes us feel good – a process that also involves neurotransmitters, the chemical messengers of thought, mood and motivation.

Neurotransmission: getting the message across

You and I communicate with words. The brain communicates with neurotransmitters manufactured in factories in the brain called neurons. Neurons, the principal working units of the brain, are tiny, complex nerve cells that send and receive messages about conditions inside and outside the body. They also serve as mood-control centres that determine the nature and intensity of our feelings and as action centres that largely control our behaviour.

Neurons are scattered throughout the body, but they are most highly concentrated in the brain, followed by the gut (more on this later). They form the 'road map' of our nervous system, and there are trillions of them. Neurons connect to one another via branches called dendrites. The average neuron will make 10,000 connections to other neurons, all linking together like a mass of interconnecting highways.

Delivering the messages

Neurotransmitters are the couriers on these highways, delivering messages from one neuron to the next. When the neuron is stimulated by something we hear, see, touch, smell, taste, think, feel or perceive, it releases some of its neurotransmitters. To get from one neuron to the next on the highway, neurotransmitters have to cross small gaps called synapses. The 'sending' neuron produces the chemical neurotransmitter, propelling it toward the 'receiving' neuron, which has a 'receptor site' to receive it. There's a slight complication though. The neurotransmitter is like a letter that only fits into a certain letterbox. If the neurotransmitter does not fit, it is not received by the receptor site. If it does, the message is delivered – that is, the receptor is activated. An electrical signal then travels along the dendrites until it reaches the next synapse, where it triggers the release of more neurotransmitters.

How this makes us feel good

The actions of neurotransmitters play a significant role in feelings of pleasure and well-being. They mediate mood, emotions, thought, motivation and memory. When neurotransmitters are present in optimal amounts, we feel good, we feel satisfied.

> **N**eurotransmitters work together to create feelings of pleasure to reward us for behaviours that keep us alive and comfortable.

The goal of this whole process is to reward us for doing what will keep us alive and functioning well. What produces these rewards is different for different people. Chocolate may produce more reward for one person whereas crisps may produce more reward for someone else; reading an interesting book may be rewarding for one person, whereas skiing may produce more reward for another. We all differ in what gives us satisfaction and in the depth of satisfaction we experience; but we are all motivated by chemical actions in the brain that nature uses to keep us alive, motivated, fully functioning and reproducing by rewarding us with good feelings.

We need feelings of pleasure

Neurotransmitters determine how you think and feel as they whiz around your brain and nervous system. Your mood, alertness, enthusiasm, ability to relax – your love of life – are all affected by the different kinds of neurotransmitters, or different levels of their activity. We all seek physical and emotional comfort. We want to feel good. The action of neurotransmitters plays a significant role in feelings of pleasure and well-being, hence a deficiency or excess of any neurotransmitter will give rise to uncomfortable feelings.

We choose actions for the rewards they give us

The interactions of neurotransmitters have an incredibly powerful effect on our emotions and thinking. Some of them act as stimulants. Some act as relaxants, stopping us from getting too hyper or stressed. As these stimulators and inhibitors act upon one another, a chemical cascade is formed, intended to result in a feeling of pleasure. This is how our brain rewards us. Most of the actions we take are chosen to produce this feeling of reward. We eat because it produces a reward of good feelings. We eat *certain* foods because they produce a better reward than others (chocolate produces more reward for most people than broccoli, for example). We have sex because it produces a powerful release of pleasurable chemicals. We work because the work itself is rewarding for us or because the end result produces a reward. We refrain from certain actions because they do not produce the feeling of reward we are seeking.

A word of praise for a job well done acts as a stimulus that activates a chemical reaction in the brain that feels good. A hug from a loved one sets off a brain chemical interaction that acts as a reward. The way we think, feel and behave results from chemical interactions in the brain and, in turn, produces additional chemical reactions in the brain. When the result of an action is positive, it reinforces that behaviour and motivates us to repeat it. So we tend to repeat actions that cause us to feel relaxed, happy, satisfied, complete and fulfilled.

The most important neurotransmitters

Although there are hundreds of neurotransmitters, the following are the main ones:

Dopamine, adrenalin and noradrenalin (adrenalin's cousin) are the 'feel-good' neurotransmitters, making you feel energised and in control. When you have adrenalin, dopamine and noradrenalin in balance you feel stimulated and energised. (Noradrenalin is called norepinephrine in the US.) Adrenalin is also the 'motivator', stimulating you and helping you respond to stress.

Endorphins and enkephalins promote a feeling of bliss, giving you a sense of euphoria. They are also painkillers, relieving both physical and emotional pain. They make you feel good.

Serotonin is the 'mellow' neurotransmitter, improving your mood and sleep, and banishing the blues. With an adequate supply of serotonin, you feel more confident, emotionally stable and connected.

GABA (gamma-aminobutyric acid) is the 'chilled' neurotransmitter, reducing anxiety, relaxing you and calming you.

Taurine helps promote GABA and also promotes calmness, helping you to relax and to sleep.

These are the key players in the orchestra of your brain and nervous system. The simple secret of feeling great is to have the right balance of these neurotransmitters. The trick to doing this is to eat the right foods and supplement the right nutrients from which your brain makes and controls these neurotransmitters.

The balancing act: why we might take harmful substances

The problem is that if you have an insufficiency in one or more of these neurotransmitters, your brain will be out of kilter, like a car out of tune. For example, 82 per cent of people with depression have very low levels of serotonin and 73 per cent have very low levels of noradrenalin.[14]

Instinctively your brain will crave anything that corrects a deficiency. This can be provided by nutrients, but too often we take other substances instead.

As you will see, that is why we end up using other substances that mimic or enhance the feel-good factor of our own natural neurotransmitters.

Amino acids:
the tools for unaddicting our brain

Neurotransmitters are manufactured in the neurons from amino acids, the building blocks of protein. Different amino acids produce different neurotransmitters, as seen below:

L-phenylalanine increases dopamine and noradrenalin

Tryptophan, and 5-hydroxytryptophan (5-HTP) increases serotonin and melatonin (melatonin helps you relax and sleep)

Tyrosine increases dopamine and noradrenalin

Glutamine increases GABA and glutathione, which in turn increase enkephalin levels

GABA is an amino acid and also a neurotransmitter

Taurine is an amino acid and also a neurotransmitter

Cysteine increases levels of glutathione

The two forms of amino acids: D- and L-

Most of the amino acids have two forms, the chemical structure of one being the mirror image of the other. These are called the D- and L- forms. Foods generally contain the L- forms. All of the amino acids recommended in this book for the management of addiction are the L- form, with one important exception: phenylalanine, which is used in both forms.

The chart below lists the neurotransmitters, the feelings that they provide for us and the essential amino acids that they need to function properly.

NEUROTRANSMITTERS AT A GLANCE

Neurotransmitter	What it does	Amino acid it's made from
Adrenalin, noradrenalin	Arousal, energy, stimulation, mental focus	L-phenylalanine, tyrosine
Dopamine	Pleasure, comfort, satisfaction and a sense of fullness after eating	L-phenylalanine, tyrosine
Endorphins, enkephalins	Physical and emotional pain relief, euphoria, pleasure, good feelings, sense of well-being	D-phenylalanine, DL-phenylalanine
Serotonin	Emotional stability, self-confidence, pain tolerance, quality sleep	tryptophan or 5-HTP
GABA	Calmness, relaxation and seizure control	GABA, glutamine
Taurine	Calmness, promotion of sleep, and digestion seizure control	taurine

Remember these amino acids, because these are the tools you are going to use to un-addict your brain, to give your brain what it really needs to stay in balance and to reward you with good feelings.

A good example of the relationship between amino acid intake and how we feel is demonstrated by an experiment on the effects of tryptophan. In the preceding list you can see how the neurotransmitter serotonin is made from the amino acid tryptophan, which gives us emotional stability, self-confidence, pain tolerance and quality sleep. A lack of tryptophan has marked effects, as was shown very clearly by an experiment carried out at Oxford University's Department of Psychiatry. Fifteen women were given a diet devoid of tryptophan (found in turkey, dairy products, green leafy vegetables, bananas, pineapple, avocado, soy, lentils, sesame seeds and pumpkin). Within eight hours, most of them started to feel more depressed. When tryptophan was added to their diet, their mood improved.[15]

Essential fats: making sure the message is received

Your brain, if you discount water, is 60 per cent fat, so eating the correct fats is essential for a healthy brain. In our explanation about neurotransmitters so far we've been looking at 'talking' – the way neurotransmitters deliver messages. If we now look more closely at 'listening' – how the receiving neuron gets the message – it soon becomes clear how vital the correct fats are for your brain.

At the synapse, brain cell membranes are also composed in part of essential fats and cholesterol, surrounding and supporting receptor sites – we can think of receptor sites in this context as the ears receiving the messages. So, to get the correct message from one brain cell to another, you need a good supply of essential fats and cholesterol.

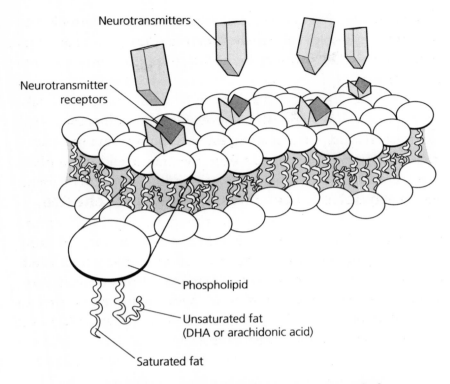

The synaptic membrane of neurons is composed of phospholipids and fats

Essential fats and phospholipids: helping you to crave less

Looking even closer at the brain cell membrane we find that it is made out of cholesterol and a type of nutrient called a phospholipid, with two fats attached: an unsaturated fat and either DHA (docasehexaenoic acid), a type of omega-3 fat, or arachidonic acid, a type of omega-6 fat.

By eating and supplementing the perfect amount and combination of essential fats, cholesterol and phospholipids you become much more receptive to your own neurotransmitters, which means you crave less. Eggs contain cholesterol and are very rich in phospholipids, as are brains and offal. You might not fancy eating brains or offal, but the smartest animals do. A fox, for example, will eat the heads and leave the rest unless very hungry. (Do you suppose they eat the heads because they are as smart as a fox or do they get smart as a fox by eating brains?)

We'll show you how to achieve the perfect intake of both essential fats and phospholipids (without eating brains) in Part 2.

Methylation: the conductor of the orchestra

How can your body's chemistry ebb and flow, creating harmony with your thoughts and emotions? The complexity and intelligence of your body's design is incredible. Probably the single most important conductor of your brain's orchestra is a process called methylation.

Your mood isn't just dependent on how much tryptophan or phenylalanine you eat; it also depends in part on how efficient you are at turning amino acids into neurotransmitters. That's mostly determined by methylation. Methylation reactions happen a billion times every couple of seconds and are totally dependent on nutrients. The process helps make, break down, and balance neurotransmitters, build nerve cells and protect your brain from damage (even slowing down the ageing process).

Methylation is the conductor of your orchestra so if you want to make sure you are in tune – feeling good, happy, alert and connected – you need to ensure you are a good methylator. Most people who need a substance to feel good are not good methylators.

Having the right connections

For us to feel well, our bodies need to be efficient at methylation, because that ensures the chemical connections are made quickly, and when that is working we will crave less. Here's an example of how fast chemical connections can be made in our body. If you have a near miss while driving your car, within 0.2 of a second your body begins to pump adrenalin. This is how it works: noradrenalin, the chemical cousin of adrenalin, is floating around your bloodstream all the time; by adding on a tiny molecule called a 'methyl group' it turns into adrenalin. By the time you've read this sentence you've already done about a billion of these methylation reactions, but in a stressful situation this process is greatly speeded up so that you can act quickly. The ability of your body to do this literally determines how well 'connected' you feel.

How being a good methylator reduces cravings

To reduce your cravings for unhealthy substances you need to raise the equivalent of your methyl IQ. First, you need to find out what your methyl IQ is at the moment by measuring a substance called homocysteine in your blood (don't worry, this is explained in detail in Chapter 9). If your homocysteine level is high, you're not firing on all cylinders. See the case of Chris below for an example of what happens if you have a high homocysteine level.

Normally, homocysteine is converted into the amino acid S-adenosyl methionine, nicknamed SAM (sometimes called SAMe, pronounced 'sammy'). SAM does all this methylation – it's called a methyl donor and literally whizzes around the motorways of your mind donating methyl groups, building or changing one neurotransmitter into another. This conversion process, from the 'bad' homocysteine to the 'good' SAM, depends on B vitamins (B_2, B_6, B_{12} and especially folic acid), plus zinc and something called tri-methyl glycine (TMG). Now, when you eat your broccoli (which is high in folate), you can perhaps visualise your methyl donor whizzing to the scene of the crime, perhaps to raise your serotonin and dopamine levels and make you feel happier.

Case study   CHRIS

Chris was feeling brain-dead. His mood and motivation was lousy. His memory was appalling – he kept losing his car in multi-storey car parks. His sex drive was non-existent. His homocysteine was 119. After a year taking all the right homocysteine-lowering nutrients his homocysteine has dropped to 9 and he's a trans-formed man. 'My memory and concentration are better than ever. My mood is great. My energy levels are amazing – in fact I now exercise each morning for an hour because I feel so good.' Last time we spoke to Chris, who is now 60, he was telling us about his new young girlfriend – so everything's working in that department. The key is getting your homocysteine down.

Poor methylation equals addiction and cravings

There's no question that just about everything we associate with addiction and cravings is related to poor methylation, reflected by high homocysteine and low SAM levels. So, what you want in your brain and bloodstream is low homocysteine and high SAM levels. How do you raise your methyl IQ? There are three answers:

1. Stop doing the things that tax the system, raise homocysteine and mess up methylation – and that includes cigarettes, excessive caffeine and, especially, coffee, alcohol and other drugs. (A double espresso raises your homocysteine level by 11 per cent in four hours.)

2. Take B vitamins (B_2, B_6, folic acid, B_{12}) and the minerals zinc and magnesium – these are the co-factor nutrients that methylation depends on.

3. Make sure you've got the building blocks of SAM in the first place – that means enough methionine from protein, tri-methyl glycine (TMG) from root vegetables, and folate from green leafy vegetables. (Exactly what to eat, what not to eat, and how to supplement is explained in Chapter 9.)

Helping your brain help you to feel good

Putting together everything you've learned so far, you'll see that there are three ways to improve your neurotransmission, and hence reduce your cravings and recover your natural energy, mood, get-up-and-go, mental clarity and alertness.

1 Better talking

To ensure 'better talking' your body must make large enough quantities of the neurotransmitters you need. This means supplying the body and brain with the amino acids and co-factor vitamins and minerals (needed to help the amino acids work) that are the building blocks of the desired neurotransmitters (explained in more detail in Chapter 7).

2 Better listening

To ensure 'better listening' your brain's cell membranes and receptors need to be in tiptop condition. This means consuming optimal amounts of the building materials for these receptor sites: essential fats, especially omega-3s, phospholipids (explained in more detail in Chapter 10) and the right amount of cholesterol.

3 Prevent down-regulation

Avoid addictive substances that make you less sensitive to your own feel-good brain chemicals. This process of becoming less sensitive is called down-regulation (see page 52).

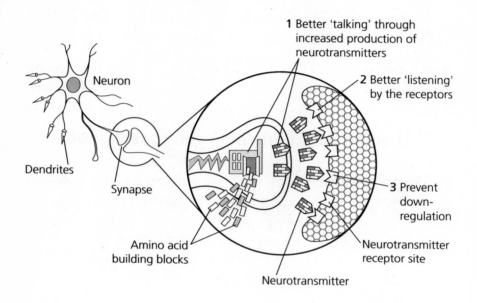

1 Better 'talking' through increased production of neurotransmitters

Neuron

2 Better 'listening' by the receptors

Dendrites

Synapse

3 Prevent down-regulation

Amino acid building blocks

Neurotransmitter receptor site

Neurotransmitter

Three ways to improve neurotransmission

Case study JANE

Jane lives alone and doesn't eat a very well-balanced diet. She's lacking the amino acid tryptophan and feeling lonely. As a consequence she is often depressed. She uses alcohol to relieve her depression. She decides to stop drinking alcohol, improves her diet, and supplements tryptophan (or its cousin, 5-hydroxytryptophan). As her serotonin levels improve, so does her mood.

She starts to eat more fish (high in omega-3 fats) and adds a spoonful of lecithin granules (high in phospholipids) to her breakfast. Her mood becomes more stable and she starts to experience a consistently higher level of mental energy. She feels more confident. Following our recommendations in Part 2, including eating a great diet high in essential fats, and taking specific supplements of amino acids, vitamins and minerals, plus regular exercise, which naturally boosts serotonin, Jane is off antidepressants and no longer feels she needs mood-boosting drugs.

As we have seen, addiction and cravings are the result of chemical changes in the brain, so what happens to cause us to become dependent? Why can't we just stop taking the substance? In Chapter 3 we explain how we get hooked.

SUMMARY

▶ The brain passes messages from one brain cell (neuron) to the next by way of chemicals called neurotransmitters.

▶ Neurotransmitters work together to create feelings of pleasure to reward us for behaviours that keep us alive and comfortable.

▶ Neurotransmitters are manufactured in neurons from amino acids, the building blocks of protein.

▶ Neuron cell membranes at synapses contain receptors that receive messages sent from another neuron.

▶ The brain cell membrane is very high in fat, so to receive the message we need a good supply of essential fats in our diets.

▶ Methylation is required for the process of turning amino acids into neurotransmitters.

▶ A substance called S-adenosyl methionine (SAM) – converted from a substance called homocysteine, which is made from

continues ▶

the amino acid methionine – is a 'methyl donor', because it is a fully loaded amino acid that can help balance neurotransmitter levels as needed.

▶ To increase methylation, stop taxing your system with harmful substances, then get enzymes working at peak efficiency by optimising your intake of B vitamins, zinc and magnesium.

3.

HOW YOU BECOME DEPENDENT

Now that you've got a basic understanding of how your brain works to change how you feel, let's look closely at how you get hooked on addictive substances. No one intends to become addicted. No child says, 'I'm going to be an alcoholic when I grow up.' No adolescent who experiments with drugs thinks, 'I want to become a junkie.' No one, when taking the first puff, drink, sniff, pill or injection, plans on getting addicted to cigarettes, marijuana, caffeine, alcohol, cocaine, speed, prescription medication or heroin. Yet for a great number of people, that first drink, smoke or hit leads, deceptively and often slowly, to physical dependence.

> Mood-altering substances change the balance of the neurotransmitters in your brain and nervous system. They sensitise the brain to drug-related stimuli, and alter brain 'organisation'.

Why the brain gets hooked

It is impossible for anyone who has never been chronically addicted to comprehend the power of addiction. It seems logical and reasonable to stop doing something so harmful to yourself and others, especially those you care about most. But the addiction process does not involve the part of the brain that is reasonable and logical. It involves a part of the brain called the limbic system. This is the brain's pleasure and reward centre; concerned with our survival, it is the part that tells us to eat, drink, fight or take flight. It monitors the body's need for survival, and when it senses our survival is dependent on a certain behaviour it creates a compulsion so strong that it becomes extremely difficult to resist taking that action. Without it we might forget to breathe or eat or reproduce.

How addiction becomes like survival

As you become hooked on any substance, this part of the brain begins to react to the presence or absence of the substance as it does to the need to eat or breathe, as though it is a substance necessary for survival. The reward systems of the brain may become hypersensitive ('sensitised') to drug-associated stimuli so that anything associated with drug use sets off a craving for the drug, even after the drug experience is no longer pleasurable.

We should point out that in the later stages of addiction to some substances, such as alcohol, withdrawal can be so serious that it is possible to die as a result. In the case of nicotine, caffeine or sugar you will not die, but the reward system doesn't distinguish between those circumstances when we might die and those when we *feel* that we might.

How the brain is tricked

To understand this process completely, it is important to know that the neuron's receptors will also accept mood-altering chemicals that mimic natural brain chemicals: dopamine, seroto-nin and endorphins. In other words, mood-altering chemicals can sneak into the letterbox (as we described on page 34) intended for neurotransmitters like dopamine and serotonin and fool the brain into acting as though they are the real thing. For example, cocaine docks onto the receptor for dopamine; heroin mimics endorphins, fitting into the same docking port; and alcohol mimics GABA. That's why these substances make you feel stim-ulated, motivated, euphoric or relaxed. They are taking over the role of the natural substances.

> **A**ny substance you crave, or any substance that makes you feel good, is either promoting your ability to make or restore the balance of your neurotrans-mitters, or it can mimic the neurotransmitter, docking onto its receptor site.

A short explanation of addiction

Probably none of us would become addicted if nature had not built in a mechanism whose goal is to prevent us from being too elated for too long. Remember the kick from your first cigarette, alcoholic drink or coffee? Have you ever wondered why you don't experience that any more? Why do you need more and more caffeine, nicotine, alcohol or drugs to get the same effect, or at least to keep thinking that if you only had a little more you would get the same effect?

When we boost our feel-good neurotransmitters, as we do with a cup of coffee, a cigarette or a drink, the dopamine released causes a feeling of well-being. However, in response, the receptors gradually shut down, deflating our high. A key concept in the body and brain, as in all of nature, is balance. Much as a thermostat keeps our home at a desired temperature, our body has ways of maintaining a state of equilibrium. It doesn't want us to be too high for too long! Is nature a killjoy? A likely explanation is evolution. Blissed out, happy monkeys get eaten. It's the paranoid, edgy, pessimistic ones, who are always on the lookout, who survive!

Why you become dependent

In response to an increase in the amount of neurotransmitter available – for example dopamine from drinking coffee – there is a 'down-regulation', a desensitising of the receptor sites. This means that some receptor sites shut down, making the neuron less responsive. Consequently, you need more of the substance – caffeine, nicotine, cocaine or whatever – to release neurotransmitters into the synapses and get the message across. It's as if, in order to block out the yelling of the neurotransmitters, the receptors put on earplugs, leaving the neurotransmitters no alternative but to yell even louder.

The body's self-regulation process, then, makes it impossible for us to gain any long-term benefit from the mood-altering substances. Herein lies the rub. The net result of addiction is that once the initial effect has worn off, the body's normal 'talking voice' just isn't loud enough to get the now-somewhat-deaf neighbouring cells excited. So you need more and more. No longer will that regular cup of coffee (around 100mg of caffeine) give you the kick-start you need. You need a large 'special' coffee (around 400mg), perhaps with a cigarette thrown in, or even a mochaccino (chocolate plus coffee – two different sources of caffeine), or some coke or a stimulant drug.

The desired effects get less and less

Of course, the more you have and the more often you have it, the more your brain cells 'down-regulate' by shutting down receptor

Normally we release enough neurotransmitters to feel good. But not too many to cause down-regulation.

Over-stimulation, which is what stimulant drugs cause, leads to too many neurotransmitters being released. The body fights back by shutting down receptor sites, and ultimately producing fewer neurotransmitters, making you more tolerant to stimulant drugs, which is why you crave more.

If you quit stimulants, to begin with you feel low because you don't have enough neurotransmitters. The body helps you recover by opening up more receptor sites, making you more sensitive to your body's own neurotransmitters.

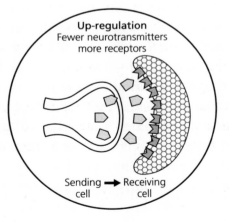

Down-regulation and up-regulation

sites. Continue along this slippery path for long enough and the effects of the substance become nothing like they used to be. The cup of coffee that gave you a rush of energy, now only relieves your ever-increasing fatigue. You need it just to feel normal. You've been trying to cheat the system and it's fighting back.

So why don't you stop? For most of us wanting the substance becomes the driving force, not necessarily liking it. Your desire for the substance becomes almost irresistible when you're in the setting or situation, or with friends that you associate with the substance, or even when you see something that you associate with it. This makes you crave the substance even though it doesn't really work for you any more.[16]

What happens when you stop?

Unfortunately, by the time you realise this and stop using the substance, your body's chemistry doesn't give you an unconditional pardon. Two things have been occurring. The reward system has become sensitised to the regular intake of the addictive substance to the point that anything associated with drug use can trigger severe craving and the sense that life depends upon continued use. For example, if you have associated smoking with a cup of coffee, then a cup of coffee following a meal may trigger a craving for a cigarette so strongly you can feel you might die without it. In addition the brain has adapted to the intake and punishes you with withdrawal when you stop using the substance. In effect, the withdrawal period is the time it takes from the moment you quit using stimulants until your neurons 'up-regulate' to hear your neurotransmitters' normal speaking voice once again. In the case of caffeine this is only a matter of days. For nicotine or heroin it can take weeks. In many cases it never recovers unless you follow our How to Quit programme, which provides an adequate supply of nutrients that nourish and repair the brain.

Does this happen to everyone?

Before we go on, we need to point out that this does not happen to everyone who drinks alcohol, smokes cannabis, tries cocaine or drinks coffee. Some people have a form of a gene that causes the reward receptors in the brain to become rapidly sensitised to the drug.[17] Other people may have a form of a gene that causes them to be deficient in certain neurotransmitters or receptors.[18] There may be other genes or combinations of genes or environmental factors that cause other people to be more susceptible to becoming addicted.[19]

Case study JAMES AND RICHARD

James and Richard are brothers. As teenagers they took drugs together. They used the same drugs in the same quantities. But as they reached college age James began to see that his drug use was interfering with what he wanted out of life. He quit using illegal drugs, though he continued to drink infrequently and always in moderation. But by the same age Richard realised that what he wanted out of life was drugs. James enrolled in college, established a career, had a family and became politically active and a respected member of his community. Richard enrolled in college, too, many times; but he never completed a term before some drug-related incident interfered. He got married a couple of times, but when each of his wives asked him to choose between them and drugs, he chose drugs. He is now in prison, serving an 18-month sentence for possession of cocaine.

What was different in these brothers? To answer this we need to look at what happens in the brain of some people that predisposes them to be more susceptible to becoming dependent on mood-altering substances.

Reward deficiency can lead you to addiction

Remember that in the last chapter we said that when your brain is working properly it rewards you? It creates a sense of well-being, pleasure and satisfaction with normal activities. But what happens when the brain is not working like this? When there is too much of one neurotransmitter or not enough of another, it sends out a powerful message to correct the imbalance. We become restless and anxious, feel empty, unsatisfied and have vague or specific cravings.

When your brain does not provide the normal reward, you will often feel as though you are constantly in need of something to fill the emptiness, reduce the anxiety, soften the environment, elevate the mood, quiet the restlessness or satisfy the cravings. People in this state are reward-deficient and look for something to relieve the imbalance and help them feel good. This is the brain telling us to take action to correct the imbalance. When you do not find healthy ways to do this, you will find unhealthy ones. You might think that the reward-deficient person would crave what is good for them (like broccoli) rather than what is not good for them (caffeine). Much of the time they don't know what it is they are craving. They are just seeking something to satisfy the lack, to fill the feeling of dissatisfaction, like when we eat something when really we are thirsty. Broccoli, for example, doesn't provide the almost-instant lift that coffee does, even though in the long run broccoli might help correct the imbalance – but coffee works in just 15 minutes. For some of us, however, that isn't fast enough and we find that cocaine does it better and faster – in 15 seconds. Crack, on the other hand, does it instantly. Now you're in heaven, heading for the hell of reward deficiency.

What causes reward deficiency?

There are many causes of reward deficiency, and it's worth going through a few of the major ones.

Genetics Some people are born with a genetic make-up that interferes with normal brain chemical balances so that mood-altering substances become more appealing. Studies have shown that numerous genes are associated with conditions that manifest as symptoms of reward deficiency.[20] There's growing evidence that if you inherit fewer receptors for dopamine you will be more likely to choose substances such as alcohol, and to become addicted.[21] It's a hot and complicated area of research.[22] Among the inherited conditions linked to reward deficiency is ADHD. In fact, there's a strong link between ADHD symptoms in a child and addiction as an adult[23] and people with ADHD are more likely to have the genetic tendency to reward deficiency.[24] Many ADHD kids are reward-deficient and so they seek stimulating behaviour such as being hyperactive and taking risks to stimulate their brains into giving them what they don't have naturally. Alternatively, they may become addicted to sugar and caffeinated drinks, and in adolescence they may begin using nicotine and alcohol and, frequently, illegal substances.

> **P**eople born with the genetic predisposition to reward deficiency are more likely to become addicted.

Case study **TWILA**

Twila's father was an alcoholic. Although she didn't realise it while she was growing up, looking back on it, Twila realises that her father also had symptoms of adult attention deficit disorder. She was diagnosed with ADHD as an adult recovering alcoholic. In remembering her childhood, she recalls that she was always restless, had difficulty concentrating, felt high levels of anxiety, was easily stressed and was distracted by noise and competing sounds. She remembers that she never felt comfortable, at ease or satisfied. She believed there was something seriously wrong with her, but she had no idea what it was. She just knew from an early age that she was different. It wasn't until she discovered alcohol in her early teens and began using it to change her brain chemistry that she began to fit in and feel comfortable and satisfied. Twila was probably born with reward deficiency that she inherited from her father. And her reward deficiency put her at risk of addiction.

One way in which your genes could tip you towards reward deficiency is fewer receptors for the feel-good neurotransmitter dopamine because of an abnormal form of the D2 receptor gene. In effect, this form of the gene renders the dopamine system inefficient.[25] The number of dopamine D2 receptors are consistently lower among substance abusers.[26] Inheriting this tendency is associated with more severe problems with alcohol.[27]

Non-genetic causes of addiction

Although the risk of addiction is very high among those genetically predisposed, reward deficiency can also result from non-genetic causes.

Prenatal conditions such as malnutrition or use of alcohol or drugs by the mother during pregnancy can result in conditions related to reward deficiency. Plenty of research has linked drinking during pregnancy with the risk of numerous problems in children, including behaviour, attention and impulse problems, alcohol disorders and even criminal behaviour.[28]

Malnutrition As we have already explained, neurotransmitters are produced from amino acids, vitamins and minerals, many of which are derived from food. So if you eat poorly over an extended period of time this can weaken the production and interaction of brain chemicals. Malnutrition can result from very low-calorie dieting, anorexia or bulimia, an unidentified food allergy (perhaps to gluten), or a diet simply lacking in adequate nutrition (due to any number of causes). When these 'building block' nutrients are lacking, the neurotransmitter system breaks down.

Severe or ongoing stress can do long-term damage to the reward system of the brain. This may be in the form of a single traumatic event (such as if you were in an earthquake or witnessed a murder), intermittent or chronic stressful events (such as child abuse), a series of highly stressful situations (a death followed by a serious injury followed by the loss of your job), or an ongoing condition of unrelenting stress (if you live with an alcoholic or drug-addicted person). It's important not to underestimate the relationship between extreme stress and altered brain chemistry. When you are under normal stress, your brain's neurotransmitter balance returns to normal as the stress passes. But when stress is severe or prolonged, these chemical levels may never return to normal without the correct nutrients to repair the damage. And when you are in a state of chronic stress you are more likely to turn to the use of mood-altering substances to lower it.

Lack of sleep If you go without sufficient sleep on a continuous basis this can also lead to reward deficiency. As you'll see in Chapter 13, sleep is a vital component of health. In fact, it's how the limbic system (the part of the brain involved with addiction) discharges negative, unexpressed emotions from the day before. Without enough sleep the stress and tension builds up and upsets the brain's normal night-and-day cycle of feel-good neurotransmitters.

Physical trauma Damage to the head can also lead to an imbalance in the brain's neurochemistry. Damage to the brain caused by the brain slamming against the skull results in many of the symptoms we have been describing and is frequently diagnosed as some other condition such as ADHD.

Heavy or long-term use of mood-altering substances can alter brain chemistry. So people who may not have the gene or be malnourished or traumatised may develop reward deficiency just by their excessive use of mood-altering substances. This is especially true if the chosen substance is a super-addictive substance (discussed below).

Not all drugs are equal

Your risk factors for reward deficiency are not all there is to consider. Although your genes are a strong risk factor, the risk of addiction also depends upon which drug you use and how you use it.

> **H**ow susceptible you are + the addictiveness of the substance + the frequency and quantity of use = your risk of addiction

But then, of course, there are social factors too: the company you keep, the availability of the drug and other triggers in your life. Addiction is a complex business.

The super-addictive substances

There are some substances that are addictive to almost anyone who uses them. Nicotine is a good example. The majority of people who smoke for any length of time become addicted and find it very difficult to give it up. Nicotine has been reported by many researchers to be more addictive than crack cocaine. (This is unlike alcohol, which is only addictive to a minority of people who drink.) However, there are a few people who smoke without becoming addicted. These people may be able to quit cold turkey and can't understand why other people cannot do the same.

There are other people, usually those with a certain genetic make-up, for whom smoking is extremely addictive, who start smoking at a younger age and find it so difficult to quit that repeated efforts usually prove futile. Other substances that are super-addictive include the benzodiazepines (tranquillisers), which are exceptionally difficult to get off. If you are one of these people it does not mean that you are weak willed. It means that you need extra help to reset your brain's chemistry and unaddict your brain. That's where the nutritional approach contained in the How to Quit programme in this book will be able to help you.

Why we seek feel-good substances

Whether the cause of reward deficiency is genetic or environmental or a combination of both, it puts you at a higher risk of beginning to use a substance to relieve the discomfort of the deficiency and of becoming dependent on it. To understand this better let's look at what happens when people with reward deficiency discover a substance that provides what they are missing.

When the normal process of neurotransmission is impaired, the discomfort that results can lead you to the use of mood-altering substances to self-medicate the discomfort. Remember that mood-altering substances fit into the same receptors as neurotransmitters or increase the amount of neurotransmitters in the synapse. So, if there is a deficiency, the appropriate substance becomes a substitute for the natural chemical and temporarily corrects the deficiency. Suddenly your anxiety, restlessness, emptiness, hypersensitivity and craving have gone. You may feel good for the first time in your life. But the substance does more than allow you to feel normal. The brain is flooded with the substance, which produces feelings of intense pleasure and euphoria.[29]

Are people who are reward-deficient more likely than the average person to continue using a mood-altering substance once they have found one that 'works' for them? Of course. It is highly unlikely that, having discovered a way to feel better instantly, you will not do it over and over again. And the reward is immediate. It works, it works now, and it works every time (at least in the beginning). It relieves your discomfort and gives you pleasure. You are no longer reward-deficient. You feel good – and perhaps you never knew that you could feel this good.

How mind-altering substances affect reward-deficient people

If you have reward deficiency you are likely to become addicted because the continued and regular use of the mind-altering substance *works* for what ails you. Also, if you have the genetic tendency to reward deficiency you are more susceptible to becoming addicted because it seems the very same genes that predispose reward deficiency also cause something different to happen in your brain when you use mood-altering substances. The experience for you is not just pleasant, but exhilarating. You get a higher high.

This is common, for example, among alcoholics. People with a genetic predisposition to become alcoholic do not metabolise alcohol in the same way as other people. Many people prone to alcoholism produce more of a liver enzyme called alcohol de-hydrogenase II (or II ADH).[30] This means they metabolise acetaldehyde (the by-product of the breakdown of alcohol by the liver) more slowly, allowing more of it to build up in the bloodstream.

The early warning signs

It is very difficult to detect addiction in the early stages because, for the people most susceptible, it is more beneficial to their daily lives than harmful. It provides what their brains lack normally. Just as Ritalin (a mood-altering substance) can allow some children with ADHD to function better, other substances are beneficial for other reward-deficiency conditions and allow improved functioning and performance. With alcohol, in spite of a common belief that as the quantity of alcohol consumed increases the ability to function decreases, some people may actually be able to perform some tasks better when a little intoxicated than they can when totally sober.

This early warning sign that addiction may be occurring (i.e. the ability to function well) makes it difficult for people affected to recognise they have a problem. The ability to 'hold your drink' (or drug) actually conceals the problem and creates the belief among early-stage addicts that they are immune to the painful consequences that they see others experience. It is difficult for a person who gets so much pleasure from a cigarette, or someone who gets such comfort from a piece of cake or someone who gets a much-needed lift from a cup of coffee, to believe the beloved substance can be harmful. Addiction is a condition that appears in the early stage to be a benefit, allowing you to experience the good feelings without paying any of the penalties.

Addiction: a gradual process

This is the process you will probably go through:

1. **Tolerance** You can consume larger quantities than other people without becoming impaired. You gradually increase the amount you use to get the same effects, still without becoming impaired.

2. **Painful consequences** You begin to experience the consequences of using the substance but often do not connect the consequences with use. You then use the substance to relieve the pain of using.

continues ▶

3. **Dependence** Now you need the substance to function, so regular use is necessary. When you don't use it you experience withdrawal symptoms. So now you need to use it to relieve the pain of *not* using.

4. **Tolerance decreases** It is impossible to consume the same amount as before without suffering. The magic is gone and the painful consequences are worse. Now there is pain whether you have it or not. At this point many people choose to do something about the problem.

5. **Abstinence symptoms** Even after the acute withdrawal symptoms are gone, there are lingering abstinence symptoms that don't improve with time.

Developing tolerance

Your brain changes and adapts to you taking the substance regularly. If you are becoming addicted to alcohol you can gradually tolerate larger and larger quantities without becoming intoxicated and without experiencing harmful consequences. If you are becoming addicted to caffeine you can gradually increase the amount of coffee you consume without becoming overstimulated and jittery. This is tolerance. But, over time, continued heavy use, especially if you have a genetic predisposition, will lead to addiction.

The more you consume, the more your brain adapts to the presence of these large quantities until you must use larger and larger quantities to get the same effect, causing more and more changes in the brain.

Case study **TWILA**

Twila knew from the first drink that she would continue to use alcohol to feel good. She knew immediately that it took away all the things about her that always made her feel different. At first she could drink with no problems. She could drink larger quantities than her friends could without getting drunk. She was able to function better when she had a few drinks than she could sober. She felt freer to express herself. She started writing poetry and thought she had found or released the creative part of her. She found that as she drank more, she was able to drink even more, then began to find that the amounts she had used before no longer did for her what they used to, and she increased the frequency and quantity of her drinking. She was unaware that neurochemical changes were taking place that were setting her up for problems. She thought she was in no danger of becoming addicted because she could 'hold her drink' better than anyone she knew. She was not aware that this was an early warning sign of alcoholism. Alcohol was her best friend and, she thought, her friend for life.

Although Twila's story is about an addiction to alcohol, this same progression applies to other addictions.

Painful consequences

When you are into heavy and continuous use of addictive substances, the good feelings produced at first are eventually negated by the painful consequences. This can come in many forms: weight gain from excessive sugar, indigestion from too much caffeine, the frustrated response of trying to function while waiting for a cigarette. Problems may arise from drinking and driving or other encounters with the law. Or there may be problems from a 'nagging' family who want you to cut down. Or there may be any number of physical complications. Whatever the problems are, you know a way to make the pain of them go away. So you are now using addictive substances to relieve the painful consequences of using addictive substances. The more pain, the more use. The more use, the more pain. The substance blocks the awareness of what is really causing the pain. It's a vicious cycle.

What is happening in the brain at this point, is that the mood-altering substance is interfering with the release of neurotransmitters and/or blocking the receptors. So, with heavier use, there are fewer neurotransmitters being produced and released than before. And it takes more and more of the substance to fill the receptors and get high – and now the receptors may no longer be working properly.

Case study TWILA

So what happened to Twila? To her surprise, she began to have problems while she was still a teenager because of her drinking. At first she did not realise that these problems had anything to do with drinking. She began skipping school and thought she was just having a good time. When she was caught and punished at home and suspended from school, she told herself everyone was just over-reacting to her free spirit. She felt misunderstood, and she comforted herself by drinking more.

Becoming dependent

When dependence is increasing most people are unaware that physiological and biochemical changes are occurring as long as they are able to drink, smoke or get their 'fix' of sugar or caffeine. They think they are functioning normally. And they may believe they are drinking, smoking or taking drugs responsibly. When enough problems occur, they may attempt to cut back. But by the time they are aware that use of the substance is the problem, they cannot choose to use it in moderation. As the brain adapts to higher levels of the substance, the body accepts this as normal and demands that this 'normality' be maintained.

So while tolerance is increasing, so is dependence. 'Want' becomes 'need'. There is a growing need to use the substance. Craving for the substance leads to continued substance use in spite of the painful consequences. The person cannot function without it.

> **A**s neurons in the brain adapt to larger and larger quantities, the brain becomes reliant upon the mood-altering substance and shuts down its own production of neurotransmitters.

The hijacked brain

Your brain does not need to keep producing its own feel-good neurotransmitters because the receptors are being filled by copycat substances. When the brain does not get its supply from an outside source, it does not snap into production and start supplying the needed chemicals. Instead, it screams out for more of the ingested substance. This is when the survival part of the brain takes over. It believes it must have the substance to survive. It overpowers the rational part of the brain, and getting the substance becomes as strong a need as breathing. This has been called the 'hijacked brain' – the drug has stolen your ability to make rational choices.

Case study **TWILA**

So how did Twila's drinking affect her? When she got married, her husband objected to her heavy drinking, so she decided she would cut back. But her attempts were short-lived. She would cut back for a few days and then find that she was back to her regular amount. As this became more and more of a problem in her marriage, she tried many ways to drink in moderation. She would set rules and break them. She would promise herself she would drink only during certain times of the day. Or she would drink only at weekends. Or she would drink only beer. Or she would drink only with other people. But all her promises to herself and to her husband were broken. Fearing her husband was going to leave her, she promised to quit entirely. And she did. For two days. She was sick and miserable for those two days. She never stopped thinking about drinking. She was obsessed with the idea of having 'just one'. The compulsion to take that one drink was overpowering. Finally, convinced she could have one and stop, she gave in and soon her drinking was out of control again. Her husband did leave her and then she felt she had a real reason to drink, and alcohol took over her life.

The pain of abstinence

Your great friend now becomes your enemy. The substance now creates pain instead of producing pleasure, and now instead of being able to tolerate more, you can tolerate less and less. You have pain when using the substance and pain when not using it. The drug has depleted the brain's supply of natural feel-good chemicals, the receptors are not working as they should and the drug is no longer a satisfactory substitute. You might continue to use food, alcohol, nicotine or other drugs, prescribed or otherwise, not for any substantial pleasure, but only because the survival part of the brain has taken over and believes it must have the substance. You find your attempts to stop are usually short-lived and futile and you suffer from severe anxiety when an unexpected situation interferes with the substance use or the source of supply.

When you continue to use despite serious consequences, other people believe you to be behaving irresponsibly, unaware that you are not consciously choosing the behaviour. It is being dictated by the survival part of the brain. You may go immediately from the pain of needing the drug to the pain of using the drug. The magic is gone. The pleasure is gone. There is nothing but pain.

Case study TWILA

Twila doesn't remember when the pleasure stopped and drinking brought her only pain. At first she thought she was so miserable because her husband had left her. Gradually she became aware that drinking was giving her no comfort. She was getting drunk more and more often. She could drink less and less before getting sick. Where had the magic gone? She was convinced she could find it again if she could just find the secret door. She tried to work at several jobs but was too sick most of the time to go to work. She was lonely and started going out with friends with whom she previously drank, those people who used to talk about her ability to hold her liquor. But now she was passing out and they were driving her home. They didn't like being with her any more. Every day she would promise herself that tomorrow she would stop. But tomorrow she only remade the promise.

Quitting becomes impossible

Sometimes seriously addicted people may have a moment of sanity when they realise that if they keep doing what they are doing they are going to damage themselves seriously or even die. They may ask for help. People with a nicotine addiction may go to some kind of stop-smoking programme. People who are diabetic or overweight because of an addiction to sugar might join a weight-loss programme. People with an addiction to alcohol, illegal drugs or prescription drugs may enter a treatment centre. If it is a treatment centre without medical detoxification, the pain of abstinence can be so severe that they leave before they have made it all the way through the detoxification process. If they get medical detoxification, many stick it out even though they are uncomfortable. But what happens now to the poor brain, totally depleted of natural brain chemicals and unable to produce an adequate supply? Usually nothing. It stays that way – perhaps for months, but often for years. It is reward-deficient, and more extremely so than before use of the substance began.

The discomfort, prior to substance use, is now even more intense. And the brain continues to crave the substance upon which it has come to depend. After struggling through months of pain and craving, many addicts give up in despair, and, believing there is no way out, go back to what they know will at least relieve the craving, if not the pain.

Case study IRENE

For 35 years sugar and weight controlled Irene's life. She was over-weight as a child and still remembers the pain of hearing people say, 'She has such a pretty face,' knowing that they were thinking, 'It's a shame she's so fat.' Throughout childhood, adolescence and adulthood, her life revolved around feeling the pain of being overweight and eating sweets to assuage that pain. She always knew she could ease it with her tried-and-true friend: sugar.

The first time she went on a diet her doctor told her that she could eat anything as long as it contained no white flour or white sugar. She immediately went home and baked a lemon meringue pie using brown sugar and wholewheat flour. Needless to say, it wasn't as good as the 'real' thing, but she soon got used to the taste – and rapidly gained five pounds.

Later that year she decided to take the bull by the horns and just stopped eating altogether. The bathroom scales kept her on course for four days; it was saying great things. When her mother pleaded with her to be more sensible, she got out the cottage cheese, took a few bites, then reached for the biscuits.

Diets came and went, each beginning with strong determination and ending in despair. She tried commercial programmes, liquid protein, diets of the stars, diets of her friends, hypnosis and fasting. For a time she felt invincible. The world was her apple and that apple would always be eaten raw, never again in a pie. Despite her unceasing hunger for sweets, each time she dieted she lost weight. And sometimes she kept it off for a period of time through vigilant self-deprivation and icy determination. Then the ice would melt and the sugar craving would win. She watched her weight come back as if it had a life of its own.

Each time the craving was stronger than before, and she was more irritable and more easily stressed. Each time the unfairness of her plight, the burden of never-ending hunger, and never-ending vigilance overwhelmed her. Sweets called her name and she would eventually answer, 'I'm back.' She would reach out to her old friend, always there to soothe and comfort her.

Now, many people will tell you that Irene was just not motivated. But why would she do the same thing over and over again unless she really wanted to free herself from her addiction to sugar? She had controlled it over 20 times for a period long enough to lose weight. Why would you do again what you had failed at 20 times previously unless you wanted it very badly? Some people will tell you that Irene just did not have any self-discipline. How many of us have the self-discipline to endure ongoing, unrelenting pain – with no relief in sight – without looking for some source of pain relief?

How our How to Quit programme can help

Let us be clear here that many addicted people do make it and find ways to remain free of their addiction. Many find a better life through practising the principles of Alcoholics Anonymous (AA), Nicotine Anonymous, Overeaters Anonymous, or Narcotics or

Cocaine Anonymous. Thousands of ex-smokers or drinkers or drug addicts are living proof that recovery from addiction is possible.

Through their experience of addiction and recovery they find meaning and purpose, and are able to live a happy life. Sadly, this is a minority. Some people are able to stop with the help of a counsellor or counselling programme. As important as counselling is, the majority do not achieve abstinence on a long-term basis, and those who do, often experience ongoing abstinence symptoms. Most treatment is helpful in that it helps addicts *cope* with the craving and pain of abstinence, but it does not take it away.

This is the missing link

With our How to Quit programme this can change for you and you can avoid relapse. Even those who have already been able to quit their addiction and stay off with the help of a 12-step support group or treatment programme can reduce the severity of their abstinence symptoms and improve the quality of their life. With our programme you can quit and begin to feel your abstinence symptoms improve in a matter of days. Some addictions are more serious and more difficult to overcome than others, but all addictions – whether to illegal drugs, prescription drugs, alcohol, nicotine, caffeine or sugar – have in common a need for restoring the brain to optimal functioning. Wherever you are along the road to addiction, you will find our How to Quit programme provides the missing link: when you fix the brain, you will find quitting and staying free of the need for substances so much easier.

SUMMARY

- ▶ We use drugs to compensate for a lack of, or imbalance in, or dysfunction of, neurotransmitters.

- ▶ When the reward system of the brain is working properly it creates a sense of well-being and satisfaction. Craving, dependence and addiction occur when the reward system goes wrong.

- ▶ Many people born with the genetic predisposition to reward deficiency are also genetically predisposed to becoming addicted.

- ▶ The more you have of a mood-altering substance the more insensitive your brain becomes to your own neurotransmitters. This is called down-regulation – it makes you more tolerant to larger amounts.

- ▶ The more you consume the more your brain adapts to the presence of large quantities until you *must* use larger and larger quantities to get the same effect, causing more and more changes in the brain.

- ▶ As neurons in the brain adapt to larger and larger quantities, the brain becomes reliant upon the mood-altering substances and shuts down its own production of neurotransmitters.

- ▶ You now crave the substance and, if you don't have it, you get withdrawal or abstinence symptoms.

- ▶ Any substance you crave, or any substance that makes you feel good, is either promoting your ability to make or restore the balance of your neurotransmitters, or is mimicking the neurotransmitter, docking onto its receptor site. Now you're hooked.

4.

ARE YOU AVOIDING PAIN?

It's not just the buzz we go for in mood-altering substances, it's the anaesthetic. If you've had a tough week, or a bust-up with a girlfriend or boyfriend, or are dead bored with your career choice or have no idea what direction to go in life, one way to relieve the pain is to get drunk, get stoned or get out of it. It works. Temporarily you forget whatever it was that was eating you up. Using a substance to blot out emotional pain may or may not lead to addiction. But the more you do it, the higher your risk. Although it is very normal to want to escape pain, it's important to understand why you are using chemical substances to do it – and to find a safer way.

How pain comes and goes

All thoughts and feelings have a corresponding change in your brain's chemistry. In Chapter 2 we learned about how our brain's neurochemistry rewards us for certain behaviours with good feelings, by stimulating the release of serotonin, endorphins and dopamine. The opposite is also true. When something happens that makes us feel bad, it sets up a corresponding craving for something to make us feel better and get those pleasurable endorphins flowing. 'Hugs not drugs', says an AA slogan, since both do have the power to up our feel-good neurotransmitters.

These are part of the brain's natural painkillers. The reason why morphine or heroin, for example, kill pain is precisely because they lock into the brain's receptors for its own natural painkillers – endorphins. They are released, for example, when you are dying. They make you blissfully unconscious of any hassles in life.

The same thing happens, although to a lesser extent, with alcohol, cannabis and tranquillisers. They switch off anxiety, helping you to chill out and temporarily forget about whatever was such a big deal a minute ago.

> The longer you go on using the drug, the less pain relief you get, and the more pain you experience the next day as a consequence.

Pain relief becomes more pain

In the short term drugs all 'work'. They relieve the pain and make you feel good. But soon they bring their own pain – the pain of withdrawal, largely due to endorphin, serotonin and dopamine depletion, leaving you wanting more of the same.

But that's just the chemistry of it. As a consequence of learning to avoid painful circumstances by 'numbing out' with drugs, situations that you need to deal with often get worse, or you make them worse by saying or doing the wrong thing 'under the influence'.

What are you avoiding?

Apart from this immediate pain, what are you avoiding when you are using drugs?

- Are you bored or unfulfilled in your work or relationship?

- Are you betraying yourself by not being who you are, or not standing up for what you believe in?

- Are you stuck in a rut and need a change, a new challenge to absorb your desire to learn or make a difference?

- Have you accumulated so much 'stuff' (fears, disappointments, anger, relationship problems)?

- Are you imbedded in your negative patterns and negative self-talk? (Self-talk is how we talk to ourselves, in our minds or out loud. Some of our self-talk is encouraging and constructive. Some of it is negative and discouraging. When you are imbedded in your negative self-talk you behave as if it is true whether or not it is.)

- Are you drowning in your sorrows?

- Is your depression really accumulated anger without enthusiasm ('Don't get sad, get mad!')?

- Are you lonely?

- Are you searching for something – something that gives meaning to life – in drugs?

- Is it time you did some work on yourself and where you are going, rather than numbing out with one substance or another?

This kind of emotional healing – getting the past out of your future – is for many a vital component of breaking an addictive habit. Finding meaning and purpose in life without drugs is a vital key for some people. For this reason it's part of our 12 Keys to Unaddicting Your Brain, explained in Part 2. We outline a variety of options to explore, from one-to-one counselling to intensive life-changing training courses (see Chapter 18).

AA has a 12-step process towards recovery; step four is to 'make a searching and fearless moral inventory of ourselves'. If you follow this, you may better understand what it is that makes the use of a particular drug so attractive to you. In Appendix 1 (which is on our website www.how2quit.co.uk) you will see a list of questions. This is designed to help you identify what it is you're compensating for, and whether there's a better way to achieve peace or fulfilment than using your drug of choice. The combination of unaddicting your brain with optimum nutrition (as we explain later), and resolving the issues that leave you feeling unfulfilled, is a powerful step away from a pattern of addiction.

Understanding why you use substances

One incredibly useful way of understanding the natural behaviour of wanting to escape pain is the model of the Doors of Compensation®, described by the psychologist and philosopher Oscar Ichazo.

In an article on drug abuse he says,

Drugs (all of them) can be characterised as 'energy consumers', consuming energy at a rate much greater than our natural ability to replace it. As drugs burn all our accumulated vitality in short periods of time, the brief exaltation is inevitably followed by depletion of vital energy, felt as the 'down', the depressant effect of drugs. Nothing can replace a natural, clean body capable of producing natural and clean vital energy.

The order of damaging drugs

Oscar Ichazo rates the drugs most damaging to our vital energy (explained on page 81) in the following order, from most damaging to the least: alcohol, heroin and opiates, tobacco, cocaine, barbiturates, antidepressants, amphetamines, marijuana and caffeine.

How we keep ourselves psychologically in balance

Ichazo's model describes nine different ways that we dissipate energy. Stimulants and drugs are just one of these. Compensating in one way or another is completely natural and can be seen as the way we attempt to keep ourselves psychologically in balance. Think of your consciousness – your psyche – as a container. When we react to situations with emotional charge (when things don't go the way we expected, or when we experience stress in one form or another) the pressure on our psyche increases. To release the pressure we compensate by behaving in a particular way – using one or more of the Doors of Compensation. That's why, for example, people go boozing on a Friday night as an escape from a stressful week, or take their stress out on the family by being bad tempered, or stuff themselves full of food. Each of these is a way of dissipating energy and reducing the psyche's tension.

The Doors of Compensation

Understanding how we use these doors of compensation helps to identify sources of stress and allows us to develop healthier ways of staying in balance to support a productive and happy life. Ichazo has developed a one-day training session to help you understand how we all use doors of compensation (see Resources, page 486).

The nine Doors of Compensation

1. Toximania The use of toxic substances, including cigarettes, alcohol and cannabis.

2. Psychosomatic illness Being overpreoccupied with one's mental and physical health and illness.

3. Overexertion, which might manifest as workaholism or excessive sport.

4. Crime Ways of getting even because you didn't feel you got a fair deal.

5. Phobia, from dislikes to aversions.

6. Panic Always being in a high-anxiety state and then spreading it to others.

7. Debauchery (excess), which could manifest as excessive intake; for example, with food.

8. Cruelty, which includes being mean, using abusive language and behaviour.

9. Sensuality, which includes excessive sex and over-preoccupation with the pleasures of the senses.

The doors and their domains

Each door of compensation relates to a particular domain where a specific psychological imbalance occurs. For example, when we have stress in the work domain we go into panic. Toximania (the excessive use of toxic substances including cigarettes, alcohol and cannabis) is associated with the domain of our sentiments and feelings. So, having the objectivity to notice which 'doors' are attractive to you also shows the aspects of your life where you are generating internal pressure.

Whereas we all use these ways of compensating at different times during every day, the degree to which we use them is also significant. The first degree of use is just occasionally, for temporary satisfaction; the second degree is regularly; the third degree habitually to excess. Using drinking as an example:

- **The first degree** is the odd occasion when you have a couple of drinks after a stressful week.

- **The second degree** is when you drink every day and you are anaesthetised by it.

- **The third degree** is when you habitually drink with drunkenness as the outcome, which is debilitating.

By the third stage such behaviour denotes addiction and represents a continual dissipation of energy and consequent brain chemistry imbalances, which are worsened by poor nutrition.

Foods and drinks that dissipate energy

From the point of view of nutrition, the foods and drinks that are associated with dissipating energy, if used regularly or habitually, are sugar, alcohol, coffee and chocolate. To generate and maintain a good level of energy it is best to either avoid these completely, or at least to get to the point where they are an occasional treat and not a daily prop. (An exception is green and black teas, which have many reported health benefits.)

Overeating

Another way of dissipating energy is to eat too much. Indian lore says we should fill our stomachs with one-half food, one-quarter water and leave one-quarter for the *prana*, or vital energy. In other words, eat to the point where you are satisfied but not full. This has the effect of energising you, whereas overeating has the opposite effect.

Vital energy

Energy isn't just about the process of eating food and metabolising it with the aid of oxygen from the air you breathe. There's another factor, called *chi* in China, *ki* in Japan and *prana* in India, which we explain in Chapter 17. It is also called 'vital energy' and it can be experienced through certain exercises and meditations. These exercises can leave you feeling alive and energised, with a delicate sense of vitality that can be directly experienced as heat in the palms of the hands, the feet and in the belly.

Deal with the issues first

So, nutritionally, it is best to avoid all the energy consumers and not to overeat. This will certainly give you more energy to deal with the stress in your life. However, from the psychological point of view, these 'doors' are used to relieve internal pressure. So by dealing with the issues that generate the psychological pressure, the need to use energy-depleting third-degree doors of compensation becomes less. In other words, you would need to change how you deal with situations in your life as well as changing what you eat and drink. The two go hand in hand.

SUMMARY

▶ Through the depletion of neurotransmitters and unhealthy changes in brain cell membranes, drugs produce 'morning after' pain.

▶ Excessive use of drugs often attracts more problems in life and increasing levels of emotional pain.

continues ▶

▶ In serious addiction the drug no longer delivers pleasure but becomes a source of pain.

▶ Identifying the sources of the pain you seek to avoid, releasing accumulated emotional charge, and finding fulfilment without drugs is an important part of the way out of an addictive process, together with optimum nutrition for restoring the brain's non-addictive chemistry.

▶ All drugs deplete energy.

▶ We often use drugs to release internal pressure or pain, to compensate.

5.

THE STRESS-SUGAR-CIGARETTE-STIMULANT TRAP

'Man is a knackered ape', said one child in an exam howler (it should have been 'naked ape'), but it can so easily be true. When we are under too much stress and we find it hard to unwind and switch off, relaxants such as alcohol, cannabis, or even sleeping pills, sound attractive. It's so easy to get caught in that trap.

For many people the first taste of addiction comes from seeking something that will increase their energy or decrease their stress, depression and anxiety, which is often caused by sub-optimum nutrition, a lack of sleep and working or playing too hard. At some point you'll taste the sweetness of sugar and feel its energy-giving effects; or have a strong tea or coffee and feel the lift; or have a cigarette and feel the elevating and relaxing buzz; or the unwinding effect of a glass of wine. Stress itself is a stimulant, promoting the release of adrenalin and cortisol, and many of us become addicted to stress, panic and living on the edge. At least you feel alive – kind of.

When occasional use becomes a need

To begin with this is no big deal – just the occasional use of a substance to change how you feel. But, as we learned in the last chapter, your brain's chemistry is already changing. You become less sensitive to the substance and therefore need more of it to feel good. Some stop at that one or two coffees a day, or that occasional cigarette, but others don't. Many people end up hooked and 'needing' 20 cigarettes or a dozen cups of tea or coffee to feel kind of normal. For some, even this isn't enough and the combination of down-regulation (becoming increasingly insensitive to the substance and needing more) and consequent reward deficiency (craving a dopamine high) leads to the desire to try something stronger – maybe cocaine for that extra kick or a more potent relaxant such as more alcohol, or even Valium or heroin if that isn't enough.

Then there's the other side of the fence, when you've quit something you had become extremely addicted to, such as alcohol, but have substituted it with loads of sugar, stimulant drinks and cigarettes. Although this appears to be a step in the right direction this means your brain chemistry is still out of balance.

The more you have, the more you want

For many people the slippery road to dependency starts with stress, sugar, cigarettes or stimulants such as caffeinated drinks. These all have similar biochemical effects by stimulating the brain's trio of inbuilt stimulants: dopamine, noradrenalin and adrenalin. These stimulants give you get-up-and-go – at least temporarily – but in the long run they make you more stressed and exhausted.

They are actually 'worker drugs', and only really became popular and excessively consumed in the Industrial Revolution, as people started to work harder and harder, driven by the culture of capitalism and competition.

The trouble is, as we have already explained, the more you have the more you want. That one cup of coffee turns into two, then three, then there is the 'speciality' coffee that you make yourself in an elaborate ritual that, behind the scenes, means you knock back a triple espresso. That occasional cigarette turns into ten, then 15, then 20 or more. Sweet foods become a constant craving. You become more tired, more stressed and more in need of a fix. Then you need alcohol to relax.

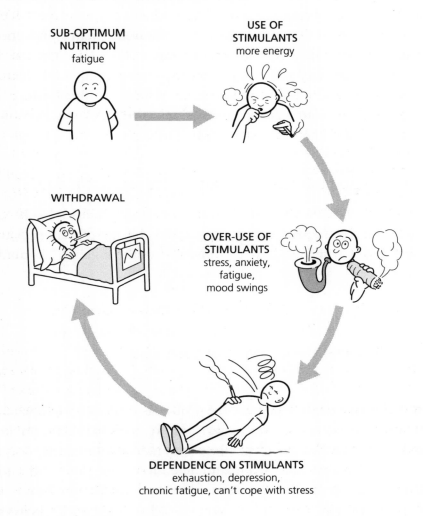

The vicious cycle of stress, stimulants and fatigue

The exhaustion epidemic

Never mind the Industrial Revolution, the technological revolution we live in today has spawned a world that never sleeps. Television, the Internet and even the stock market call to us 24 hours a day, seven days a week. When we shave an hour off our sleep, we feel we've gained some small advantage.

Many of us are also trying to keep impossible schedules of work and family responsibilities. And it has a cumulative effect. You struggle to find time with your children, friends and colleagues, not to mention your partner. You're less alert than you'd like, feeling drowsy as the day wears on, dozing off if you sit down to read or watch TV in the evening. When you finally do get together with your partner at bedtime, neither of you has the energy for anything more than falling asleep.

We turn to chemicals to help us through the day

Too often today we become reliant on chemical 'helpers' to keep us going: the frequent coffee breaks, the chocolate bar to satisfy our hunger when we have no time to eat, the cigarette to calm our nerves.

> **H**eavy use of substances like coffee, chocolate and cigarettes can lead to reward deficiency.

Although we might recognise the problems that are created when we use illegal drugs such as heroin, or if we drink to excess, smoke or become hooked on strong prescription drugs, we usually don't recognise that we can become addicted to caffeine or sugar and that these too can have serious repercussions for our health – dominating our lives and making us feel under par. We believe that we just need a little boost sometimes to get us through the day – despite the fact that if we're low on energy it might be because we are dependent on stimulants.

How dependent are you on stimulants?

To get an idea of how depleted your natural energy might be and how dependent you are on stimulants, check yourself out in the following questionnaire:

QUESTIONNAIRE: check your energy

	Yes	No
1. Do you have trouble getting up in the morning?	☐	☐
2. Do you rely on a cup of coffee to get you going in the morning?	☐	☐
3. Do you feel tired all the time?	☐	☐
4. Do you often feel foggy, fuzzy or dull?	☐	☐
5. Do you have trouble concentrating?	☐	☐
6. Do you use sugar, caffeine (tea, coffee, caffeinated cola drinks) or a cigarette as a pick-me-up throughout the day?	☐	☐
7. Are you often irritable or angry, for no apparent reason?	☐	☐
8. Do your moods seem to go up and down for no apparent reason?	☐	☐
9. Are your mood swings often relieved by food, especially sweets?	☐	☐
10. Do you have trouble falling asleep at night?	☐	☐
11. Do you have headaches or shaky feelings that are relieved by sugar, caffeine or cigarettes?	☐	☐

	Yes	No
12. Do you suspect you're addicted to coffee, caffeinated cola, or cigarettes?	☐	☐
13. Do you find yourself operating from crisis to crisis?	☐	☐
14. Are you drawn to thrills, danger and drama in your life?	☐	☐

Score 1 for each 'yes' answer.

Total score: ☐

Score

Below 5
You're doing fine. We all have our moments – bad moods, feeling tired or foggy – when we are in need of a pick-me-up.

Between 5 and 10
You are showing signs of an overdependence on stimulants to keep you going. This next section will explain what is happening in your body, and how to make healthier choices.

More than 10
You are seriously hooked on stimulants, and it is affecting your mental and physical health. It's important for you to take yourself off them. We will show you how in Part 2.

The see-saw of stimulants and relaxants

If you give in to your cravings for stimulants, it does not necessarily mean you are weak or 'bad', but simply that your chemistry is controlling you. You need the right fuel – foods, vitamins and other micronutrients – to run your body's engine (see Part 2). You also need sufficient sleep to restore body and mind and maintain your energy level. When you turn to stimulants to give you energy, however, they further deplete your already bankrupt system.

The reason they work in the short term but not in the long term is because of what they do to your blood sugar balance, as well as the balance of your neurotransmitters and hormones.

> **S**tress, sugar and stimulants all raise your blood sugar, which can give you a short-term boost in energy. But, in time, your blood sugar level becomes more and more unstable.

One of the reasons for this is that the body becomes less and less sensitive to the hormone insulin, which controls your blood sugar level. So now you need more stimulants to keep you going. Eventually you become dependent on stimulants. It's a vicious cycle of stress, overuse of stimulants and fatigue. The end result is daily craving – and exhaustion.

Some people start using more potent stimulants such as amphetamines and cocaine to get an extra lift. The more stimulants you use, the harder it is to relax and sleep soundly. Then you need relaxants such as alcohol, sleeping pills, tranquillisers and marijuana to bring you down. This see-saw lifestyle affects performance, promotes stress and depletes your energy.

Handle with care: popular stimulants

As you can see from the diagram on page 90, all stimulants work by mimicking or triggering the release of the three neurotransmitters: dopamine, adrenalin and noradrenalin. That's what makes you feel motivated and upbeat. We learned in Chapter 3 how down-regulation in the brain eventually puts a stop to the fun of getting high. That's exactly what happens with stimulants. This overstimulation leads to down-regulation, as receptor sites for dopamine, adrenalin and noradrenalin start to shut down. You keep needing more of the product to feel the same effect. But how much is too much, and are there some stimulants we can take safely in moderation?

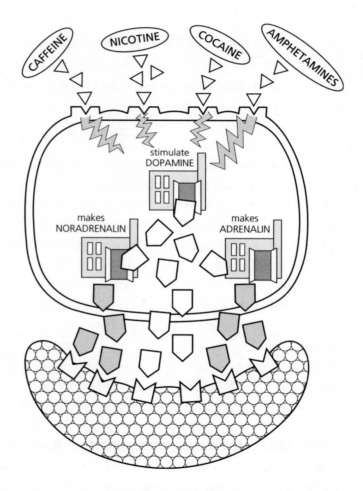

How stimulants work

Although a substance can be good in one context, it can be harmful in another. In one short-term experiment, coffee was shown to heighten alertness, but you already knew that, didn't you? And now you know that something can have benefits in the short term but be harmful in the long term.

We'll deal with these issues as we discuss each substance in detail. But for now let us say that some stimulants are never recommended, whereas others can be acceptable in moderation, depending on the situation.

Sugar: toxic treat

Sugar is a fairly recent entry into the stimulant game. Of course it's always been available in natural sources such as fruit, with its slow-releasing fructose and fibre. Refined sugar, however, only came in with the Industrial Revolution. Yet today, we can hardly picture a celebration without sweet treats – birthday and wedding cakes, Christmas puddings, Easter chocolates.

How can such a delicious, seemingly harmless children's treat be so damaging? Rapidly absorbed and broken down into molecules of glucose, it quickly reaches the brain, producing feelings

The downside of sugar

- Sugar is bad for you. Although a valuable fuel for our cells, it can be toxic when consumed in excess, often causing damage to the arteries, kidneys, eyes and nerves.

- The body tries to get it out of the blood as quickly as possible, but this can then cause a 'rebound' low blood sugar with its own set of problems. Some people feel stimulated immediately after eating it, then become cranky and finally go into a low blood sugar slump.

of 'comfort' or 'energy'. Sugar bingeing looks a lot like any other addiction: tolerance develops, and you need more to get the same effect. How serious is that? Furthermore, there's a strong link between sugar addiction and alcoholism. An illustration of this is a study by addiction researchers from University of North Carolina at Chapel Hill.[31] In one study they asked 20 abstinent alcoholic men and 37 non-alcoholic men to taste five sugar solutions. The solutions ranged from not sweet at all to very sweet. Sixty-five per cent of alcoholics preferred the sweetest solution compared to only 16 per cent of non-alcoholics. In another study they found that 19 pairs of twin brothers shared a similar liking for sweets and alcohol despite having quite different life experiences.

> Individuals who reported drinking more alcohol on occasion and having more alcohol-related problems also had problems controlling how many sweets they ate.

They were more likely to report urges to eat sweets and craving for them. They also were more likely to report this craving when they felt nervous or depressed, and they believed eating sweets made them feel better. This suggests that the craving for sweets and the urge to drink may stem from the same genes, possibly reward deficiency genes.

Caffeine: brewing up trouble

Found in over a hundred plants, caffeine is consumed primarily in drinks. A half-dozen caffeine-containing plants are more widely used than all other herbal materials combined!

Over a thousand years ago, Muslims used coffee for religious rituals. When the stuff finally reached Europe in the seventeenth century it was seen by the authorities as a dangerous drug. Nonetheless, coffee houses spread, as did dependence on this new drug. The rest is history. Together with tea, it comprises 97 per cent of worldwide caffeine consumption. Some parts of the world use other forms of caffeine – mate, guarana and kola nut – which are now becoming more popular in the West.

Caffeine was first isolated from coffee in 1821. The effects of coffee are more potent than those of caffeine alone since it contains two other stimulants: theophylline and theobromine.

How does it work?

Caffeine boosts mood and energy by blocking the receptors for a brain chemical called adenosine, whose function is to stop dopamine release. With less adenosine activity, you increase dopamine and adrenalin. You then feel alert, motivated and stimulated, although some people will feel uncomfortable and jittery. In 30 to 60 minutes, caffeine reaches its peak concentration. It is then inactivated by the liver, with only half its peak level left after four to six hours. Of course, if your liver function is poor you don't do this so well.

So where's the danger? Caffeine is highly addictive. Research shows that consuming as little as 100mg a day can lead to withdrawal symptoms when you stop, including headache, fatigue, difficulty concentrating and drowsiness. It's worth knowing that while a small cup of instant coffee may contain less than 100mg of caffeine, a large 'designer' coffee can contain as much as 500mg – five times the 'addictive' dose. Decaf has much less – less than 1mg in a cup.

The downside of caffeine

- Overstimulation of the central nervous system, leading to increased risk of heart attacks, irritability, insomnia and rapid and irregular heartbeats.

- Elevated blood sugar and cholesterol levels.

- Heartburn and other gastrointestinal problems.

- Increased risk of fibrocystic breast disease.

- Diuresis (excessive urination), which can lead to dehydration.

- Used during pregnancy, it increases the risk of birth defects.

- Contains tars, phenols, and other carcinogens.

- Pesticides are used during growing most coffee beans, and these contain cancer-causing compounds (so choose organic if you choose it at all).

At best, we can say that coffee has minor short-term mental and emotional benefits, but these are not sustained. A study published in the *American Journal of Psychiatry* observed 1,500 psychology students divided into four categories depending on their coffee intake: abstainers, low consumers (who drank one cup or equivalent a day), moderate (one to five cups a day) and high (five or more cups a day). On psychological testing, the moderate and high consumers had higher levels of anxiety and depression than the abstainers, and the high consumers had a higher incidence of stress-related medical problems coupled with lower academic performance.[32]

The bottom line? Use in moderation, but preferably not at all.

Tea: not always refreshing

In Britain three times more tea than coffee is drunk every day. In the US the figures are reversed. You can guess why by recalling the historic Boston Tea Party, which preceded the American Revolution. Rather than pay a tea tax to their oppressors across the sea, the colonists dumped boxes of imported tea from British ships into the harbour – and haven't had much taste for it since.

Tea's stimulating effects come from caffeine, theobromine and theophylline, the same compounds as in coffee. Because of different methods of preparation and the many varieties of the cultivated plant, the average caffeine content of tea ranges widely. Tea contains less caffeine than coffee. However, even when caffeine levels are matched, the effects of tea and coffee on mood are very different, suggesting that there is another component in tea that may be responsible.[33] This may be because tea also contains the natural amino acid L-theanine, a relaxant. Early research suggests that 50mg L-theanine naturally stimulates activity in the brain, known as alpha waves, which are associated with a relaxed but alert mental state.[34] A typical cup of tea contains 14–18mg of L-theanine.[35] Green tea contains even more, and also has much higher levels of health-promoting antioxidant polyphenols. In addition, green tea may help prevent liver damage and lower the risk of death from a number of diseases, including heart disease and strokes.

Case study PAUL

Paul is a good example of what happens when you have too many stimulants. He was drinking 20 cups of tea a day, each with two sugars, and smoking over 20 cigarettes a day. He had no drive or motivation in life and lacked confidence in himself. After following a low-GL diet (as explained in Chapter 11), plus the right supplements, he has given up cigarettes and caffeine. 'I feel 100 per cent better. My energy is great. I'm not tired. I feel motivated. My skin is transformed. It's made a major difference.'

The downside of tea

- A strong cup of tea contains as much caffeine as a weak cup of coffee – with all the attendant risks (see page 94).

- The tannin content interferes with absorption of minerals.

We recommend tea in moderation, meaning two cups a day, or three cups of green tea.

Colas and caffeinated drinks: 'cocaine in a can'

A cola drink contains about half the caffeine found in a cup of coffee. The original Coca Cola even contained small amounts of coca (cocaine) – hence the name. Today's drinks usually contain sugar and colourings, which also act as stimulants. Maybe worse, diet drinks contain the artificial sweetener aspartame (Nutra Sweet), which can be toxically overstimulating to the brain. We have seen people who thought they were 'going crazy' with anxiety, insomnia and disordered thinking magically recover when they stopped their diet drinks. Ironically, although touted as a diet product, they can actually cause weight gain. (See www.dorway.com/blayenn.html for information on this chemical.)

However, caffeinated soft drinks that are even stronger, with names such as Jolt or Red Bull, can contain up to 80mg of caffeine per can (that's more than a weak cup of coffee) and that increases their kick and addictiveness. Shades of the tobacco industry! Red Bull shot to fame in the UK after a newspaper article described it as 'cocaine in a can'. Children and young people are drinking large amounts of these drinks, especially relative to their weight, thereby exposing their developing brains and bodies to a hazardous substance. Their use, together with alcohol, allows a person to drink more because they stay awake. Never mind illicit drugs, consuming too much junk food and high-sugar, high-caffeine drinks can lead to serious health problems and addictions in children. We often encounter diet cola addicts.

Case study **DENISE**

Denise became so addicted to Diet Coke she bought a small fridge to keep by her bed so that when she woke up at night she could reach out and grab a can! Coca Cola's corporate agenda has been to have their products 'within a hand's reach of desire' and, in the case of Denise, they had certainly achieved their goal! At her worst she was knocking back 20 a day. She had irritable bowel syndrome (IBS), frequent colds, low energy, poor sleeping and a desire to lose some weight. Her periods were also irregular, often heavy, with cramping. She had headaches twice a week and took painkillers regularly. After three months of following our nutritional programme not only is she caffeine-free, but all her health problems have resolved – and she has lost weight.

The downside of colas

- Colas contain caffeine – with all its attendant risks (see The Downside of Caffeine, page 94).

- Sugar and colouring are added stimulants, whereas aspartame in diet versions can toxically overstimulate the brain.

- New drinks aimed at young people have even higher levels of caffeine.

Other sources of caffeine

Another source of caffeine is guarana, which is sold as a herbal stimulant. The seeds and leaves of the climbing shrub native to Brazil and Uruguay are high in caffeine. A dried paste made chiefly from the crushed seed of guarana has a relatively high caffeine content, ranging from 2.5 to 5 per cent and averaging about 3.5 per cent. To determine how much caffeine there is in any product, you must do your maths. You multiply the total weight of the capsule or powder by the percentage of caffeine or guarana to get the number of milligrams of caffeine per dose. The conclusion regarding its use? Like coffee, it can be over-stimulating, and have the same ill effects.

Some medications for the relief of headaches, such as Anadin, contain caffeine. Other caffeine tablets such as Pro Plus and the herb guarana are sold outright as stimulants. With the exception of a moderate intake of caffeine in tea we recommend you limit your intake of caffeine to no more than 100mg a day.

Here are the caffeine levels of some common products:

CAFFEINE BUZZOMETER

Coca-Cola Classic 350ml (12fl oz)	35mg
Diet Coke 350ml (12fl oz)	47mg
Red Bull 250ml (8.3fl oz)	76mg
Hot cocoa 150ml (5fl oz)	10mg
Coffee, instant 150ml (5fl oz)	40–105mg
Coffee, espresso, cappuccino, latte	50–175mg
Coffee, filter 150ml (5fl oz)	102–200mg
Coffee, Starbucks (grande)	150mg
Decaffeinated coffee 150ml (5fl oz)	0.3mg
Tea 150ml (5fl oz)	20–100mg
Chocolate cake (1 slice)	20–30mg
Bittersweet chocolate 28g (1oz)	5–35mg
Pro Plus	50mg
PEP	30mg

(Source: Centre for Science in the Public Interest www.cspinet.org/new/cafchart.htm, American Beverage Association, 2005, and Journal of Agricultural and Food Chemistry, 2003)

Death by chocolate?

Chocolate's major active ingredient is cocoa, a significant source of the stimulant theobromine. Research by British psychologist Dr David Benton at the University of Wales in Swansea, showed chocolate to be an excellent mood elevator.[36] When he played sad music to a group of students, their mood sank. He then offered them milk chocolate or carob (a natural chocolate substitute that is similar in taste), although they did not know which one they had chosen. The participants found that the chocolate raised their mood, whereas the carob didn't. Moreover, as their mood fell, their cravings for chocolate increased.

In addition to theobromine – also found in tea and coffee, as we've seen – chocolate contains the mood-enhancing stimulant, phenethylamine. Both of these stimulate dopamine production. Even experimental alcohol-loving rats, when given the choice, will replace some of their alcohol intake with chocolate.

The downside of chocolate

- Too much chocolate, especially the highly sweetened kind, causes all the problems of going overboard on sugar, including weight gain.

- It is often high in the wrong kinds of fats.

- The addictive nature of it suggests the development of tolerance, so 'just one chocolate' becomes 'just one *more*'.

- Cocoa beans, like coffee, are grown in countries where pesticide use is unregulated, exposing the consumer to cancer-causing compounds.

However, chocolate does have some redeeming qualities. It is very high in antioxidants. Of all the stimulant vices it's probably the least bad, provided you eat the pure, dark, preferably organic stuff, not cheap bars full of fat and sugar. Eat chocolate with a minimum of 70 per cent cocoa solids. But, as with any stimulant, if you eat it every day, or find yourself craving it, you've gone too far. Keep chocolate as a special treat, not a daily ritual.

Addicted to adrenalin and cortisol

Stress itself is a stimulant, promoting high levels of adrenalin and cortisol, which keeps you alive and alert. Many people get almost addicted to the buzz of adrenalin and have to keep going, fuelled by additional adrenalin and cortisol-related stimulants such as coffee and cigarettes.

Case study KATHY

Kathy was an adrenalin junkie. She was drinking up to 30 cups of coffee a day to keep herself going. She also smoked 10 to 15 cigarettes a day. She was gaining weight and losing sleep. She wasn't fully awake when she was awake, nor peacefully asleep when she was asleep. Within six weeks of starting our recommended diet, however, plus taking the specific supplements explained in Part 2 (combined in our How to Quit Action Plan), she had given up all caffeine, had stopped smoking, and was feeling loads better. She went to bed at 11pm, instead of 2am, and was waking up feeling refreshed. Three months on she had lost a staggering 20kg (3 stone/44lb) without going hungry. Her energy was greater, her skin looked much clearer and she hadn't suffered from any colds. 'I feel so much better. My energy levels are improved, I sleep like a baby, I don't miss coffee at all and I'm not smoking.'

Nicotine

Alongside caffeine and alcohol, nicotine is one of the three most widely used psychoactive drugs in our society. With no redeeming value 'smoking will continue as the leading cause of preventable, premature mortality for many years to come', says the US surgeon-general. According to the World Health Organization nearly 5 million people a year die prematurely as a result of smoking.

> **N**icotine, the primary stimulant in cigarettes, has a significant effect even in small doses.

If you have ever smoked, can you recall the sensation of your first cigarette? It probably tasted terrible, burned your mouth and lungs (if you actually inhaled), and made you nauseated and dizzy. Those are some of its toxic effects in action. A few more smokes, and for most people the body no longer rebels. In fact you rather like it. In short: you're hooked.

Nicotine has a complex series of actions, both stimulating and relaxing. For many people it is more addictive than heroin – and is often the hardest addiction to break. It stimulates the adrenals to release adrenalin and cortisol, raising blood pressure and heart rate, and increases gastrointestinal activity. It also acts as a muscle relaxant. (We'll explore this more in Chapter 21.)

In the brain, nicotine activates the release of dopamine, exhibiting a stimulant effect similar to that of caffeine. It also has a short-term antidepressant effect, although this is most often followed by a rebound depression. In larger amounts, nicotine acts as a sedative, probably because of its effect on serotonin. People trying to kick the tobacco habit describe the accompanying tension and irritability as 'feeling like you want to jump out of your skin'. They often experience low blood sugar problems, which leads them to overeat and gain weight. The trouble is that smoking keeps your brain's chemistry hooked in to needing stimulants.

Case study **AMANDA**

Eleven years ago, after years of drug abuse, Amanda quit heroin, but still felt lousy, with constant low energy, and occasionally got the shakes if she hadn't eaten. She 'managed' her state by smoking up to 40 cigarettes a day, plus caffeinated drinks and sugar or sugary snacks. She often felt anxious and irritable and didn't sleep well. Within a month of following our recommendations in Part 2 (combined in our How to Quit Action Plan), her energy had rocketed. Twelve weeks later she had quit smoking, avoided caffeinated drinks and sugary foods and definitely felt the benefits. 'My energy is so much better. I go to bed at 11pm and wake up feeling refreshed. I no longer suffer from mood swings, and I feel much more motivated and less stressed.' Even after 11 years she was able to 'rebalance' her brain's chemistry in just a few weeks with the right intake of nutrients, both from food and supplements.

The How to Quit programme

Whether you are reading this book because you want to give up caffeine or cigarettes, or have stopped using drugs or drinking alcohol, but still 'rely' on stimulants, if you really want to feel great you have to go the whole hog and break out of the sugar-stress-stimulant trap. Just quitting one addictive substance, but continuing others rarely works. You need to eat a diet that balances your blood sugar and take supplements that help 'reset' your brain's chemistry. How to do this is explained in Part 2.

SUMMARY

▶ Nicotine, caffeine and sugar are all stimulants.

▶ The more stimulants you have, the more stressed and tired you become.

▶ Your brain becomes increasingly less sensitive to your own natural stimulants – dopamine, noradrenalin and adrenalin. As a consequence you need more stimulants just to feel normal.

▶ Anyone who has quit an addictive substance but continues to rely on stimulants still has an addicted brain.

6.

PRESCRIPTION DRUGS ARE NOT THE ANSWER TO ADDICTION

Some of the most widely prescribed drugs are antidepressants, tranquillisers, sleeping pills and stimulant drugs. You might have been prescribed these drugs because you were feeling depressed, anxious or unable to sleep – and then became addicted to them. Or you might have started taking these drugs to help you deal with the withdrawal effects associated with coming off another addictive substance. But using an addictive substance to relieve the pain of getting off an addictive substance is not the answer.

It is true that when most people give up using a feel-good substance because it is creating problems for them, they quickly find another substance to relieve the discomfort of abstinence. When alcoholics stop drinking they increase their intake of nicotine, caffeine and sugar. People who give up smoking frequently relieve their stress by eating – usually junk food. In order to control their weight, some sugar addicts take up smoking. Some marijuana users start drinking or increase their alcohol consumption.

Switching one addictive substance for another is not the answer; it is part of the problem. Swapping one drug for another doesn't unscramble your brain.

The rise of prescription drugs

In recent years, medical professionals have become part of this problem: by prescribing prescription drugs to relieve the pain of abstinence symptoms. Of course they are not aware that this is what they are doing. They believe they are prescribing drugs for depression, or anxiety, or sleeplessness or lack of energy. And frequently the outcome for the patient is trading one addiction for another. Most of these prescribed drugs are addictive, sometimes more so than the original addictive substance.

While these drug approaches may be a short-term stepping stone to staying clean or sober, the need for alternative stimulants or relaxants is a sure sign that your brain chemistry is still out of balance. Substituting one drug for another doesn't correct the underlying imbalance. Until this fundamental factor is addressed, any approach to quitting any addictive substance, from cigarettes to cocaine, becomes several times harder.

The main point of giving these prescription drugs is to minimise, in the short term, abstinence symptoms. However, as you will see, if these abstinence symptoms can be more effectively reduced by our nutritional approach (using nutrients and amino acids), the need for substitute medications, with their own withdrawal effects, becomes unnecessary, thus removing this curious paradox: using a drug to correct a biochemical imbalance in the brain caused by using a drug.

How mental-health conditions are diagnosed

You might think that a scientific approach would be to check whether a person actually has a biochemical imbalance, and, if so, exactly which neurotransmitters (see Chapter 2) were low. The correct amino acids or other nutrients could then be prescribed to help restore the brain's chemical balance. But that is not what happens. Instead, the diagnosis of almost all mental-health conditions, addiction being one, is based solely on a checklist of symptoms that doesn't tell you anything about what is going on with the brain or its chemistry.

Checking neurotransmitter balance

At the Brain Bio Centre, our outpatient treatment centre, one of the first things we check for in anyone experiencing problems with depression, anxiety or sleep is the balance of neurotransmitters. We do this based on the tests first developed by Professor Tapan Audhya, from New York University Medical Center, who found very low levels of serotonin in the blood of depressed patients.[37] Noradrenalin levels are also often low in those with depression.

Knowing that this neurotransmitter is made directly from amino acids found in food, Audhya then gave his patients 5-hydroxytryptophan (5-HTP), the amino acid that's a direct precursor to serotonin. This corrected the deficiency and resulted in major and rapid relief from depression.

The usual route with prescribing

We're sure you would agree that the above is a logical approach: to identify the imbalance, then provide the brain with the nutrients necessary to allow it to rebalance. But this is not what happens in most medical practices or recovery centres. When the abstinence symptoms (depression, anxiety, insomnia) are severe, many people are given more drugs (antidepressants, tranquillisers and sleeping pills) that compound the problem. Many addicts then get hooked on these. Heroin addicts are given methadone, and then get hooked on that. For many, it's harder to get off methadone than heroin, and incredibly difficult to get off certain tranquillisers and antidepressants.

In our experience, some of the new drugs on the market, which were launched on the premise that they were less addictive or had fewer side effects, have proven to be just as bad, if not worse. Let's take a look at these, starting with antidepressants.

Are you addicted to antidepressants?

Depression is an extremely common symptom in those with addiction problems, especially among alcoholics, both while drinking and when sober. One in six people in Britain between the ages of 25 and 44 suffers from depression, according to a report by the Royal College of Psychiatrists.[38] If you are, or have been, one of these people, the chances are you will have been offered antidepressant drugs. If you've taken them, the chances are you'll have a hard time getting off them, especially if you are taking one of the more recent generations of drugs.

Understanding antidepressants

Back in the 1980s the most prescribed drugs were called 'tricyclic' antidepressants, the most popular being amitriptyline. In the 1990s these were largely replaced by a new class of drug (with new patents affording them higher prices) called SSRI (which stands for selective serotonin reuptake inhibitor) antidepressants, with names like Prozac, Seroxat and Lustral, and SNRI (which stands for serotonin and noradrenalin reuptake inhibitor) antidepressants, like Cymbalta and Efexor. The marketing of these drugs suggested they were safer and more effective. The so-called 'cessation effects' (symptoms experienced when you stop taking the drugs) were downplayed until, in 2003, the Medicines and Healthcare Products Regulatory Agency (MHRA) said that these should be called 'withdrawal' effects. (In the US, these are euphemistically called 'discontinuation' effects.) SSRIs and SNRIs have largely replaced tricyclic antidepressants, although a review of the research in 2005 noted that most studies show little difference in effectiveness.[39]

SSRIs and SNRIs are more 'selective' in the sense that, in the case of SSRIs they only target the enzyme that clears away serotonin, the key mood neurotransmitter; and in the case of SNRIs, they target enzymes that clear both serotonin and noradrenalin. Their major advantage was supposed to be fewer side effects, and it is not as easy to overdose on them as on tricyclics. The most commonly prescribed SSRIs are fluoxetine (Prozac), paroxetine (Seroxat) and sertraline (Lustral, Zoloft); and the most commonly prescribed SNRIs include venlafaxine (Efexor) and duloxetine (Cymbalta). However, they appear, in some ways, to be more dangerous. We have heard of many patients who have failed to quit Efexor because the 'discontinuation' effects are so severe.

The side effects

The risk of suicide in both children and adults for many of these SSRIs is, at least, doubled. A major review in the *British Medical Journal* of 702 studies on SSRI antidepressants showed that people taking an SSRI were more than twice as likely to attempt suicide compared with those taking a dummy pill.[40] The researchers also noted that the actual number of suicide attempts is likely to be much higher, because many of the studies did not gather information on suicide. SSRIs can also cause patients to feel 'fuzzy' and can cause major sexual dysfunction, resulting in an inability to climax in both men and women. This can prevent the intimacy that might help someone come through depression and addiction. On top of this, research published in 2006 suggests that SSRIs might dramatically increase the risk of death in those with cardiovascular disease.[41] Despite these risks, UK doctors wrote out 31 million prescriptions for antidepressants in 2006, at a cost of £291 million.

All these drugs have side effects, such as nausea, headaches, insomnia, sleepiness, dry mouth, dizziness, constipation, weakness, sweating, nervousness and sexual dysfunction. Many people also report memory loss with continued use. But most worrying are the withdrawal symptoms when you need or want to stop taking them. Consider the case of Nancy:

Case study NANCY

'When I came to treatment 15 months ago I had been on Seroxat for ten years, clonazepan and Adderall for five years each, and smoking marijuana for ten years. Of all the drugs I was coming off, the antidepressant Seroxat had by far the worst withdrawal problems. I had been taking it for so long that my body did not know what to do without it. I experienced severe withdrawal effects such as panic attacks, the feeling of crawling out of my skin, brain zaps, nausea, dizziness and restlessness, as well as uncontrollable emotions (laughter and crying). I tried to stop taking it all at once and my body could not handle it, so Dr Braly and I decided I would taper slowly off it. The thing that helped me the most was taking the amino acids GABA and tryptophan during the day as needed to ease my anxiety and panic.

'I truly believe that your approach to treating addiction disease is the best out there. I definitely feel that I would not have been able to successfully come off drugs had I not gone through this programme. I'm extremely grateful to have come off the drugs I was on and especially to have given up Seroxat. I feel great today and I know it's a result of the treatment I had and my continuing to eat the right foods and take supplements (especially eating fish and taking fish oil supplements), as well as exercising.'

Taking it slowly

In our experience, supported by scientific literature, antidepressants like Seroxat and Efexor are very difficult to come off. It is essential to taper off these drugs slowly, over at least three months, but, for some people, withdrawal symptoms continue for much longer.[42] The organisation CITA (see Resources page 484 for details) gives precise, day-by-day, withdrawal charts for all antidepressants and tranquillisers. If you are on an antidepressant and have tried and failed to come off, Chapter 24 explains how to minimise withdrawal symptoms if you want to quit. But don't try to get off an antidepressant suddenly and do not make any changes in your antidepressant medication without consulting and cooperating with your, hopefully, nutritionally informed doctor.

> **I**f you are taking more than one prescription drug it is very important to withdraw them one at a time, with a gap of ideally three months between them.

Benzos, the Zs and the frying pan

If you've been consuming large amounts of stimulants – caffeine, nicotine, amphetamines or cocaine – and you stop, it's often hard to stay awake when you're awake or asleep when you're asleep. You might find yourself drinking more alcohol to help you relax and sleep. When you stop drinking you find it hard to switch off the anxiety and go to sleep. As a consequence you may have either been prescribed some kind of sleeping pill or tranquilliser. You are not alone. In the UK over 16 million prescriptions for what are called hypnotic (sleeping) and anxiolytic (anxiety-reducing) drugs were written out in 2004, at a cost of £37 million.

Remember the Rolling Stones' song 'Mother's Little Helper'? Back in the 1960s the new miracle drugs for curing anxiety and insomnia were the benzodiazepines (the 'Little Helper' referred to in the song), said to be safer and less addictive than their predecessor, the 'non-addictive' meprobamate (Miltown), which was later shown to be as addictive as the old drugs it had replaced. We now know that the replacement 'benzo' drugs are among the most addictive, and hard to get off, substances – for many people, harder than heroin.

The benzos

Benzodiazepines include diazepam (Valium), chlordiazepoxide (Librium), clonazepam (Klonopin) and then the shorter-acting alprazolam (Xanax), lorazepam (Ativan) and temazepam. In the UK, 16 million prescriptions are still written annually for these so-called 'minor tranquillisers' to treat anxiety, insomnia, seizures and muscle spasms. Their calming effect is due to their action on GABA: by increasing GABA receptors, the most common receptors in the brain. The benzodiazepines dull both awareness and overall brain activity. However, they also have turned out to be nearly as addictive as what they replaced. Addiction to Xanax has been reported to occur in some people in as little as three days. And, in our experience, benzodiazepines may be the most difficult drugs to withdraw from, sometimes taking months.

CAUTION You should never stop taking benzodiazepines suddenly. It is dangerous. Give yourself plenty of time to taper them off gradually.

The Zs

Then (as the patents and consequently the profits run out) along come the Zs, with names such as zolpidem (Ambien), zaleplon (Sonata) and zopiclone (Zimovane). They were introduced in the 1990s amid claims that they were a safe and non-addictive alternative to earlier drugs. Guess what? They too are every bit as addictive.

A major review in 2005 by the National Institute for Clinical Excellence (NICE) concluded that 'there was no consistent difference between the two types of drug [benzodiazepines and Zs] for either effectiveness or safety.'[43] They too can cause tolerance and withdrawal. Dependence can develop after as little as one week of continuous use. Similarly, you are also advised not to take nonbenzodiazepines for more than a few weeks at most. A bulletin regarding the drug zopiclone advises:

> This medicine is generally only suitable for short-term use. If it is used for long periods or in high doses, tolerance to and dependence upon the medicine may develop, and withdrawal symptoms may occur if treatment is stopped suddenly. For this reason, treatment with this medicine should usually be stopped gradually, following the instructions given by your doctor, in order to avoid withdrawal symptoms such as rebound insomnia or anxiety, confusion, sweating, tremor, loss of appetite, irritability or convulsions.[44]

But these are the sleeping pills you are more likely to be offered on prescription these days, especially if you can't sleep because you've stopped smoking or drinking or you have come off a stimulant drug. In 2004, there were close to 4 million prescriptions made for Zimovane (zopiclone) in the UK alone. They will certainly help if you have a short-term problem with sleeping due to a crisis, but in the long term they are not what's needed. 'If you have chronic insomnia,' says Professor Jim Horne of Loughborough University's Sleep Research Centre, 'it's because you have an underlying problem and just getting an extra half an hour's sleep, which is about all the drugs give you, is not going to help tackle it.'

Nutrition can create an escape route

Both benzodiazepines and the Zs can be very difficult to come off, and near impossible without the nutritional support we recommend in Chapter 23. In that chapter you'll find the story of Pauline, who was hooked on Zimovane: 'I tried so many times to come off it and failed. Once I didn't have any for three days, couldn't sleep and drove into the back of a car!' Pauline finally got free using our nutrition-based approach. 'To this day I still take these nutrients and I feel great. Goodbye Zimovane!'

We don't recommend benzodiazepines and the Zs, except for very short-term use. It's a case of out of the frying pan into the fire. Of course, there are newer drugs now on offer, which are claimed to be non-addictive, although this remains to be seen. First in the ring was eszopiclone (Lunesta), licensed in 2005 for long-term use after studies apparently showed no addiction and no need for an increased dose after six months. It is a variation on zopiclone and is little different in effect. In controlled trials, this drug increased the amount of sleep time by between 15 and 21.5 minutes, compared to a placebo. So why risk potential addiction for so little benefit? In the US you can barely turn on the television without seeing ads for drugs such as these vying for the market of an estimated 1.7 million benzo addicts and probably just as many Z addicts. We don't recommend you join them. If you have already, or you are tempted to because of abstinence symptoms from other substances, the 12 Keys to Unaddicting Your Brain in Part 2 will dramatically reduce your need. If you have already developed a dependency, also read Chapter 23 to find out the most effective ways to get off these drugs.

Methadone madness

Finally, a word on methadone. Many treatment approaches for heroin addiction involve replacing the heroin with methadone, a similar drug that can be, and is, prescribed to the hundreds of thousands of methadone addicts in the UK alone. If your thinking is that heroin addiction is 'incurable' and your goal is to keep an addict away from crime and dodgy needles, then switching to a prescribable, controllable substance may sound like a good thing. But if the ultimate goal is to get clean, methadone is not the answer. A methadone user is still addicted. And methadone is usually harder to get off than heroin. Neither the quadrupling of methadone prescriptions in Britain between 1982 and 1992, nor the doubling of them in the US between 1999 and 2001, has had any effect on the scale of the problem of opiate addiction. Many addicts become addicted to both heroin and methadone. Substantial numbers of people are killed by methadone. Between 1993 and 2004 there were 7,072 deaths involving heroin or morphine and 3,298 deaths involving methadone.[45] Currently, about 1.5 million prescriptions for methadone are written every year.[46] Some doctors recommend switching to other opioid drugs such as buphenorphine, but these carry the same kind, although possibly not the same scale, of risks.[47]

In Chapter 27 we look at the most effective ways to get off heroin or methadone or any opioid drug for good.

None of these drugs correct the underlying imbalances that lead to addiction and dependence even though they can temporarily relieve the abstinence symptoms. Even if they do get you out of the fire, you're still in the frying pan.

The way forward

In the next part we explain the 12 Keys to Unaddicting Your Brain, many of which, on their own, have already been shown to be more effective than prescription drugs and, in combination, are substantially more effective without any of the associated risks of addiction and side effects. There is also nothing to stop you doing these keys to recovery while you are still on a prescription drug.

And as you start to feel better, discuss with your doctor gradually tapering off the drug as it becomes increasingly unnecessary. How to do this is explained for each kind of drug in Part 3.

SUMMARY

▶ Drugs prescribed for depression, anxiety and sleeplessness are usually highly addictive.

▶ These drugs are often prescribed when people are experiencing abstinence symptoms.

▶ Swapping one addictive drug for another – even if prescribed by a doctor – is not an answer.

▶ It is very important to taper off any prescription drug under the supervision of a doctor.

▶ You can begin using the keys to unaddicting your brain listed in the next section while you are tapering off prescription drugs.

PART 2

THE 12 KEYS TO UNADDICTING YOUR BRAIN

In this part we explain the 12 Keys that have proven most helpful to people kicking their addiction. Think of it as a boot camp for your brain. The 12 Keys are simple steps you can take to give your brain, and your psyche, the equivalent of a trip to the health farm. And it works. By eating healthy foods and taking the absolute optimum amount of key nutrients you reprogramme your brain and body chemistry so that you quickly start to experience a state of natural energy, clarity and steady mood – in effect an enjoyable *natural* high. Because of this, you'll find the desire to use an addictive substance far less strong.

Don't underestimate the power of your brain

It is important to remember that there is no '1 Key' solution to addiction. If you've been using addictive substances for many years, possibly in large quantities, your brain will not simply be 'reset' by eating a so-called well-balanced diet. Similarly, if you've experienced major stresses and traumas in life you don't just recover by leading a balanced life. There is damage that needs to be undone. You have to reprogramme your mind and rebuild your brain. If you've seriously scrambled your brain, just sitting in a room and talking about your past isn't going to unscramble it.

The bottom line is that if your brain is programmed for addiction, with all the will in the world, and the best counselling, and even some of the new addiction drugs that make you feel sick if you use the drug of your choice, *nothing* is stronger than the impulse of your brain telling you that your survival depends on having this substance. Biological urges are immensely strong. You try not breathing, or not peeing, for example. We take our hats off to those who have quit when all the cells in their body are screaming for a cigarette, a drink or a drug. That's definitely the hard track.

The easier track is to work with your brain's natural design, not against it, by restoring the imbalance, not with drugs, but with the very nutrients that your brain has evolved to use over millions of years. This approach not only reprogrammes your brain and your body's chemistry to make you feel good naturally, but it also reprogrammes how you react to the triggers that lead you to take an addictive substance. As your brain, mood, concentration and energy start to come back to life so does your capacity for learning and resolving psychological or life conflicts that may be part of you getting stuck in some level of addiction. Hence counselling is much more effective in optimally nourished people. Although psychological issues, such as feeling completely stressed or depressed, can lead you into addiction, once you are in it, the brain's chemistry becomes reprogrammed, and simply solving the reason for your stress or depression, and avoiding the substance, doesn't reset your brain's chemical balance. The best way to achieve this is through the programme presented in this book.

Success is proven

This isn't just talk. Our approach works in the real world. For example, in one treatment centre, Bridging The Gaps in Winchester, Virginia, which has incorporated these 12 Keys into their treatment agenda, along with intravenous nutrient therapy, the success rate has gone through the roof. We followed up 23 clients one year after they had started the equivalent of this How to Quit approach to quit their serious drug and alcohol addictions, and found that of the 23, 21 were clean and sober. That's an incredible 91 per cent success rate! The usual one year success rate (meaning still clean and sober) for other methods of quitting is around 20 per cent. Of the 23 participants, 16 (70 per cent) had not even had a brief relapse – not a single drink or use of any drug.

Using the 12 Keys

The 12 Keys to Unaddicting Your Brain are designed to help you understand the solutions that are right for you. The first six define what 'optimum nutrition' really means in terms of unaddicting your brain: how to find out which amino acids will most rapidly reduce your abstinence symptoms; the kind of foods and supplements to take to get the best intake of essential fats, vitamins and minerals; and how to improve your ability to digest and absorb these nutrients. The next three chapters on getting a good night's sleep, solving hidden food allergies and rejuvenating your liver, will be more applicable to some readers than others, but please read them all to see if they address issues that relate to you. The last three chapters explain what you can do to raise your feel-good endorphins naturally, generating vital energy and emotional healing – all have the effect of increasing your energy.

Get support

Although everything in this programme can be done at home, if you have a serious addiction we encourage you to work with a team of health professionals, including a nutritional therapist and psychotherapist, or a treatment centre that uses most of these 12 Keys to Unaddicting Your Brain. If your treatment centre of choice does not incorporate our How to Quit nutrition approach you can always also attend, as an outpatient, the Brain Bio Centre in Richmond, Surrey (see Resources) to find your ideal nutrition prescription.

Add value to your programme

Whereas the optimum nutrition approach to reversing addiction is a vital missing piece we do not believe that it is the only piece of the jigsaw and recommend you do anything and everything that works for you. There is no contradiction to adding our How to Quit programme to any other method or technique for reversing your addiction. (If you are on prescribed medication please make sure you read Chapter 7 as there are some amino acids that should not be taken alongside certain drugs.)

Moving on

In Part 3 you'll find out which of the keys we outline here will make the biggest difference to you, depending on which substances you want to quit.

7.

REBALANCE YOUR BRAIN WITH AMINO ACIDS

We've got some very exciting news for you. Contrary to what you might believe, it is possible for you to get almost immediate relief from the symptoms you experience when you stop taking a substance. The answer is to supplement the amino acids that are right for you. We explained in Chapter 2 that it is the transmitters in your brain that make you feel pleasure, but that these can be depleted through using mood-altering substances such as drugs, alcohol, caffeine, nicotine and even sugar. When we stop taking the mood-altering substances we suffer abstinence symptoms because our brain chemicals remain unbalanced. In this chapter we explain how to rebalance your brain by taking amino acids – among the tools that un-addict our brain. The extraordinary effect of amino acid therapy is, in our view, one of the most important new discoveries in the fight to maintain a commitment to quit. Our scientifically based How to Quit programme will guide you through.

As we have already pointed out, it is the imbalance of neurotransmitters that gets your brain out of kilter. When you use a mood-altering substance this creates or intensifies an imbalance by causing the brain to lose its ability to help you feel good naturally. Because neurotransmitters are made from amino acids,

> **S**upplementing with specific amino acids is the fast track to restoring normal brain chemistry and becoming free of cravings.

your brain starts to recover its own natural high when you nourish it with specific amino acids. This chapter will explain how to do this in detail to find the combination of nutrients that is just right for you. However, Parts 3 and 4 bring all this information together to give you the supplement dosages for your particular addiction and abstinence symptoms.

When healthy eating alone is not enough

Some people will tell you that you get all the amino acids you need from eating protein, and that is true – provided you are in optimal health, you are not reward-deficient and you have no history of addiction or cravings. But that probably is not true for you.

Case study   DAVID MILLER

'I have found that the story of my recovery from alcoholism is very similar to that of other people, whether theirs is a story of addiction to nicotine, caffeine, sugar, or some other substance. I had over ten years of abstinence from alcohol when I first heard of amino acid therapy. Although I had learned to cope with the discomfort after I had given up drinking I had found nothing that truly gave me relief from the symptoms I experienced after I had given up. I especially struggled with hypersensitivity to noise and the stress related to that. I used to say that a fly on the wall down the hall could drive me crazy. Another addiction professional told me about an amino acid supplement and suggested I try it.

'I did, more because he asked me to than because I really expected a positive result. I noticed the effects almost immediately. Everything seemed toned down. Life was less shrill. I felt less bombarded by sounds and things going on around me. In a word, I felt relief. My internal molecules seemed to quiet and stop fighting me. I felt at ease. It felt as if I had taken a stone out of my shoe.

'The effect was so dramatic that my wife noticed it right away. She said I seemed more relaxed and easy to be around. In fact, over time I discovered that any time I failed to take the amino acid supplement she would say, "Did you take your nutrients?" sometimes before even I realised that I had forgotten. For the first time in my life I was functioning at a comfort level that seemed to begin in my brain, filter throughout my body, and affect my behaviour. Even though I still had some ups and downs with mood, this level of comfort became my normal state, and the ups and downs are now much easier to deal with.'

Your brain depends on amino acids

You will probably be amazed at the relief you can get if you begin nourishing your brain with amino acids. Every cell in your body is produced in large part from them. Reproducing, altering or growing any type of cell requires a balance of many different amino acids. Any behaviour or function you have – concentration, memory, mood, sleep, thirst, appetite, alertness and emotions – involves the functioning of your whole nervous system. The nervous system is regulated almost entirely by amino acids and their biochemical companions: vitamins, minerals and essential fats.

Everything you think, feel and do, as well as everything you eat, drink or smoke, has a direct effect on your neurotransmitter balance and brain function. Amino acids and brain functioning go hand in hand. Amino acids nourish the brain with what should be there. Neurotransmitter balance – and imbalance – are related to amino acids; so too is neurotransmitter production and depletion. So, in a way, it is a no-brainer (or go-brainer):

> **Y**ou must restore neurotransmitters and receptors to their normal state with amino acids.

Getting to grips with the effects of amino acids

Because different amino acids and combinations of amino acids – with their helping vitamins and minerals – produce different effects, finding the correct balance is quite complex, but we now have over 30 years of research to prove that amino acid therapy is not a theory or a gimmick, but that it actually works in practice and makes a big difference in addiction recovery.

Accessing amino acids

In the US many addiction treatment centres now include amino acid therapy, but hardly any use this in Europe. In fact, EU legislators, if anything, are making it harder to access these essential nutrients. GABA and SAM, two important amino acids that we described in Part 1, are no longer available over the counter in Europe because they've been reclassified as medicines. But you can ask your doctor for a prescription.

How will amino acids help you?

As we have said, drug craving and other abstinence symptoms are a result of malfunctions of the reward centres of the brain involving the neurotransmitters and the enzymes that control them. We now know, as a result of studies carried out with amino acids, that it is possible to reduce stress, depression and anxiety as well as increase glucose and neurotransmitter receptor sensitivity, and to restore serotonin, dopamine, enkephalins, taurine and GABA with amino acid supplementation, which will give you a generally improved feeling of well-being.[1] If this sounds too good to be true or a dream for the future, let us assure you that it is already happening.

Essential and non-essential amino acids

It is generally agreed that there are 21 amino acids necessary for the creation of proteins in the body (protein is required for cell building). The body normally produces most of these 21 amino acids. These are called non-essential, not because they are not essential to the functioning of your body and brain but because under ideal circumstances it is not essential to get them from the diet or oral supplements.

But the body does not manufacture all of the amino acids needed to form neurotransmitters. Some are derived only from food or supplements and come to the brain by way of the blood supply. These are called essential amino acids.

Amino acids for times of stress

There's an important third category: conditionally essential amino acids. These are amino acids that are non-essential during periods free from illness and excessive stress. But during periods of illness or chronic stress (injury, surgery, excessive physical exertion, cancer therapy or addiction) they become essential. The body's machinery is simply unable to generate adequate levels, so additional sources are required from food or supplementation. Examples of conditionally essential amino acids that often become essential as a consequence of addiction are glutamine, tyrosine and taurine.[2]

Most experts agree that there are nine essential amino acids, seven non-essential and five conditionally essential amino acids.

ESSENTIAL AND NON-ESSENTIAL AMINO ACIDS

Essential amino acids	Non-essential amino acids	Conditionally essential amino acids
Histidine **	Alanine	Arginine
Isoleucine	Aspartic Acid	Cystine/cysteine
Leucine	Glutamic Acid	Glutamine
Lysine	Glycine	Taurine
Methionine	Proline	Tyrosine
Phenylalanine	Serine	
Threonine		
Tryptophan		
Valine		

** Histidine is essential only in children

Amino acids that are also neurotransmitters

Some amino acids are already neurotransmitters, and therefore don't have to be made from other amino acids. These are glycine, GABA and taurine. We mention this here so that you will be aware that when we talk about GABA, for example, we are sometimes referring to it as an amino acid and sometimes as a neurotransmitter.

Addiction-busting aminos: your allies

As we learned in Chapter 1 there are certain amino acids that help produce the stimulating and relaxing neurotransmitters that are most often involved in addiction. If you are finding your abstinence symptoms are particularly uncomfortable or you experience repeated relapse, these amino acids will become important allies for you. The more you understand what they do and how they help relieve your symptoms the better able you will be to manage your own intake and help keep your brain in tune and in balance. These are:

L-phenylalanine (increases dopamine and noradrenalin)

D-phenylalanine (increases enkephalin)

Tyrosine (increases dopamine and noradrenalin)

Tryptophan and 5-HTP (increases serotonin and melatonin – a neurotransmitter-like compound that helps us sleep)

Glutamine (increases GABA and glutathione)

GABA (is already a neurotransmitter)

Taurine (is already a neurotransmitter)

Now, let's explore each one in more detail:

The feel-good factor: phenylalanine[3]

Phenylalanine is a vital brain booster. It elevates mood, increases confidence and motivation, increases energy, improves alertness and wakefulness, decreases pain, indirectly decreases cravings, sharpens your memory and ability to learn and decreases your appetite. It comes in three different forms:

1. **L-phenylalanine** (LPA), the most common form, which (with vitamin B_6) is converted into tyrosine. From this you can make dopamine and noradrenalin – the feel-good and motivating neurotransmitters.

2. **D-phenylalanine** (DPA) inhibits an enzyme that breaks down enkephalin, making more of it available at the reward sites in

the brain. Enkephalin is a natural, morphine-like substance that reduces pain and increases feelings of pleasure.

3. DL-phenylalanine (called DLPA) is a combination of both.

CAUTION L-phenylalanine has been reported to cause hypertension in some people. DO NOT TAKE L-phenylalanine if:

- You are pregnant or nursing.

- You suffer from panic attacks or severe anxiety (both may be aggravated by making more adrenalin, which can be made from L-phenylalanine).

- You suffer from skin cancer melanoma or phenylketonuria (PKU).

- If you are taking monoamine oxidase (MAO) inhibitors, a class of antidepressant.

The motivator: tyrosine[4]

Tyrosine, which can be made from L-phenylalanine, is one step closer to dopamine and noradrenalin: the neurotransmitters that make you feel upbeat and motivated. It is also an important building block for the thyroid hormone, called thyroxine, which revs up your energy-producing cells. If you need a physical, mental or emotional lift, this is the best amino acid to take. Break a 1g capsule in your mouth so that it will be quickly absorbed in order to provide an immediate boost. Taken with vitamin B_6 and zinc, it can really help concentration.

For good mood and sleep: tryptophan[5]

Tryptophan is mostly a relaxing amino acid. It's the essential building block for serotonin, the mood-boosting neurotransmitter, and melatonin, which reduces cravings and helps you relax and sleep. We recommend that tryptophan be taken in doses of 1,000–2,000mg. It is completely safe, and until 1988 there was no limit on how much you could buy. But then one batch manufactured in Japan was contaminated and went untested, causing 1,500 people to become ill, resulting in 37 deaths. It was not the tryptophan itself that was the problem but a new processing method that resulted in the contamination. It was taken off the shelves but it is now back, with manufacturers required to sell only pure trytophan. In the UK it is limited to 220mg per tablet, which is too low.

Alternatively you can try the derivative of tryptophan called 5-hydroxytryptophan (5-HTP). Tryptophan is a precursor to 5-HTP, which immediately becomes serotonin, and as a consequence, can give you the same good feelings as tryptophan. 5-HTP is one step closer to serotonin.

Signs of tryptophan deficiency

When your tryptophan intake is deficient, serotonin levels drop, causing depression, anxiety, carbohydrate craving, insecurity, irritability, suicidal thoughts, insomnia and a lowered pain threshold. This happens quickly. A study at Oxford University gave 15 women a diet devoid of tryptophan. Within eight hours ten of the women started feeling depressed.[6] A deficiency in serotonin is strongly linked to alcohol or drug abuse, craving and bingeing on carbohydrates, hyperactivity, rage, violence, sexual promiscuity and uncontrolled gambling.

How to take the supplements

Both tryptophan and 5-HTP are safe, natural relaxants, mood boosters and sleep aids. When supplementing with either, it is important also to include vitamin B_6 and zinc: essential in the conversion of both to serotonin.

Only a few foods contain high amounts of tryptophan; most foods contain more tyrosine or phenylalanine, which compete with tryptophan for entry into the brain, and generally win. So take tryptophan or 5-HTP on an empty stomach or with a carbohydrate snack such as a piece of fruit or an oatcake, away from a main meal. As well as supplementing with tryptophan or 5-HTP, make sure your diet gives you at least 1g (see page 138).

The mood boosters: tryptophan and 5-HTP

Researchers in England compared the effects of tryptophan and the popular prescription drug Tofranil on two groups of patients with depression. (Tofranil, or imipramine, is a drug commonly used for depression.) Both groups of patients improved. Tryptophan was just as effective as Tofranil and there were no side effects. However, the side effects for the Tofranil group included blurring of vision, dryness of mouth, low blood pressure, urinary retention, heart palpitations, hepatitis and seizures.[7] Donald Ecclestone, professor of medicine at the Royal Victoria Infirmary in Newcastle, UK, reviewed the available studies and concluded that supplementing tryptophan leads to an increase in the synthesis of serotonin in the brain, improving mood just as well as some antidepressant drugs.

In a similar play-off study between 5-HTP and an SSRI antidepressant, 5-HTP comes out slightly better. One double-blind trial headed by Dr W.P. Poldinger at the Basel University of Psychiatry gave 34 depressed volunteers either the SSRI fluvoxamine (Luvox or Faverin) or 300mg of 5-HTP. At the end of the six weeks, both groups of patients had experienced a significant improvement in their depression. However, those taking 5-HTP had a slightly greater improvement, compared to those on the SSRI, in each of the four criteria assessed – depression, anxiety, insomnia and physical symptoms – as well as their own self-assessment.[8] There have been 27 trials on 5-HTP,[9] including 11 double-blind placebo-controlled trials, and six of those measured depression using the HRS (a standard measure of depression called the Hamilton Rating Scale). The average improvement is double that of antidepressants.

CAUTION

- DON'T COMBINE antidepressant drugs with tryptophan or 5-HTP. The drug blocks the normal breakdown of serotonin whereas the amino acid helps you make the amount you need. The combination of the two could theoretically induce serotonin excess and the results could be the same as an overdose of antidepressant medication. Serotonin overdose can be fatal, although this has never been reported in association with 5-HTP on its own, or in combination with an antidepressant.

- Some people experience mild gastrointestinal disturbance on 5-HTP, which usually stops within a few days. Since there are serotonin receptors in the gut, which don't normally expect to get the real thing so easily, they can overreact if the amount is too high, resulting in passing nausea. If this happens, just lower the dose.

To reduce cravings: glutamine[10]

Glutamine is an anti-craving amino acid.[11] Whatever you crave – whether it is food, alcohol or cocaine – glutamine will reduce the craving and help you feel more satisfied and content by directly increasing brain levels of GABA and indirectly increasing levels of enkephalins. This makes you feel good and relaxes you.

As a bonus, glutamine is your gut's best friend.[12] This is because the cells that make up your intestinal lining – the barrier between your body and everything you ingest – literally run on glutamine. This barrier, which is the size of a small football pitch and the thickness of a quarter of a sheet of paper, is replaced every three days. If you drink alcohol most days, or often take painkillers or antibiotics, this 'inner skin' becomes more permeable. Glutamine powder, ideally taken in water last thing at night, or first thing in the morning on an empty stomach, helps to heal the gut.[13] In Japan glutamine is one of the most popular and effective anti-ulcer medications. Four grams (a level teaspoon) of glutamine also increases the growth hormone, a common deficiency in addiction.

There is a lot of glutamine in uncooked protein, but the chances are you probably eat meat, fish and poultry cooked, but don't eat enough raw nuts and seeds to provide all the glutamine you need. Up to 95 per cent of glutamine is inactivated by heating it. So your best source is a powdered supplement. Glutamine is tasteless and mixes easily with liquid (which should be cool) and is basically non-toxic. We recommend 4g, which is one heaped teaspoonful, two to three times a day, taken ideally first thing in the morning, at midday and at night.

CAUTION Although it helps the liver detoxify, we do not recommend that glutamine be taken in cases of advanced cirrhosis of the liver or kidney disease, or by people with elevated creatinine or ammonia.

The relaxer: GABA (gamma aminobutyric acid)[14]

GABA is both an amino acid and a neurotransmitter. It is the calming amino acid, which alleviates anxiety and provides a mental and physical lift. As stated earlier, glutamine works as an anti-craving substance because it stimulates the production of the neurotransmitter GABA. People who are GABA-deficient will probably have high levels of anxiety, tension and sleep problems. A recent study indicates that GABA enhances alpha-wave production in the brain, which promotes relaxation.[15]

Although the scientific literature states that GABA does not pass through the blood brain barrier into the brain very well, reports from many people suggest otherwise. You can take GABA or you can take glutamine to stimulate the production of GABA.

Some people take both GABA and glutamine. Whichever you use, take vitamin B$_6$, magnesium and zinc along with it. GABA comes in capsules, but may be taken as a powder, with ⅛ teaspoon equalling 250mg. Mixed in water, GABA powder is mildly unpleasant-tasting. It is inexpensive to buy, but is not available over the counter in the UK.

CAUTION The beauty of GABA is that it is a naturally occurring substance that has few side effects in reasonable amounts. Too much GABA, however, may cause odd sensations such as flushing and/or tingling in the face or fingers.

- Do not take more than 3,000mg GABA in any one day. Shortness of breath, a drained feeling and mild anxiety have been reported by those who have used GABA in very large doses. These sensations and side effects soon stop when you lower the dosage.

- People addicted to alcohol and benzodiazepine drugs are very commonly GABA-depleted and hence prone to seizures during the period of acute withdrawal. Therefore, they should be under a doctor's supervision while acute withdrawal is going on. GABA depletion is so serious with any benzodiazepine medication that anyone using them for any reason, whether or not they believe they are addicted, should not attempt to get off suddenly. The drug should be gradually tapered over a period of time.

The calmer: taurine[16]

Taurine is an inhibitory, calming neurotransmitter. During periods of stress or illness, it becomes an essential amino acid and needs to be supplemented. It enhances GABA activity in the brain, and has many direct uses: treating migraine, insomnia, agitation, restlessness, irritability, obsessions, depression and even mania (the 'high' phase of bipolar disorder or manic depression).

Because different amino acids and combinations of amino acids – with their helping vitamins and minerals – produce different effects, finding the correct balance is quite complex, but we now have over 30 years of research to prove that amino acid therapy is not a theory or a gimmick, but that it actually works in practice and makes a big difference in addiction recovery.

It's also a potent antioxidant, and helps regulate concentrations of calming minerals such as magnesium – hence the combination of the two. Magnesium taurate is especially beneficial. Taurine is normally derived from the amino acid cysteine, provided you are good at the process of methylation (page 42), which depends on your intake of B vitamins.

(Remember, you will find full details of the dosages for your addiction in Parts 3 and 4.)

So that's the family of amino acids you need to know about. They each have an effect on particular neurotransmitters, deficiency of which leads to particular symptoms and cravings. The table on pages 135–36 summarises the action of neurotransmitters that are most often related to addiction.

ACTIONS OF NEUROTRANSMITTERS AND AMINO ACIDS

Neurotransmitter	Amino acid it's made from	What it does	Symptoms of deficiency	Substance used to compensate for deficiency
Adrenalin, noradrenalin	L-phenylalanine Tyrosine	Arousal, energy, stimulation, mental focus	Lack of energy, depression, poor concentration	Caffeine, cocaine, speed, tobacco, marijuana, alcohol, sugar
Dopamine	L-phenylalanine Tyrosine	Good feelings, satisfaction, comfort, alertness	Emptiness, lack of pleasure and reward, fatigue, depression, lack of motivation, over-eating	Alcohol, marijuana, cocaine, caffeine, amphetamines, sugar, tobacco
Endorphins, enkephalins	D-phenylalanine DL-phenylalanine	Physical and emotional pain relief, pleasure, good feelings, euphoria, sense of well-being	Hyper-sensitivity to emotional and physical pain, inability to feel pleasure, feeling of incompleteness, craving for comfort or pleasure, craving for certain substances, feeling down	Heroin, alcohol, marijuana, sugar, chocolate

continues ▲

Neurotransmitter	Amino acid it's made from	What it does	Symptoms of deficiency	Substance used to compensate for deficiency
Serotonin	Tryptophan or 5-HTP	Emotional stability, self-confidence, pain tolerance, quality sleep	Depression, obsessiveness, compulsiveness, worry, low self-esteem, sleep problems, craving for sweets, irritability, fearfulness, tantrums, violence, sexual promiscuity	Alcohol, sugar, chocolate, tobacco, marijuana
GABA	GABA, Glutamine	Calming, relaxation	Anxiety, panic, tenseness, insecurity, sleeplessness, seizures	Valium, alcohol, marijuana, tobacco, sugar
Taurine	Taurine	Calmness, promotion of sleep and digestion, seizure control	Proneness to seizures, sleeplessness, anxiety, poor digestion	Benzodiazepines, alcohol

How to choose which amino acids you need

Your current symptoms are probably your best guide when deciding which amino acids are most likely to help you. Rather than determining which amino acids are appropriate for you based on which substance you have used, ask yourself what effect you get from the substance and what symptoms you experience when you don't use it: your abstinence symptoms. The table below shows you which amino acids you are most likely to benefit from, depending on your abstinence symptoms. Highlight those that are ringing big bells for you. Sometimes you need to experiment a little to find out what works for you. If you try GABA to relax and sleep better, for example, and you don't get the result you are seeking, try 5-HTP and taurine instead.

ABSTINENCE SYMPTOMS AND THE AMINO ACIDS TO RELIEVE THEM

Abstinence symptoms	Amino acids
Anxiety, stress, tension	GABA, taurine, 5-HTP
Low energy, apathy	Tyrosine
Poor concentration, poor memory, mental fuzziness	Tyrosine
Hypersensitivity	L-phenylalanine, D-phenylalanine
Sleeplessness	Tryptophan or 5-HTP, GABA, taurine
Irritability, negativity, worry	Tryptophan or 5-HTP
Cravings	Glutamine, GABA, tryptophan, 5-HTP
Depression – tense, agitated	5-HTP or tryptophan
Depression – passive, low energy	Tyrosine

Supplementing amino acids

Eating protein is the best way to get the essential amino acids for a normal healthy person, but taking amino acid supplements is the best way to guarantee you are receiving optimal amounts for rebalancing neurotransmitters, which is essential if you are suffering from an addiction. One of the advantages of taking supplements containing individual amino acids is that they are more easily absorbed this way. The reason for this is that certain amino acids compete for absorption, so if you supplement with tryptophan, for example, you will absorb more into the bloodstream if you take the tryptophan supplements without eating protein-rich food at the same time. Taking the supplements with a carb such as fruit may be even better because carbohydrates promote insulin release which helps deliver tryptophan to the brain.

How much to take

The minimum effective starting dose for most of these amino acids is 500mg per day, which can be increased gradually to 3,000mg per day (except for 5-HTP, which ranges in dosage from 50 to 400mg per day, and L-glutamine, which ranges in dosage from 500 to 15,000mg per day). It is best to start with a lower dose and increase it until you feel the benefits. Most people respond to the daily dose being divided into two or three doses a day. (We'll let you know exactly what you need to take in Parts 3 and 4, depending on your addiction.)

In addition, try to boost your amino acid intake through diet. The box below gives some examples of meals that provide substantial amounts of amino acids.

Five meals rich in amino acids

1. Oat porridge, soya milk and two scrambled eggs.

2. Baked potato with cottage cheese and tuna salad.

3. Chicken breast, potatoes au gratin (potatoes with a white sauce and cheese) and green beans.

4. Wholewheat spaghetti with a bean, tofu or meat sauce.

5. Salmon, quinoa and lentil pilaf with green salad and yogurt.

Some people start with a supplement powder containing a balance of 'free-form' amino acids. This can be taken on its own, sprinkled on cereal or added to a fruit smoothie. Or you can get it in formulated complex capsules, usually taken three times a day. These free-form amino acids don't require digestion in the same way that protein does, so they are easily absorbed. They do, however, compete with each other, so they are not as effective as taking individual amino acid supplements.

A good protein powder should provide the following key brain-boosting amino acids, and more, in these kinds of amounts in a daily serving:

Glutamine/glutamic acid	2,000mg
Tyrosine	1,000mg
GABA/taurine	1,500mg
Tryptophan	1,000mg
Phenylalanine	1,000mg

NOTE The amount of tryptophan in supplements is restricted in some countries; in the UK it is restricted to 220mg per serving.

Many people find their perfect solution by having a daily amino acid complex, and then add specific amino acids depending on their need. For example, Carol, who has quit smoking and also has attention deficit hyperactivity disorder, has found that if she takes a formulation of D-phenylalanine, tyrosine, glutamine and important vitamins and minerals three times a day, she still has a down time in the afternoon when she has difficulty concentrating and feels slightly irritable. Some additional tyrosine at those times gives her a lift, improves her mood, increases alertness and improves concentration. Trial and error will probably result in the reward you are seeking.

When you are especially stressed, you may want to take more

than your normal dose to help bring you back into balance. If you don't get the benefits you are seeking from the appropriate amino acid, gradually increase the dose until you have reached the maximum dose. But if you are combining a complex and individual amino acids, be careful not to overdo it. In Part 4 we help you find your own most effective amino acid solution.

Are amino acid supplements for life?

Experts do not agree on how long a recovering person needs to take amino acid supplements. People with less severe addictions may be able to stop taking daily supplements after a relatively short period of time. But people who find themselves going back to their feel-good substance time and time again, people with pre-existing conditions such as attention deficit hyperactivity disorder, and people who continue to be uncomfortable when abstinent need all the help they can get, possibly for life. This means giving the brain daily what it cannot produce naturally with nutritious foods. Your best guide as to whether you need to keep going with supplemental amino acids is your score on the Scale of Abstinence Symptoms Severity (page 26).

A few guidelines

Medication If you are currently on any medication you should use these amino acids only under medical supervision. You should not use them if taking MAO inhibitors (antidepressants such as Nardil or Parstelin) or any drugs affecting the particular neurotransmitters listed in the table, Actions of Neurotransmitters and Amino Acids (page 134). Tryptophan and 5-HTP are also contraindicated when you are taking antidepressant drugs. Always read the small print and never take anything that is contraindicated for any condition you may have.

How to take the vitamins Always take amino acids with a good multivitamin–mineral. Vitamins and minerals are not only important for their individual roles but also because they help the amino acids make it to the brain and help their conversion into neurotransmitters. In creating brain neurotransmitters, amino acids rarely act alone. Apart from those that are already neurotransmitters (for example, taurine and glycine) amino acids need the help of vitamins and minerals before the formation can take place. For example, vitamin B_6 and magnesium are needed for the manufacture of dopamine and serotonin, whereas vitamin C assists in the conversion of dopamine to noradrenalin. There's more on this in the next chapter.

Use educated trial and error Rebalancing brain chemistry is not just a matter of taking one amino acid to produce serotonin and another for endorphin release. The brain is a complex biological matrix with different neurotransmitters stimulating and inhibiting signals across it. Although a single amino acid may be involved in the formation of a given neurotransmitter, it may require a combination or formulation to correct the problem. We'll guide you towards your ideal balance in Part 4. With educated trial and error you'll find out what works best for you.

Side effects Occasionally people do experience mild side effects or an unusual reaction such as an upset stomach, especially to large doses of amino acids. In these instances no permanent harm will be done, as the amino acids leave the body within one to four hours. If this should happen to you, and you are taking multiple amino acids, stop taking all of them and reintroduce them one by one until you can determine which one is causing the problem. Sometimes if the reaction is mild you might want to persist in taking it to see if the situation gradually improves. Frequently, the reaction occurs only in the first few days as the body adjusts. The benefits may prove to be worth the persistence.

Taking the correct amino acids Sometimes you can have a problem because you are taking the wrong amino acid. For example, if you want to quieten your nervous system and you take tyrosine, you will not get the desired response. Learn as much as you can about which amino acids usually produce which results. Nevertheless, finding the right amino acids or combination of amino acids for you is not an exact science and may require some experimentation on your part.

Adjusting the supplements If you have sleep problems, don't take the stimulating amino acids, tyrosine or phenylalanine, after 2pm. If you become jittery or 'hyper', stop taking tyrosine or phenylalanine. Take the inhibitory, calming glutamine, taurine or GABA to reverse the effects. If that is not enough, take tryptophan or 5-HTP. On the other hand, if you become too relaxed or spacey, stop taking GABA, taurine, glutamine and/or 5-HTP. Take tyrosine to counteract the effects. If you get a headache, check you are also supplementing magnesium, vitamins B and C, and drink water.

(You will find full details of the dosages for your addiction in Parts 3 and 4.)

Consult a qualified practitioner

Ideally, we recommend seeking the guidance of a nutritional therapist or suitably qualified health-care practitioner (see Resources) to help you find the winning formula for you. Please do not give up if you do not attain the desired response immediately.

What if you find no benefit?

Sometimes oral supplements don't work well enough because of absorption problems or other physical problems. In which case we strongly suggest that you work with a health-care practitioner and seriously consider bypassing the digestive tract with intravenous nutritional therapy, which we discuss in Chapter 30. This is especially relevant for those with serious addiction and many failed attempts at quitting.

Freedom from addiction: amino acids not drugs

No drug currently in wide use, medical or recreational, addresses the root cause of neurotransmitter imbalance. Drugs merely stimulate temporary excessive release of pre-existing neuro-transmitter stores or block the action – for example, of adrenalin. They do not increase production of neurotransmitters. How can they without supplying the building materials, which are amino acids? Optimising your intake of the relevant amino acids, vita-mins, minerals and essential fats is the way out of addiction, not more drugs.

Since the inception of amino acid therapy in the mid 1980s, tens of thousands of people have taken them safely with few side effects. There have been almost no complaints to government watchdogs. The one exception was the contamination problem with tryptophan we mentioned on page 129. If you stick within our guidelines, amino acids are very safe to supplement.

Combine supplementation with a healthy lifestyle

We do not want to give you the impression that amino acid therapy is an instant cure-all. Although we are definitely fans of amino acid supplementation, it is not a substitute for good nutrition or other aspects of healthy living. (That is why it is called supplementation, not substitution.)

> **Y**ou must combine your amino acid supplementation with a healthy diet and lifestyle, for best results.

So make sure the rest of your nutrition is up to scratch by following the total programme recommended in this book. The more pieces you put in place the better the results.

You will be surprised at how much better you will feel when taking the appropriate amino acids at the right dosage for you. You will not feel 'high'. You will just feel more 'normal', happier and less irritable, more calm, rested and alert, and you will notice that your cravings for mood-altering substances will be much reduced.

SUMMARY

► Specific amino acids help reduce cravings and make you feel better.

► Supplementing the right amino acids for you will rapidly reduce cravings for particular substances.

► You may already have a sense of which ones are likely to help you from your cravings and abstinence symptoms.

► We will tell you which ones are important for you to supplement, depending on your main addiction, in Part 3.

► You don't need to supplement amino acids for ever, just until your abstinence symptoms are relieved.

8.

A HEALTHY BRAIN NEEDS
A HEALTHY GUT

Did you know that your digestive tract actually makes neuro-transmitters and sends signals to your brain? Yes, cells in the digestive tract make neurotransmitters that have a direct effect on your brain. You will remember from Chapter 2 that neurotrans-mitters become depleted and out of balance when you become addicted, so it's vitally important to restore these so that you will enjoy freedom from addiction without abstinence symptoms. Your gut's job is to extract the nutrients your body needs from digested food, such as the amino acids from protein, so having a healthy gut is key to getting your brain working properly. Over half the serotonin and melatonin made in the body, for example, is made in the gut. And therein lies the rub.

> **M**any addictive substances mess up how your gut works, either by damaging it or shutting down the digestive process.

This is especially true for alcohol, caffeine, painkillers and heroin. If you consume a lot of these substances, and especially if your diet isn't great, you will not be good at getting the correct nutrients to your brain.

QUESTIONNAIRE: how's your digestion?

Tick the boxes if your answer is yes to the following questions:

1. Do you have a poor appetite? ☐

2. Do you eat too fast and fail to chew your food thoroughly? ☐

3. Do you sometimes suffer from bad breath? ☐

4. Do you often get a burning sensation in your stomach or regularly use indigestion tablets? ☐

5. Do you often have a feeling of fullness in your stomach? ☐

6. Do you often get diarrhoea? ☐

7. Do you often suffer from constipation? ☐

8. Do you often get a bloated stomach? ☐

9. Do you often feel nauseous? ☐

10. Do you often belch or pass wind? ☐

11. Do you often get stomach pains? ☐

12. Do you fail to have a bowel movement at least once a day? ☐

13. Do you feel worse, or excessively sleepy, after meals? ☐

Total score: ☐

Score

5 or more

There's a very good chance that your digestion needs some additional support. Focus on improving your diet and taking the necessary supplements (see below) to repair any damage to your digestive tract. We'll show you exactly how to do this in Part 4.

Healing your digestive tract

There is a lot you can do to heal the gut and improve your ability to digest and absorb nutrients. Along with avoiding gut destroyers such as alcohol, the foundation for healing your gut includes:

- Taking digestive enzymes with meals to help digest your food completely.

- Glutamine powder to heal the gut lining.

- Probiotic supplements to re-inoculate it with friendly bacteria.

These are all available in health-food stores.

Digestive enzyme complexes

Take digestive enzyme complexes (lipase, amylase and protease), which help digest fat, protein and carbohydrate. Since stomach acid and protein-digesting enzymes rely on zinc and vitamin B_6, it may help to take 10mg of zinc and 25mg of vitamin B_6 twice a day, as well as the digestive enzyme with each meal.

Powdered glutamine

Take 4–8g (one or two heaped teaspoons) of powdered glutamine mixed with water at bedtime and again first thing in the early morning to help heal the gut lining. This is because those gut wall cells (mucosal cells) literally run on glutamine. Since glutamine is also so vital for calming down your brain with GABA, having extra glutamine is a double whammy in your favour. (Glutamine powder should not be taken if there is severe, end-stage liver damage.)

Probiotics

Beneficial bacteria such as *Lactobacillus acidophilus and Bifido-bacteria* can also help to calm down a reactive digestive tract and help heal the gut. This is because the gut depends on having a healthy 'garden' of these beneficial bacteria, which are easily destroyed by a poor diet, chronic stress, alcohol and, especially, overuse and abuse of antibiotics. It often takes three months to restore healthy gut bacteria after a course of antibiotics. These bacteria help prevent and reverse allergies, help repair your digestive tract, which helps reduce food intolerances, and may even boost neurotransmitter levels.

> Recent research has found that healthy gut bacteria are capable of activating neurons in the brain that make serotonin.[17]

For how long should you take them?

You don't need these gut supplements for ever, but including them for the first month after you are free of alcohol, heroin, heavy caffeine and sugary food consumption is an excellent idea. We also recommend you do this if you do have suspected food allergies (see Chapter 14) or digestive problems, such as viral and bacterial infections of the gut, irritable bowel syndrome, ulcerative colitis,[18] bloating, abdominal pain, intermittent diarrhoea or constipation. (Probiotics have even been reported to lower total cholesterol, reduce the risk of colon cancer, help prevent infections, and protect the liver from alcohol damage.)[19]

Eliminating foods you are allergic to is a prerequisite to improving gut health, a subject we examine in detail in Chapter 14.

As a Harvard professor of gastroenterology once said, 'A good set of stomach and bowels is more important to human health and happiness than a large amount of brains.' Our How to Quit Action Plan includes a healthy diet (see Chapter 28) that will ensure your gut is kept in optimum condition to help you towards recovery.

Intravenous nutrients – bypassing the gut

If you have a serious addiction, you may benefit from the new intravenous treatment that is soon to begin in the UK and is available in the US. An incredible breakthrough in the treatment of addiction was made with the discovery of simultaneously giving, intravenously and orally, a person-specific cocktail of amino acids, vitamins, minerals and nutrient derivatives to jump-start recovery. This causes an immediate and dramatic reduction in abstinence symptoms, achieving a reduction in one week that oral supplements alone cannot match in four weeks.

The digestive tract easily gets damaged (by poor nutrition, stress, alcohol, caffeine, painkillers and other drugs) and this prevents proper digestion and absorption of nutrients. With IV nutrient therapy the brain directly receives most of the nutrients it needs because they bypass the gut. Because the nutrients are received intravenously and orally they promote rapid healing of the gut, so, within one week of IV nutrient therapy, you can substantially restore gut health if you abstain from alcohol and drugs and get proper nutrition.

In Chapter 30 we discuss this option in more detail for those with serious addiction problems.

SUMMARY

▶ Your digestive tract makes neurotransmitters just as your brain does.

▶ The gut's job is to digest food protein into amino acids ready for absorption, so having a healthy gut is key to a properly working brain.

▶ Addictive substances can damage or shut down the digestive process, so your brain will not be nourished properly.

▶ Heal your digestive tract by taking digestive enzymes, zinc and vitamin B_6, powdered glutamine, and beneficial bacteria and by eliminating foods you are allergic to.

▶ For people who have damaged digestive systems because of addiction, short-term intravenous nutritional therapy is available in order to bypass the gut.

9.

RAISE YOUR METHYL IQ WITH VITAMINS AND MINERALS

In Chapter 2 we learned that just about everything that happens in your brain involves a process called methylation. It's absolutely vital for making neurotransmitters and healthy brain-cell membranes and keeping them in balance. Although the brain's feel-good neurotransmitters are made from amino acids, if you just chuck the very same amino-acid building blocks into a bucket you don't get neurotransmitters. You need the careful orchestration of the brain's building team to make, break down and keep your neurotransmitters balanced. Methylation is the conductor of your brain's orchestra.

Balancing homocysteine

We also learned that the best indicator of how good you are at this methylation business, which we call your methyl IQ, is your blood homocysteine level. There's a whole host of nutrients that help bring your homocysteine into the healthy range if it isn't, and help raise your methyl IQ. These are:

- Folic acid, folate, methylfolate
- B_{12} (methyl B_{12}, glutathional B_{12})

- B_6 (pyridoxine, pyridoxal-5-phosphate)

- B_2 (riboflavin)

- B_3 (niacin)

- Magnesium

- Zinc

- S-adenosyl methionine (SAM)

- Tri-methyl glycine (TMG)

- N-acetyl cysteine (NAC)

These nutrients turn toxic homocysteine into SAM, the amino acid that actually does methylation. (If you'd like to see exactly how these nutrients are involved in turning homocysteine into SAM go to www.patrickholford.com/methylation – the • in the live animation is the methyl group. The enzymes, dependent on these nutrients, are shown as squares.)

The first five are B vitamins. The last three are actually amino acids. By eating foods rich in these nutrients, such as beans, nuts, seeds and greens, and also supplementing the right levels (defined by your homocysteine level) you will tremendously enhance the effect of taking any supplemental amino acid. Single supplements containing all these 'methylating' nutrients are available, so improving your ability to methylate is an easy and fast track to feeling better.

What's your H score?

It's well worth knowing your homocysteine score; first, because lowering a raised homocysteine is highly likely to reduce cravings and abstinence symptoms on its own; and second, it helps you to identify what levels of these nutrients are right for you. Otherwise you are shooting in the dark. It's very easy to test your homocysteine. If your doctor won't do it for you, you can order a home-test kit and do it yourself (see Resources).

The average person's homocysteine score is 10 μmol/l (micromoles per litre), which is too high. Above 15 is very bad news. It multiplies your risk of many diseases – from strokes to Alzheimer's disease. Ideally, you want to be aiming for a homocysteine level below 7.

(If you don't know your homocysteine level, however, a good bet is to take two homocysteine-lowering supplement formulas a day in addition to eating a homocysteine-lowering diet.)

What happens with raised homocysteine levels?

- A homocysteine level above 15 doubles your risk of depression, especially if you are a woman.[20] One in three depressed people need more folate.[21]

- Smokers (20 cigarettes per day or more) on average have homocysteine levels 18 per cent higher than non-smokers.[22]

- People who drink more than one shot of spirit per day have an average homocysteine score of 10.2; those who drink more than one red wine have a score of 9.9; and those who drink more than one white wine a score of 10.[23]

- Alcoholics have homocysteine levels 40 per cent higher (9.66 vs 6.93) than non-alcoholics.[24]

- If you have the equivalent of two or more drinks a day, your homocysteine level will be significantly higher than if you have one drink a day,[25] and your risk of cardiovascular disease goes up, despite what they say about the benefits of moderate amounts of alcohol.[26]

continues ▶

- If you have a low intake of folate (found in greens and beans, which is important for a healthy homocysteine level) and also drink a moderate amount of alcohol you triple your risk of colon cancer, as a man,[27] and breast cancer, as a woman.

- Two cups of coffee raises your homocysteine by 11 per cent in four hours, according to a study by Dr Verhoef and colleagues at the Wageningen Centre for Food Sciences in the Netherlands. They also showed that caffeine tablets without coffee increased it by 5 per cent.[28] So there's something else in coffee, as well as the caffeine, that raises homocysteine. Another study found that when volunteers drank about four cups of coffee a day their H score rose to 14 after two weeks.[29]

If you don't smoke, don't drink alcohol or caffeinated drinks, and you feel great, then the chances are your homocysteine level won't be that high. But then you probably wouldn't be reading this book, would you? If your levels are raised, then don't smoke or drink alcohol heavily, as this will make the supplements less effective.

To help you identify whether you have poor methylation, complete the following questionnaire.

QUESTIONNAIRE: test your methyl IQ

Tick the boxes if your answer is yes to the following questions:

1. Are you tired a lot of the time?

2. Is your stamina, or ability to keep going, noticeably decreasing?

3. Are you having a hard time keeping your weight stable?

4. Do you often experience physical pain, be it arthritis, muscle aches or migraines? ☐

5. Do you get frequent colds? ☐

6. Is your eyesight deteriorating? ☐

7. Is your mental clarity or concentration decreasing? ☐

8. Are you experiencing more sleeping problems? ☐

9. Is your memory on the decline? ☐

10. Are you often depressed? ☐

11. Do you average two or more alcoholic beverages daily? ☐

12. Do you drink more than three cups of coffee daily? ☐

13. Do you smoke cigarettes? ☐

14. Are you a strict vegan? ☐

Total score: ☐

Score

5 or more

It's very likely that your homocysteine is moderately high to very high (that is 9 to 14, if not higher). Ideally test your homocysteine level with a home kit (see Resources).

Why supplementing B vitamins is essential

As we saw in Chapter 2, the homocysteine-lowering B vitamins, especially B_2, B_6, B_{12} and folic acid, are absolutely vital for dealing with abstinence symptoms. The big illusion is that you can get everything you need from a so-called well-balanced diet. We cover both bases with a diet high in folate, which means at least eating a small handful of seeds and nuts every day, two servings of greens a day, plus a serving of beans or lentils, then supplemental folic acid on top, giving 400–1,000mg depending on your homocysteine level.

Supplementing with B_{12}

Many people dealing with addiction are deficient in B_{12}. Any addiction that messes up digestion – alcohol or heroin for example – means the odds are you're not absorbing B_{12} very well. The older you are the more likely this is. Many older people become mildly B_{12} deficient, not so much because they don't eat the foods that produce B_{12} but because they don't absorb it well. The solution is either to take larger oral doses or have B_{12} injections.

How do you correct a B_{12} deficiency?

One study found that you needed 200 times more vitamin B_{12} than the basic RDA (Recommended Daily Amount) of 3 micrograms (mcg) to correct a mild deficiency.[30] There is no way you can eat this amount. The most absorbable and effective form of B_{12} is called methyl B_{12} (methylcobalamin).

Supplementing with B_6

The RDA for vitamin B_6 is only 2mg, yet many studies clearly show that an intake of ten times this amount (20mg) is more effective in lowering homocysteine and improving methylation. Again, this is more than you can eat. Ideally, supplement some of your B_6 as pyridoxal-5-phosphate (P5P), which is the most active form of vitamin B_6. P5P is important in the production of dopamine (and hence noradrenalin) and serotonin (and hence melatonin), so it's good for mood, motivation and sleep.

Supplementing folic acid

If you've been told that nutrients from food are always better, or more effective, than supplemental nutrients, you may be surprised to find that the reverse is true for folic acid. In one study homocysteine levels did not decrease significantly among patients given cereal containing 127mcg of folate daily. Levels did decrease, however, when the patients were given the same amount of folic acid as a supplement. They found that folic acid from oral supplements is 1.7 times more effective than the same amount from food. This means that supplementing 100mcg of folate is equivalent to eating 170mcg in food.[31]

Working together

Just as important as the dose is the combination. These vitamins are team players. No one ever becomes deficient in only one nutrient and neither should you supplement only one B vitamin. They work much better together. For example, in a Japanese study with a group of people who had raised homocysteine, they were divided into three groups: one was given either folate or methyl B_{12} alone, one group folate and methyl B_{12} together, and the third group folate, methyl B_{12} and B_6.[32] The trial lasted for three weeks. Here are the results:

Supplement group	Homocysteine change
Folate alone	17.3% reduction
Methyl B_{12} alone	18.7% reduction
Folate plus B_{12}	57.4% reduction
Folate, B_{12} and B_6	59.9% reduction

That's why we recommend that you supplement all three of these vitamins, ideally with a multivitamin also containing vitamins B_2 and B_3 (niacin), along with other vital methylation nutrients.

Zinc and magnesium: the dynamic duo

These two minerals are not only vital to keep you well methylated, but they are also two of your brain's best friends and are more commonly deficient than not in those with addiction problems. For example, up to half of all alcoholics are zinc-deficient because alcohol makes zinc harder to absorb and encourages its excretion as well.[33]

Deficiency in zinc

Zinc deficiency is extremely common in people with addiction problems, ADHD and depression. Classic signs of deficiency include loss of appetite, unintended weight loss, bad skin, poor wound healing, and proneness to and difficulty shifting infections, as well as low mood and energy, and low thyroid hormone levels. Mood and energy are low because zinc is necessary to make the stimulating hormone, thyroxine, from tyrosine – the motivating amino acid.

Diet and supplements for zinc

If a food grows, it's got zinc in it. Seeds, nuts, beans and lentils, as well as meat, fish and eggs are all high in zinc. (But nothing is as high as oysters: a single oyster provides 10mg of zinc.) You need about 15mg of zinc a day. A bad diet may give you 5mg, if that. Alternatively, it's worth making sure you supplement at least 10mg – or even two or four times this amount if you are withdrawing from any addictive substance. If you take more than 50mg of zinc a day for more than two months, make sure you supplement 1mg of copper with every 20mg of zinc, as too much zinc can knock out this other essential mineral.

Before you start to worry about all these various supplements and amounts, rest assured – what you need to take is summarised in the chapter in Part 3 that deals with your addiction.

Deficiency in magnesium

Like zinc, magnesium is often deficient in those dealing with addiction. This is partly because it's depleted by stress. It is also because, like zinc, magnesium is involved in so many vital enzyme reactions in the body and brain that make neurotransmitters and help keep you well methylated.

> **M**agnesium keeps your heart beating regularly and helps relax your mind and your muscles. You need lots if you are coming off any addictive substance.

Classic deficiency signs are anxiety, insomnia, muscle cramps and spasms, migraines, recurring kidney stones, and high blood pressure.

The more your brain chemistry is out of kilter, the more magnesium you are going to use up. The higher your consumption of stimulants such as caffeine, nicotine and cocaine, the lower will be your magnesium level. Alcohol also knocks out magnesium.

Diet and supplements for magnesium

The best foods for magnesium are dark green vegetables, as well as seeds, especially pumpkin seeds. We recommend that you eat a small handful of pumpkin seeds a day and two servings of green vegetables. Supplement between 400 and 600mg of magnesium, ideally as magnesium taurate (magnesium bound to the amino acid taurine, which is good for heart function), or as magnesium ascorbate, providing additional vitamin C.

SAM: the methylating amino

Having an optimal amount of all the vitamins and minerals we have been talking about helps increase the production of S-adenosyl methionine (SAM), which is the master tuner of your brain and a vital ally in recovery from any addiction. Without SAM, we cannot produce many of the key brain neurotransmitters needed for recovery (for example, serotonin, melatonin, dopamine and noradrenalin). Without SAM, you're at risk of suffering from depression. What is more, you cannot protect or heal the liver from the insults of alcohol, drugs, smoking, pollution, infections and other illnesses.

Your body makes SAM from the vitamins and minerals you obtain from food or from supplementing. If you get plenty of what you need to produce SAM from food and vitamin and mineral supplements, that's good. If your homocysteine level is high you are not getting enough of these nutrients to make enough SAM. But if you want to cut right to the chase, you can just take SAM. Supplementing SAM, especially for the first month after you come off any addictive substance, can be extremely helpful in rapidly healing your brain and body. It helps the liver recover from excess alcohol.

But ... sorry, it's no longer available over the counter in Europe, because SAM has been classified as a medicine. This means that your doctor could prescribe it or you can buy it for your own use on the Internet from the US, South Africa or other countries where it is still considered a nutrient. You need not worry about safety if it comes from a country where it is available to buy over the counter.

You need about 400–1,600mg a day, always taken on an empty stomach, and best first thing in the morning, on waking up, then mid-morning and mid-afternoon. Some people get mild nausea on very high doses and, very rarely, some people find it over-stimulating. If so, lower the dose or try tri-methyl glycine (TMG). There's more info on SAM given in Appendix 2 (which is on our website www.how2quit.co.uk).

TMG: another way to make SAM

Another way of upping your SAM level is to supplement its pre-cursor called TMG. This, plus zinc, is another way to lower your homocysteine. TMG and zinc turn the harmful homocysteine into the desirable SAM. Some people lower homocysteine more effectively with TMG than with the usual cocktail of B_6, B_{12} and folic acid.

In a study in New Zealand, high homocysteine levels were reduced by a further 18 per cent when 4g of TMG was given, along with vitamin B_6 and folic acid, compared to patients taking just B_6 and folic acid.[34] In another study, researchers found that 6g of TMG daily lowers homocysteine, even in so-called healthy people with 'normal' homocysteine levels. But they noted that the extent of the decrease is much smaller in 'healthy' volunteers than in high-risk patients with much higher homocysteine. For example, in patients with H scores above 50, TMG supplemen-tation can lower the scores by up to 75 per cent.[35]

TMG in partnership

On its own, TMG supplementation tends not to be as good as folic acid. However, researchers from the Netherlands have dis-covered that folic acid *and* TMG may work much better as partners, because TMG encourages homocysteine detoxification mostly in the liver, whereas folic acid supports this process in cells all over the body. To repeat, TMG works best when taken in conjunction with all the other homocysteine-lowering B vitamins.

Boosting levels of TMG may be particularly beneficial if you're overdoing alcohol and your liver is under a lot of strain. TMG helps to lower toxic levels of homocysteine, thereby protecting the liver from alcohol-provoked injury.[36]

Diet and supplements for TMG

We recommend 1–4g TMG a day, depending on your homocysteine level, as well as eating root vegetables. TMG is available in health-food stores on its own, or in formulas with other methylating nutrients.

Glutathione and N-acetyl cysteine

There's another way that your brain can lower homocysteine. In the diagram opposite you'll see another route for homocysteine, turning into the brain's most critical antioxidant, called glutathione. That sounds like good news and, in a way, it is. But it can also mean that you have less homocysteine to turn into SAM – and that's really what you want.

By supplementing a little glutathione, or its precursor, a vital antioxidant called N-acetyl cysteine (NAC), you can 'satisfy' this pathway, which ups your ability to make SAM. This pathway is, however, totally dependent on vitamin B_6, which is another reason to make sure you really are getting enough. So, if you take optimal amounts of all the nutrients shown in the diagram opposite (B_6, B_{12}, folic acid, glutathione and/or NAC) you'll get the best of both worlds: better antioxidant protection and better methyl-ation. As well as helping raise your methyl IQ these vital anti- oxidants help repair the brain and protect it from the damage of over-stimulation, which some stimulant drugs induce.

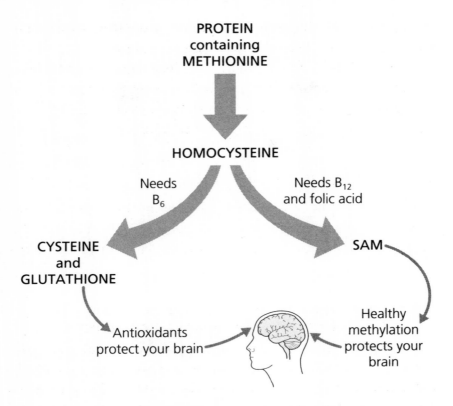

How glutathione protects your brain

Supplements at a glance

Before you get tongue-tied with all these new words and fearful that we might be asking you to pop zillions of supplements, let us explain that the reason we've told you all this is so that you will understand the importance of well-designed supplements aimed at normalising homocysteine and supporting optimal methylation. To make it easier for you, the chart overleaf shows you how much you need and how many of the better combination supplements you are likely to need – depending on your homocysteine score – to get your methyl IQ back up to scratch.

THE CORRECT SUPPLEMENTS TO TAKE FOR YOUR HOMOCYSTEINE SCORE

	OK	High	Very high	Much too high
Your H Score	7–9	9–14	15–19	>20
Supplement	1	2	3	4 per day
Folate	250mcg	500mcg	750mcg	1,000mcg
Methyl B_{12}	250mcg	500mcg	750mcg	1,000mcg
B_6	20mg	40mg	60mg	80mg
B_2	10mg	20mg	30mg	40mg
Zinc	5mg	10mg	15mg	20mg
TMG	500mg	1g	1.5g	2g
NAC	250mg	500mg	750mg	1,000mg

mcg: micrograms (also written as µg); mg: milligrams; g: grams

Stress, smoking, excess alcohol and caffeinated drinks, especially coffee, all raise homocysteine. Small amounts of alcohol don't raise homocysteine, but large amounts do. However, even five-a-day smokers have higher homocysteine levels.

SUMMARY

▶ Test your homocysteine, and take supplements at the appropriate levels of the key homocysteine-stabilising nutrients.

▶ Eat more greens, beans, nuts and seeds, which are high in folate.

▶ Cut back on tea, and especially coffee – have no more than one a day.

▶ Don't smoke.

▶ Don't drink alcohol in excess.

10.

REBUILD YOUR BRAIN WITH ESSENTIAL FATS

Most addictive substances strip the brain of essential fats. So the chances are you're deficient and/or have an imbalance – unless you eat unfried oily fish three times a week or take daily supplements of essential fats or fish oil. Essential fats are those that cannot be produced by the body and must be obtained by eating them.

About 60 per cent of the dried weight of your brain is made of fats – omega fats (omega-3 and omega-6), cholesterol and phospholipids, as we explained in Chapter 2. The major sources of these in your diet are fish, nuts, seeds and eggs. These four foods are essential for a sharp mind, mood and motivation and have been shown to ease many addiction or abstinence symptoms, including depression, anxiety, suicidal thoughts, irritability, aggression, poor school performance and poor memory.

Are you getting enough omega-3 and omega-6?

Here are the known signs that indicate you're not getting enough:

- Elevated triglycerides[37] (this can be checked in a routine blood test; ask your doctor to test if yours are elevated).

- Elevated cholesterol (ask your doctor what yours is).

- High blood pressure.

- Thickened or thinned cracked heel calluses.

- Rough skin on the back of the upper arms.

- Scaly, rough, dry skin.[38]

- Pale skin patches on cheeks.

- Dandruff, brittle or soft nails, dry, brittle hair.

- Chronic inflammation (such as colitis or arthritis, which usually results in pain, redness or swelling).

- Chronic pain syndromes (such as arthritis, fibromyalgia, migraines).

- Airborne and food allergies.

- Poor, slow healing of wounds and injuries.

- Excessive ear-wax accumulation.

- Physical weakness, low stamina, chronic fatigue.

- Excess body fat.

- Excessive thirst, frequent urination.[39]

- Dry eyes (omega-6 deficiency).

- Paper-thin skin (omega-6 deficiency).

- Skipped or dropped heartbeats.

Research has shown that relapse among cocaine- and alcohol-dependent people over the course of two years was significantly lowered with an increased intake of omega-6 and omega-3 foods.[40] But, regardless of the addiction, to ensure recovery these important fats should form a significant part of the diet, as the brain is totally dependent on them.

Omega-3 and 6: getting the balance right

Although an essential fat deficiency is something to guard against, we must also be concerned about the balance between omega-3 and omega-6 essential fats in our diet. There should be equal quantities of both, but the average Western diet has ten to 25 times more omega-6 than omega-3.

High omega-6 levels (in relation to omega-3 levels) are associated with inflammation and disease, including heart disease, strokes, cancer, diabetes, depression, anxiety, sleep disorders, ADHD, alcohol and drug dependency. Chronic abstinence symptoms are associated with an omega-3 deficiency and/or a high level of omega-6 compared to omega-3.

Which foods do these oils come from?

Omega-6 fats are found in hot-climate seeds and their oils, such as sesame and sunflower. However, most of the apparent omega-6 fats in our diet are damaged fats (those that have oxidised by high heat), found in processed food and food that has been fried, for example, in sunflower oil. A type of omega-3 fat, alpha linolenic acid (ALA), comes from cold-climate seeds and their oils, such as flax and pumpkin (as well as nuts such as walnuts). In addition to ALA you also need the more potent types of omega-3, called EPA, DPA and DHA.

All of these fats – EPA, DPA and DHA – are present in salmon, tuna, sardines, herring, mackerel and other carnivorous fish. But virtually no DHA or EPA is made in the body from the ALA that's in flax seeds and walnuts. So it's not a great idea to be a recovering alcoholic vegan.

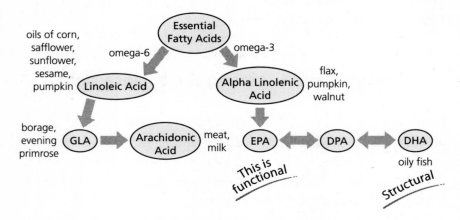

The brain's essential fats

What we should eat

In practical terms you can achieve the ideal amount and balance by doing the following:

- Eating three servings of unfried oily fish a week.

- Having a small handful, or heaped tablespoonful, of raw, ground seeds (ideally half flax, and half sesame, sunflower and pumpkin seeds) a day.

- Supplementing 1 or 2g of omega-3 EPA and DHA or 1g EPA and DHA plus one capsule of combined omega-3 and 6 (the best ones give you GLA, plus EPA, DPA and DHA). Make sure that the total milligrams of EPA + DPA + DHA is twice that of the total milligrams of GLA.

> **W**e humans, especially those in recovery, need fish and fish oils in our diet.

The chart below shows you the best fish to eat. Since larger fish contain more mercury, we've also shown the omega-3–mercury ratio. The best fish to eat are those with the highest scores – that's the most omega-3 and the least mercury. This is especially important if you are pregnant. If a pregnant woman fails to eat enough omega-3 the child is more likely to have problems that pave the way for reward deficiency and addictive tendencies. So it is important not to eliminate all fish from your diet because you are worried about the mercury. Just eat the fish with the highest scores, which we've listed in bold. In this respect wild salmon is the best and tinned tuna the worst.

FISH: HOW MUCH OMEGA-3?

	omega-3 g/100g	mercury mg/kg	omega-3– mercury ratio
Fresh salmon	2.70	0.05	54.00
Fresh mackerel	1.93	0.05	38.60
Canned sardines	1.57	0.04	39.25
Canned/smoked salmon	1.54	0.04	38.50
Herring/kipper	1.31	0.04	32.75
Trout	1.15	0.06	19.17
Fresh tuna	1.50	0.40	3.75
Canned tuna	0.37	0.19	1.95
Swordfish	2*	1.40	1.43*

* estimated figure

(Source: FSA 2004)

Essential fats, ADHD and substance abuse

As we have previously said, there's a strong link between ADHD and substance abuse. And there is much evidence that omega-3 and 6 supplements improve the most observable symptoms in children just as effectively as stimulant drugs such as Ritalin.[41]

How essential fats can help depression

Other common tendencies among those with addictions that respond favourably to an increased intake of essential fats include depression,[42] anxiety,[43] hostility,[44] aggression[45] and suicidal thoughts.[46] Surveys report a substantially greater risk of major depression, post-natal depression, bipolar disorder and homicide in countries with little seafood consumption when compared with countries that have high levels of consumption.[47]

> If you don't eat enough fish you are much more likely to be depressed.[48]

A survey of 21,000 people in Norway also found that the longer a person had been supplementing cod liver oil, a rich source of omega-3, the less likely they were to be depressed.[49]

Fish oils also give your brain's serotonin and dopamine function a boost.[50] In a study giving prison inmates vitamins, minerals and essential fats, those taking the supplements, not the placebos, became much less aggressive within three weeks.[51] Taking omega-3 supplements also reduces self-harm.[52]

The effects of alcohol on essential fats

Too much alcohol strips essential fats from the brain. This can actually decrease brain size. Having less grey matter, particularly in the hippocampal region of the brain (the part responsible for memory, learning and mood functions), is not only a common finding in alcoholics, but is also associated with depression and memory loss. When scientists from the University of Pittsburgh ran magnetic resonance imaging (MRI) brain scans they found that the more DHA a person consumed, the more grey matter there was in the areas of the brain linked to mood, especially in the hippocampus. People who had lower blood levels of omega-3 fats were also more likely to have a negative outlook and be more impulsive. Conversely, those with higher blood levels of omega-3s were found to be more agreeable and less likely to report mild or moderate symptoms of depression.[53]

Essential fats' additional benefits to the heart

As well as being good for the brain, essential fats, especially omega-3 fats, are exceptionally good for the heart and circulation. A systematic review of all the studies to date show that increased consumption of omega-3 fats from fish or fish-oil supplements (but not of ALA, which is the type of omega-3 found in flax seeds) reduces overall mortality, including cardiac and sudden death and possibly stroke.[54] In fact, doctors in Britain and the US are now actively encouraged to give patients fish oils after a heart attack, according to the National Institute for Clinical Excellence (NICE).

Intake of tuna or other poached, grilled or baked fish at least once a week is associated with a slower, healthier heart rate than eating these fish less than once a month. And eating fish at least five times per week is associated with an even healthier heart rhythm. Consumption of fish oil supplements has similar effects. However, eating fried fish is not so beneficial.[55]

Fish: the all-round healthy food

Of course you are not likely to eat fish five times a week. It may be that you're not a fan of fish at all and plan to just take fish oil supplements. We encourage you to try different kinds of fish prepared in different ways (not fried) and perhaps you will find it appealing so that you can eat it at least three times a week. We recommend fish and fish oil supplements for people in early recovery. Fish is included because it is also rich in other brain-friendly nutrients including:

- High-quality protein and amino acids.

- Taurine – an amino acid neurotransmitter that lowers cholesterol and is used in Japan in treatment of alcohol withdrawal.

- NADH – a nutrient that increases production of dopamine, noradrenalin and serotonin in the brain; studies indicate beneficial outcomes with NADH in the treatment of ADHD, Parkinson's disease, mild-to-moderate depression and, most recently, chronic fatigue syndrome.

- Vitamins D and B_{12}.

- Selenium, iodine.

- Sterols, which lower total and the 'bad' LDL cholesterol, increase the adrenal hormone DHEA and suppress cortisol levels (linked with stress).

In our How to Quit Action Plan in Part 4 (Chapter 28) you will find quick and tasty recipes containing fish to get you started.

How essential fats become phospholipids

Roughly half of the fats in your brain are essential omega-3 and 6 fats, most of which end up as phospholipids. Phospholipids are a family of 'intelligent' fats in your brain cell membrane. They are proving essential in animals and in humans,[56] vital for normal memory,[57] but haven't been granted that official title yet for the simple reason that your body can make them, but doesn't make enough.

Besides making your brain cell membranes and receptors work efficiently, phospholipids are the insulation experts. They help signals in the brain to run smoothly because they make up the insulating layer, or myelin, around all nerves (see page 41). Not only do phospholipids enhance your mood, mind and mental performance but they also protect against age-related memory decline and Alzheimer's disease.

> Alcohol, cocaine and poor nutrition help strip these vital fats, phospholipids, from your brain, making you more prone to relapse. The more you drink the more your brain will become damaged.

Which foods do phospholipids come from?

The best food sources of phospholipids are egg yolk, brains, kidneys and liver. Eating organs has gone out of fashion, and many people mistakenly avoid eggs, because they are worried about having too much cholesterol in the diet. The net result is a deficiency of phospholipids. One way to up your intake of phospholipids is to eat more eggs. But aren't they high in fat and cholesterol? As long as you don't fry them, eggs are a great brain food. Eating eggs neither raises blood cholesterol nor causes heart disease. An egg is as healthy as the chicken that laid it, so a free-range, organic, omega-3-rich egg is a superfood. We have included some recipes using eggs in our How to Quit Action Plan in Part 4 (Chapter 28), to give you variety for breakfasts and main meals.

Using supplements

You can also supplement phospholipids. The ones you need are called phosphatidyl choline, serine and dimethylaminoethanol (DMAE). Phosphatidyl choline is found in lecithin capsules (take two 1,200mg capsules) and granules (have one tablespoon a day; for example, sprinkled over cereal). Lecithin is available in health-food stores. Alternatively, take a supplement that provides all these (see Resources).

Essential oils and phospholipids at a glance

Here's what you need to eat and supplement to ensure an optimal intake of both essential fats and phospholipids:

- Eat an egg a day, or seven eggs a week – preferably free-range, organic and high in omega-3s. These are high in phospholipids.

- Eat three servings of unfried, unbreaded oily fish a week.

- Have a small handful or heaped tablespoonful of raw, ground seeds (ideally flax, sesame, sunflower and pumpkin) a day.

- Supplement 1 or 2g of omega-3 EPA and DHA or 1g EPA and DHA plus one capsule of combined omega-3 and 6 (the best ones give you GLA plus EPA, DPA and DHA). Make sure that the total milligrams of EPA + DPA + DHA is twice that of the total milligrams of GLA. Alternatively, supplement 1 or 2g (1 or 2 large capsules) of omega-3-rich fish oil.

- Add one tablespoon of lecithin granules, or a heaped teaspoon of high PC lecithin, to your cereal every day, or a supplement containing phospholipids.

In Chapter 29 of Part 4 you will find prescriptions for your particular addiction and abstinence symptoms.

SUMMARY

▶ Most addictive substances strip the brain of essential fats and create an imbalance of fatty acids.

▶ Restoring the omega-3 and omega-6 fats and phospholipids stripped by addiction requires a diet rich in fish, seeds, nuts and eggs.

▶ Supplementing with EPA, DHA, omega-3 and omega-6 capsules is also necessary to restore essential fats.

▶ Part 4 gives you the correct dosages to take for your particular addiction.

11.

BALANCE YOUR BLOOD SUGAR TO GAIN ENERGY AND REDUCE CRAVINGS

In Chapter 5 we saw how easy it is to get caught in the sugar-stimulant trap and how addiction to other substances usually goes hand in hand with underlying blood sugar problems. If you simply avoid one addictive substance – for example cigarettes or caffeine – but do nothing to correct the underlying blood sugar imbalance your chances of success are much less. The best way to overcome cravings is to feel satisfied by eating the foods that will keep your blood sugar levels balanced.

So, your best chance of success is to go the whole hog and sort out once and for all your blood sugar control. This has many advantages. Firstly, within a matter of days your energy level goes up. Secondly, your craving for stimulants and sugar goes down. Then, if you need to, you start to lose weight, seemingly without effort. If you are underweight or have a lack of appetite, you'll find your healthy appetite returns as you reset your 'appestat' by eating a low glycemic load (low-GL) diet, providing low GL foods that release their natural sugar content very slowly, making you feel more satisfied.

> **S**ymptoms such as fatigue, irritability, dizziness, insomnia, aggression, anxiety, sweating (especially at night), poor concentration, excessive thirst, depression, crying spells, and feeling faint and shaky can indicate blood sugar dips.

The classic symptoms outlined above occur in the vast majority of people coming off an addictive substance, but they can be virtually eliminated by mastering the ability to keep your blood sugar level. If you are overweight, or diabetic, this will change too, as this tale of two diabetics, Linda and Adrian, who followed our low-GL diet, illustrates:

Case study **LINDA**

'Now my energy level is incredible. I've lost 1 stone 2lb (7.25kg/ 16lb) in six weeks. My blood sugar is well under control (I'm diabetic) and I've been able to halve my medication. It's been so easy. I used to be a sugar-aholic. I have no cravings.'

Case study **ADRIAN**

'I am a totally changed person. I feel incredible. Before, I didn't have a cut-off switch. I could just eat and eat and would still be hungry throughout the day. After a month on the diet my blood sugar was stable. I've stopped all diabetes medication.' Adrian went from 145.1kg (22 stone 12lb/320lb) to 106.6kg (16 stone 11lb/235lb), losing over 38kg (6 stone/84lb) and 25cm (10in) off his belly.

The golden rules: blood sugar balance

There are three golden rules to mastering your blood sugar balance:

1. Eat low-GL foods.

2. Eat protein with carbohydrate.

3. Graze, don't gorge – eat little and often.

Eat low-GL foods

The measure of what a food does to your blood sugar is known as the glycemic load (GL). Neither protein nor fat (for example, meat, fish, cheese or eggs) have any substantial effect on your blood sugar balance, so we are talking here about sugary or carbohydrate-rich foods.

The sugars and starches in foods with a high GL (refined carbohydrates, such as white bread, sweets and biscuits) are broken down and absorbed quickly into the bloodstream making your blood glucose levels soar. You are likely to experience an increase in energy followed by an energy crash when your blood sugar drops, and you will probably reach for something sweet in order to relieve the symptoms of low blood sugar. Meanwhile, the sugars and starches in foods with a low GL (complex carbohydrates such as whole grains, vegetables, beans or lentils, or simpler carbohydrates such as fruit) take longer to digest than refined carbohydrates. As a result, the glucose released from these foods trickles slowly into the bloodstream. This means that it's used for energy rather than being stored, leaving blood glucose levels on an even keel, and preventing dramatic changes in your mood, behaviour and energy.

The carbs that keep blood sugar even

The chart on pages 179–82 gives the GL score of an average serving of a range of common foods. Foods with a GL of less than 10 (in bold) are good and should be the staple foods of your diet. A GL of 11–14 (in regular type) can be eaten in moderation. A GL higher than 15 (in italics) should be avoided.

GLYCEMIC LOAD OF COMMON FOODS

Food	Serving size in grams	Serving	GLs per serving
Bakery products			
low-carb muffin	**60**	**1 muffin**	**5**
muffin – apple, made without sugar	**60**	**1 muffin**	**9**
muffin – apple, made with sugar	60	1 muffin	13
crumpet	50	1 crumpet	13
croissant	*57*	*1 croissant*	*17*
doughnut, plain	*47*	*1 doughnut*	*17*
sponge cake, plain	*63*	*1 slice*	*17*
Breads			
wholemeal rye or pumpernickel-style rye bread	**20**	**1 thin slice**	**5**
wheat tortilla (Mexican)	**30**	**1 tortilla**	**5**
wholemeal wheat-flour bread	**30**	**1 thick slice**	**9**
pitta bread, white	**30**	**1 pitta bread**	**10**
baguette, white, plain	*30*	*⅓ baton*	*15*
bagel, white	*70*	*1 bagel*	*25*
Crispbreads and crackers			
rough oatcakes (Nairn's)	**10**	**1 oatcake**	**2**
fine oatcakes (Nairn's)	**9**	**1 oatcake**	**3**
cream cracker	25	2 biscuits	11
rye crispbread	25	2 biscuits	11

continues ▶

Food	Serving size in grams	Serving	GLs per serving
water cracker	*25*	*3 biscuits*	*17*
puffed rice cakes	*25*	*3 biscuits*	*17*

Dairy products and alternatives

yogurt (plain, no sugar)	200	1 small pot	3
non-fat yogurt (plain, no sugar)	200	1 small pot	3
soya yogurt (Provamel)	200	1 large bowl	7
soya milk (no sugar)	250ml	1 glass	7
low-fat yogurt, fruit, sugar (Ski)	150	1 small pot	7.5

Fruit and fruit products

blackberries, raw	120	1 medium bowl	1
blueberries, raw	120	1 medium bowl	1
raspberries, raw	120	1 medium bowl	1
strawberries, raw	120	1 medium bowl	1
cherries, raw	120	1 medium bowl	3
grapefruit, raw	120	½ medium	3
pear, raw	120	1 medium	4
melon/cantaloupe, raw	120	½ small	4
watermelon, raw	120	1 medium slice	4
apricots, raw	120	4	5
oranges, raw	120	1 large	5
plum, raw	120	4	5
apple, raw	120	1 small	6
kiwi fruit, raw	120	1	6
pineapple, raw	120	1 medium slice	7
grapes, raw	120	16	8
mango, raw	120	1½ slices	8
apricots, dried	60	6	9
fruit cocktail, canned (Del Monte)	120	small can	9
papaya, raw	120	½ small papaya	10
prunes, pitted	60	6	10

Food	Serving size in grams	Serving	GLs per serving
apple, dried	60	6 rings	10
banana, raw	120	1 small	12
apricots, canned in light syrup	120	1 small can	12
lychees, canned in syrup and drained	*120*	*1 small can*	*16*
figs, dried, tenderised (Dessert Maid)	*60*	*3*	*16*
sultanas	*60*	*30*	*25*
raisins	*60*	*30*	*28*
dates, dried	*60*	*8*	*42*
Jams/spreads			
pumpkin seed butter	16	1 tbsp	1
peanut butter (no sugar)	16	1 tbsp	1
blueberry spread (no sugar)	10	2 tsp	1
orange marmalade	10	2 tsp	3
strawberry jam	10	2 tsp	3
Snack foods (savoury)			
eggs (boiled)	–	2 medium	0
cottage cheese	120	½ medium tub	2
hummus	200	1 small tub	6
olives, in brine	50	7	1
peanuts	50	2 medium handfuls	1
cashew nuts, salted	50	2 medium handfuls	3
potato crisps, plain, salted	30	1 small packet	7
popcorn, salted	25	1 small packet	10
pretzels, oven-baked, traditional wheat flavour	*30*	*15*	*16*
corn chips, plain, salted	*50*	*18*	*17*
Snack foods (sweet)			
Fruitus apple cereal bar	35	1	5
Euroviva Rebar fruit and veg bar	50	1	8

continues ▶

Food	Serving size in grams	Serving	GLs per serving
muesli bar with dried fruit	30	1	13
chocolate bar, milk, plain (Mars/Cadbury/Nestlé)	50	1	14
Twix biscuit and caramel bar (Mars)	*60*	*1 bar (2 fingers)*	*17*
Snickers bar (Mars)	*60*	*1*	*19*
Polos, peppermint sweets (Nestlé)	*30*	*16*	*21*
Jelly beans, assorted colours	*30*	*9*	*22*
Kellogg's Pop-Tarts, double choc	*50*	*1*	*24*
Mars Bar	*60*	*1*	*26*

A comprehensive list of the GL values of foods is also available online at www.holforddiet.com

Healthy snack options

Try these alternatives:

- **Instead of crisps** have oatcakes, pumpkin seeds, roasted snack mix or plain popcorn.
- **Instead of biscuits** have sweet oatcake biscuits (such as Nairn's) or fruit or nut bars (such as Fruitus bar by Lyme Regis Foods).
- **Instead of sweets and chocolate** have fresh fruit (apple, pear, peach, plum, berries), dried fruits such as apricots (these are a concentrated source of natural sugars, so eat in moderation).
- **Instead of sugar** (in drinks and home baking) have xylitol (it tastes just like sugar but doesn't upset blood sugar balance or cause tooth decay).
- **Instead of sweetened drinks** drink water, fruity/herbal teas, diluted fruit juice (gradually increase the amount of water to let your taste buds adjust), diluted apple and blackcurrant concentrate, such as Meridian or cherry concentrate such as Cherry Active.

Important: stay off the caffeine

Sugar isn't the only factor in blood sugar problems. Stimulants are, too. And as caffeine is a powerful one, it can be highly disruptive to your blood sugar balance. The biggest culprits are cola and energy drinks, chocolate bars and chocolate drinks, tea and coffee. Instead, have herbal teas or rooibos (redbush) tea or green tea in moderation (maximum three cups a day). You can also have decaf tea or coffee, but these still contain some stimulants. A stimulant-free alternative, such as a grain or dandelion coffee substitute, are better. Our favourite coffee substitutes are Teeccino and Caro Extra. These are available in health-food stores. You may experience 'withdrawal' symptoms, such as headaches, when you give up caffeine, but these will disappear within a couple of days – unless you have a serious addiction to caffeine. In that case, as the first symptoms subside you may begin to experience some of the ongoing abstinence symptoms. Stabilising your blood sugar is an important part of decreasing the severity of these symptoms. (See Chapter 19 for guidelines on giving up caffeine.)

Eat protein with carbohydrate

The more fibre and protein you include with any meal or snack, the slower the release of the carbohydrates, which is good for blood-glucose balance. So, combining protein-rich foods with high-fibre carbohydrates is an excellent rule of thumb. Here's how you do it:

Ways to combine carbohydrates and protein:

- Eat unsalted seeds or nuts with a whole fruit snack.

- Add seeds or nuts to carbohydrate-based breakfast cereals.

- Top wholemeal toast with eggs, baked beans or nut butter.

- Serve salmon or chicken with brown basmati rice.

- Add kidney beans to pasta sauce served over wholemeal pasta.

- Put cottage cheese on oatcakes, or hummus on pumpernickel-style whole-grain rye bread.

- Make sandwiches with sugar-free peanut butter and whole-meal bread.

What about high-protein diets?

Very high-protein diets have proved effective in managing blood sugar (as well as providing you with an abundance of amino acids that your brain needs to restore neurotransmitter balance), but they are not great for your health in the long term. This is because too much protein, especially from meat and dairy products, can have negative effects on the kidneys and bones, as well as being associated with a higher incidence of breast, prostate and colo-rectal cancer.

You can get the best of both worlds – that is, more health as well as a good supply of amino acids – by eating protein-rich foods with low-GL carbohydrates.

> **Y**ou need some protein with every meal because protein provides essential amino acids, and you need low-GL carbs to give you energy.

For breakfast, you can achieve the correct balance and amount of protein and low-GL carbohydrate by, for example, eating some seeds, yogurt or either skimmed milk or soya milk, with your cereal and fruit. If you have an egg on toast, or kippers and oat-cakes, you've done it already.

The correct balance

The simplest way to visualise your meals, as far as lunch and dinner are concerned, is in quarters. Visualise one of the protein-rich food portions shown in the chart, Guide to a Protein Serving, overleaf, filling one-quarter on the left side of your dinner plate, and an equivalent-sized serving of any carbo-hydrate-rich food on the right, then a large salad or two servings of vegetables filling the rest of the plate. So, half of what's on your plate is vegetables, one-quarter is a protein-rich food and one-quarter is a carbohydrate-rich food.

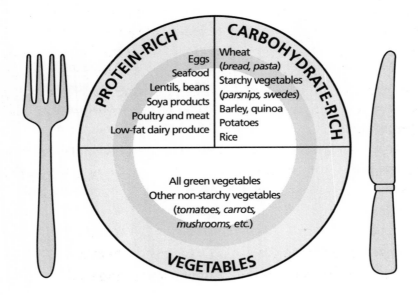

The perfectly balanced dinner plate

GUIDE TO A PROTEIN SERVING

Tofu and tempeh	160g	¾ packet
Soya mince	100g	3 tbsp
Chicken (no skin)	50g	1 very small breast
Turkey (no skin)	50g	½ small breast
Quorn	120g	⅓ pack
Salmon and trout	55g	1 very small fillet
Tuna (canned in brine)	50g	¼ can
Sardines (canned in brine)	75g	⅔ can
Cod	65g	1 very small fillet
Clams	60g	¼ can
Prawns	85g	6 large prawns
Mackerel	85g	1 medium fillet
Oysters	–	15
Yogurt (natural, low fat)	285g	½ large tub
Cottage cheese	120g	½ medium tub
Hummus	200g	1 small tub
Skimmed milk	440ml	about ¾ pint
Soya milk	415ml	about ¾ pint
Eggs (boiled)	–	2
Quinoa	125g	large serving bowl
Baked beans	310g	¾ can
Kidney beans	175g	⅓ can
Black-eye beans	175g	⅓ can
Lentils	165g	⅓ can

GUIDE TO A STARCHY CARBOHYDRATE SERVING (7 GLS)

Pumpkin/squash	186g	big serving
Carrot	158g	1 large
Swede	150g	big serving
Quinoa	131g	big serving
Beetroot	112g	big serving
Polenta (cornmeal)	116g	1 serving

Pearl barley	95g	1 small serving
Wholemeal pasta	85g	½ a serving
White pasta	66g	⅓ of a serving
Brown rice	70g	1 small serving
Brown basmati rice	80g	1 moderate serving
White rice	46g	⅓ of a serving
Couscous	46g	⅓ of a serving
Broad beans	31g	1 serving
Corn on the cob	60g	½ a cob
Boiled potato	74g	3 small potatoes
Baked potato	59g	½
French fries	47g	tiny portion
Sweet potato	61g	½

LOW-GL MEAL EXAMPLES

Protein	Carbohydrate	Vegetables
Chilli con carne*	on brown basmati rice	with a green salad
Marinated tofu	on wholewheat pasta	with steam-fried vegetables
Grilled chicken breast	with boiled new potatoes	with steamed runner beans
Cottage cheese salad	on oatcakes/rye bread	with broccoli and tomato
Venison sausages*	with sweet potato and carrot mash *	with roasted vegetables *
Spiced turkey burgers*	with avocado and potato salad *	with steamed savoy cabbage with crème fraîche
Poached salmon	with roast butternut squash and shallots *	with petits pois, lemon and mint

Low-GL versions of the recipes marked with a star (*) are given in the *Holford Low-GL Diet Cookbook*. We recommend you use this to expand your repertoire of delicious and simple low-GL meals. This cookbook also gives you many tasty low-GL snacks with the correct protein–carb combinations. In Part 4 of this book you'll find our How to Quit Diet, which includes a selection of recipes.

You will probably be eating more protein-rich foods in relation to carbohydrate-rich foods than you are used to, as well as more fresh fruit and vegetables. The GL of non-starchy vegetables (broccoli, kale, cabbage, peas, spinach, carrots and so on) is small, so eat as much of these as you like. Aim, too, for two pieces of low-GL fruit a day (see page 180).

Graze, don't gorge – eat little and often

You also want to spread your 'GLs' throughout the day. By keeping your blood sugar level you don't get starving hungry or have blood sugar overload. That means roughly:

10–15 GLs for breakfast

5 GLs for a mid-morning snack

10–15 GLs for lunch

5 GLs for a mid-afternoon snack

10–15 GLs for dinner

The chart opposite gives you an idea of three days' menus, putting this idea into practice (the recipes can be found on pages 357–74).

LOW-GL MENUS

Day 1

Breakfast: Low-GL Muesli with berries and yogurt

Mid-morning: apple with 6 almonds

Lunch: Rice, Tuna and Petits Pois Salad

Mid-afternoon: peanut butter and wholegrain toast

Dinner: Thai Green Curry with brown basmati rice and steam-fried vegetables

Drinks: unlimited water, herbal teas and coffee alternatives, plus one glass of diluted juice

Day 2

Breakfast: Smoked Salmon with Scrambled Egg on rye toast

Mid-morning: pear and 1 tbsp pumpkin seeds

Lunch: Beany Vegetable Soup

Mid-afternoon: hummus and oatcakes

Dinner: Spiced Turkey Meatballs with baked beans, grilled mushrooms and tomatoes, and wholegrain spaghetti

Drinks: unlimited water, herbal teas and coffee alternatives, plus a smoothie

Day 3

Breakfast: Scots Porridge with ground seeds and cinnamon

Mid-morning: natural yogurt with fresh berries

Lunch: Green Bean, Olive and Roasted Pepper Salad

Mid-afternoon: pear with 6 almonds

Dinner: Sticky Mustard Salmon Fillets with steam-fried spinach, red peppers and boiled baby new potatoes

Drinks: unlimited water, herbal teas and coffee alternatives, plus one glass of diluted juice

Train yourself to have two low-GL snacks. *The Holford Low-GL Diet Cookbook* gives you lots of low-GL soups, snacks, salads and light meals to choose from during the day, as well as tea-time treats to solve any energy slumps in the afternoon.

Never go without breakfast

The biggest mistake you can make is not to eat breakfast. This is when your blood sugar is lowest. If you're in the habit of having a strong coffee, a piece of toast and jam (carb plus sugar) and maybe a cigarette, you are setting yourself up for a blood sugar level that yo-yos your whole day. This will probably satisfy your immediate hunger, but it will set up a cycle of craving for the wrong foods or for the mood-altering substance you are giving up.

At first you may have to *make* yourself eat breakfast because, as you wake up, perhaps with some level of abstinence symptoms and lack of motivation, you'll be craving a quick fix. This is the time to eat a healthy low-GL breakfast (see our menus and recipes in Part 4) and to take your morning supplements.

> **A**s you get healthier and start feeling better in the morning, you will find yourself looking forward to a nutritious breakfast.

Nourish yourself with an evening meal

Having a healthy low-GL dinner is as important as having a good breakfast. This will help you wake up feeling refreshed, without rock-bottom blood sugar and a desperate need for a stimulant or something sweet to get you going. As you continue to eat a nutritious diet you will probably get a much better night's sleep. The knock-on effect is that it's easier for you to get out of bed in the morning – which in turn gives you the time and inclination to eat a decent breakfast.

Our How to Quit Action Plan in Part 4 contains full details for healthy eating, which will help you control your blood sugar level and conquer your abstinence symptoms. It includes a selection of breakfasts, lunches, evening meals and snacks (see Chapter 28).

SUMMARY

▶ Choose low-GL carbohydrate foods.

▶ Always eat carbohydrate foods with protein foods.

▶ Always eat breakfast.

▶ Have half of your main meal plate as vegetables, one-quarter as protein and one-quarter as low-GL carbs.

▶ Have two low-GL snacks a day.

12.

REPAIR YOUR BRAIN WITH ANTIOXIDANTS

Our bodies run on oxygen. We derive energy in every single brain cell by combusting glucose with oxygen. This is the fuel for all those chemical reactions that make us feel stimulated, relaxed, happy or sad. And with it comes the equivalent of exhaust fumes: oxidants (or free radicals), which are small, highly reactive molecules containing oxygen. In excess, these literally age the brain in the same way that they age our skin and, as a consequence, the brain is less able to make those mood-boosting neurotransmitters we described in Chapter 2. Most mood-altering substances – including alcohol, nicotine and caffeine – whether or not you are addicted to them, speed up this process either by directly introducing more oxidants or by over-stimulating the brain cells, forcing a massive release of neurotransmitters. This is especially true for stimulant drugs such as speed, cocaine and MDMA-based drugs, such as Ecstasy. Over-excitation damages neurons in your brain by flooding it with oxidants.

> To repair the brain, give the liver what it needs to detoxify the body of oxidants that damage the brain.

Oxidant-damaging substances

The single worst source of brain-damaging oxidants is smoking. Although it's the nicotine that's addictive, it's the oxidants in cigarette or joint smoke that kill you. Each puff contains over 50 known brain toxins, and a trillion oxidants. Cigarette smoke kills over 100,000 people in Britain every single year.

Alcohol helps create oxidants and/or interferes with the body's normal defence mechanisms against them, as oxidants are formed while alcohol is being broken down in the liver. It also stimulates the activity of enzymes that contribute to oxidant production and reduces the levels of antioxidants – those natural chemicals that can eliminate oxidants. This can result in liver cell injury, and excessive oxidants in the liver cells are an important factor in liver disease.[58]

> **D**amaged brain neurons become less and less able to produce the natural neurotransmitters that help you feel good.

By increasing your intake of vital antioxidant nutrients you gain energy, detox your body and brain, and help your brain cells recover. Antioxidants include vitamins A, C and E, curcumin, glutathione, alpha lipoic acid, selenium, zinc, and n-acetyl-cysteine (NAC), as well as vital carotenoids, flavonoids and anthocyanidins found in berries, fresh fruit and vegetables. In the diagram on page 194 you can see how these antioxidants work together as team players, along with coenzyme Q_{10} (CoQ_{10}) and lipoic acid. You need all of these vital antioxidants every day, both from diet and supplements, to maximise your good feelings in recovery.

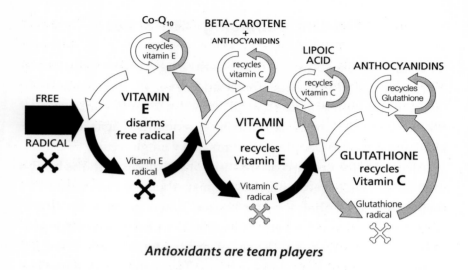

Antioxidants are team players

Repairing the damage

Increased oxidation messes up methylation and vice versa. We have found that the combination of a diet high in antioxidants and B vitamins – which means a lot of fresh vegetables and fruit – and more raw and steamed whole foods, as well as unfried, unsmoked, oily fish, helps you recover your natural get-up-and-go. Supplementing specific antioxidants helps even more.

Glutathione and NAC

In Chapter 9 we learned how methylation keeps you feeling connected, helping to reduce cravings. We also saw how one way to improve methylation was to supplement the potent antioxidant NAC. In truth, methylation and oxidation work against each other.

The single most potent antioxidant for humans is glutathione. But glutathione is made from NAC, which is a bit more stable, hence it is generally better to supplement.

Over-stimulating the brain – as alcohol, nicotine and other drugs do – usually depletes the brain of glutamate, a key 'reward' neurotransmitter. This leads to reward deficiency and the desire to use a stimulating substance again and again. NAC and glutathione not only help disarm oxidants and detoxify your liver but also help restore normal levels of glutamate in your brain. NAC and glutathione also help to promote glutamine levels in the brain, which in turn helps to make GABA – the relaxing neurotransmitter.

According to US researchers at the University of Minnesota School of Medicine (Department of Psychiatry), NAC even helps gamblers (known to have imbalances of brain neurochemistry, just like those with substances addictions) to gamble less.[59] They gave pathological gamblers NAC supplements for eight weeks. More than half of the participants reported significantly fewer urges to gamble. In the second half of this trial the gamblers were given either NAC or dummy pills. More than 80 per cent who received NAC reported even fewer urges to gamble, while more than 70 per cent who received the dummy pill resumed their previous gambling habits. The research team is now testing the effects of NAC on addiction to stimulant drugs.

Breaking the vicious cycle

The combination of excessive use of substances that deplete GABA (alcohol, tranquillisers and sleeping pills, marijuana, or stimulant drugs, from caffeine to cocaine) plus eating a diet low in antioxidants leads to a vicious cycle of flooding the brain with oxidants, damaging brain cells, changing brain chemistry, and craving substances to temporarily make you feel better. The net effect of ever-increasing brain and liver damage makes it even harder to feel as good as you need to be able to quit and stay off addictive substances.

This may also partly explain why drinkers who give up drinking but not smoking, and smokers who give up smoking but not drinking, have a much lower success rate of staying abstinent. You have to get your brain, gut and liver back to firing on all cylinders

– and antioxidants are a vital piece of the equation. So, what does this mean in terms of your diet?

Foods for upping antioxidant power

So, how can you use diet to get the antioxidants you need? Overall, you are aiming for at least five, if not seven, servings of fresh fruit and vegetables a day; for example, two or three servings of fruit, plus two servings of vegetables with your two main meals. In addition, have seeds, onion and garlic every day.

Seeds of life

Everything grows from a seed. For this simple reason seeds are jam-packed full of energy, protein and the nutrients necessary for plants to grow – and we grow from eating plants. All seeds are packed with antioxidant minerals, essential for brain recovery, such as zinc and selenium, as well as calming calcium and magnesium. Pumpkin seeds are the highest in magnesium. All seeds and nuts are rich in vitamin E, a powerful antioxidant, but it's important to eat them raw. The easiest way to do this is to add a spoonful of ground seeds to your cereal in the morning or, if you don't have cereal, have a handful of seeds, perhaps with some almonds. Make up a jar of our Essential Seed Mix (see page 357) and grind a serving to add to your cereal each day.

Eat your greens

Dark green vegetables are packed with vitamin C, folate and chlorophyll, all of which are exceedingly good for you, helping your body detoxify but also helping support healthy brain function. Of course, these are only three of dozens of vital antioxidant nutrients found in greens, but some greens are better than others. Spinach is the highest in folic acid, giving 204mcg in a cup, or a good handful. Other great leafy sources are watercress, basil and parsley.

Avocado is also excellent. Watercress, parsley and basil are exceptional sources of beta-carotene, second only to carrots, and great sources of vitamin C, second only to broccoli and green peppers. All these super-greens are packed full of bioflavonoids, which are special antioxidants that help your liver detox your body.

One excellent way to give yourself a daily shot of nutrient-packed greens is to have a serving of super-greens, made by blending a handful of spinach leaves, watercress, parsley and basil with a tablespoon of extra-virgin olive oil, and a squeeze of lemon juice. The combination is quite delicious and can be adapted to make pesto, soups, stews and salads.

Cruciferous vegetables rule

Vegetables whose leaves grow as a cross (cruciferous) are all part of a special food family that enhances the liver's capacity to detoxify and thus help heal a damaged brain. These include cabbage, cauliflower, broccoli, Brussels sprouts and kale. Cruciferous vegetables are important antioxidants and they are also essential for detoxing the liver, as we explain in Chapter 15. That's why we recommend that you have a serving of them every day.

Sulphur so good

Onions, spring onions, garlic and shallots are excellent food sources of sulphur-containing amino acids. The amino acids in these foods also give the body the raw ingredients to make glutathione which drives another critical detox pathway, as well as helping to make GABA, the brain's natural relaxer. Red onions are especially good because they are high in quercetin, which is a natural anti-inflammatory that also curbs allergic reactions and pain.

Garlic has many other benefits; a key one being as a gut protector. Alcohol, caffeine and many drugs damage the gut and often lead to dysbiosis, whereby you have the wrong balance of bacteria or an overgrowth of yeast in the gut, called candidiasis.

Garlic is a natural anti-fungal agent that helps keep your digestive tract free of unwanted fungi and yeast.

Fruits and vegetables

Certain fruits are high in antioxidants to repair the brain and they also support your liver. They are high in folic acid and zinc to help methylation, and low in sugar. Blueberries, strawberries and raspberries are the best all-round antioxidant-rich fruits. A serving of strawberries contains more antioxidant power than three apples or four bananas. Best of all are blueberries, which are especially rich in a type of flavonoid called anthocyanidins and proanthocyanidins. You can measure the total antioxidant power of a food by its ability to detoxify and disarm dangerous oxidants. This is called the ORAC score; the higher the score the more potent an antioxidant.

THE SUPERFRUITS

	Zinc	Folic acid	ORAC	Vitamin C	**Total Score**
Strawberries	3	3	4	5	15
Raspberries	2	3	4	5	14
Blueberries	3	5	5	1	14
Watermelon*	5	2	3	4	14
Cherries	0	3	5	5	13
Grapes	4	5	2	2	13
Grapefruit	0	4	3	5	12
Oranges	0	4	3	5	12

* If eaten or blended with the seeds

We recommend that you eat two servings of these fresh fruits every day. When berries are out of season you can use frozen berries; otherwise it's best to eat fresh, organic fruits. It is generally better to eat your fruit than drink it because concentrated fruit juices can contain too much natural sugar and because studies indicate that fruit juice does not satisfy one's appetite and hence may be associated with overeating and obesity. One exception, especially during the first two weeks of detoxifying your body of oxidants, is watermelon juice, made simply by blending the flesh and seeds of a watermelon. The seeds crack and the black husk of the seed sinks to the bottom, while the seed itself, rich in zinc, selenium, vitamin E and essential fats, becomes part of the drink with the vitamin C and beta-carotene-rich flesh.

In terms of vegetables, those that are orange in colour (carrots, sweet potato, butternut squash) are highest in beta-carotene, whereas tomatoes are high in lycopene and beetroot in betanene – all potent antioxidants. Have something blue, red or orange every day.

The golden rules: antioxidants

There are six golden rules for upping your antioxidant intake with food. Eat these every day:

1. Nuts and seeds (but not marijuana seeds).

2. Two servings of greens, including a 'cruciferous' vegetable.

3. Something blue, red or orange – preferably including a serving of berries.

4. Some onion or garlic.

5. Quercetin-rich green or black tea, red onions or apples.

6. Something yellow: mustard, turmeric or yellow peppers.

In Part 4 we give you a selection of healthy recipes that are rich in antioxidants – see our How to Quit Diet in Chapter 28.

Supplementing antioxidants

In addition to eating antioxidant-rich foods every day we recommend taking antioxidant supplements daily, especially during the first three months of abstinence. There are three specific supplements we recommend:

1. **An all-round antioxidant complex**, taken twice a day. This should contain a combination of vitamin A, natural beta-carotene, C and E, selenium, zinc, glutathione and/or NAC, anthocyanidins, CoQ_{10} and alpha lipoic acid.

2. **Extra NAC** A combination supplement will never provide enough NAC for maximum effect so it's well worth supplementing an additional 500mg of NAC twice a day.

3. **Extra vitamin C** As you'll see again and again, vitamin C is such a powerful ally in restoring health, detoxifying and reducing cravings, that we recommend 2g (2,000mg) taken twice a day for anyone quitting just about anything. The most you'll find in a multivitamin is 200mg, which isn't enough. Extra vitamin C is especially important if you smoke or are alcoholic.

SUMMARY

- ▶ Eat nuts and seeds every day.

- ▶ Have two servings of super-greens, plus a 'cruciferous' vegetable every day.

- ▶ Have something blue, red or orange – preferably including a serving of berries every day.

- ▶ Have some onion or garlic every day.

- ▶ Supplement an all-round antioxidant complex twice a day.

- ▶ Supplement 500mg of NAC twice a day.

- ▶ Supplement 2g of vitamin C, twice a day (or 1g, four times daily).

13.

HOW TO GET
A GOOD NIGHT'S SLEEP

You toss and turn, curl up, stretch out – but whatever you do, you can't get to sleep; and when you do you frequently wake up. In the morning, you wake tired or depressed. You're not alone. In Britain almost a quarter (22 per cent) of people suffer from insomnia at some time.[60] The vast majority of people with addictions, or in recovery, don't get enough sleep, which, in turn, makes them less likely to stop and more likely to relapse (as we explained in Chapters 1 and 3). Getting enough good-quality sleep is as vital to your health and brain function as getting enough vitamins.

You almost certainly have been given tips about what to do about your sleep problem; you've probably tried some or all of the more common remedies such as sleeping pills or perhaps cognitive behavioural therapy (CBT), or maybe you are even following a set of rules curiously named 'sleep hygiene' (see page 215). If so you are undoubtedly aware of their shortcomings. The pills can have nasty side effects, and sleep hygiene is not much more than common sense. While CBT can help some, it does not address underlying causes of poor sleep. And, while we do believe CBT can be beneficial, you may have a hard time finding it because in the UK we are around 10,000 therapists short in the NHS, although you can get treatment privately.

Sleep and addiction

'Often, sleep isn't discussed (or treated) in alcohol recovery pro-grammes, but it should be,' says Dr Conroy, whose research has found that the brains of alcoholics are often awake for a large part of the night.[61] This is true for many addictive substances, espe-cially all stimulants. In other words you are not asleep when you are asleep, and not awake when you are awake. Does this sound like you? If you don't find a solution for your sleeping problems you are more likely to stay in the addiction cycle.

A study in China found that the less well adolescents slept, the more they smoked or drank alcohol.[62] But is it the drinking and smoking that causes sleeping problems or the sleeping problems that lead to smoking and drinking? We think it cuts both ways. The worse you sleep the more likely you are to crave stimulants and relaxants, and the more of these you have, the worse you sleep.

Perhaps most important from the point of view of helping you to give up a substance is the effect that a lack of sleep has on critical brain hormones. Most addicts, while using and in early recovery, have raised cortisol levels (the stress hormone), and low levels of the important anti-ageing growth hormone. A lack of sleep promotes both of these, as well as leading to a lack of melatonin. Now your brain is looking for a fix.

Alcohol

Alcohol suppresses REM (the period of sleep when we do most of our dreaming), and decreases deep sleep;[63] and drinkers wake up more frequently in the night. But what most people are not aware of is that the lack of REM due to alcohol can also cause sleep disturbances when the person gives up drinking. When alcohol is removed, there is a rebound of REM sleep. The body attempts to make up for the REM sleep that it has missed. This results in nightmares and severe sleep disturbances in many people in early recovery from alcoholism.

Alcohol increases snoring and sleep apnoea, as does smoking.

Smoking

Smokers are more likely to sleep fewer than eight hours, have nightmares, have difficulty getting to sleep and staying asleep and more likely to use sleeping pills.

Caffeine

The effects of caffeine on sleep seem rather obvious. Caffeine is a stimulant, and excessive intake can interfere with the relaxation necessary for sleep. Caffeine, as we saw earlier, depresses melatonin for up to ten hours, and melatonin is your brain's natural sleep inducer.

The worst thing you can do if you want a good night's sleep is smoke or drink coffee or alcohol, or take sleeping pills (we look at these on page 209).

Sleeplessness makes you vulnerable

Getting enough sleep is at least as important as eating fruit and vegetables. People who don't get enough are twice as likely to become addicted to something, twice as likely to feel anxious and four times more likely to feel depressed.[64] Anxiety caused because you can't sleep adds to the problem. Anxiety and depression increase cravings and the risk of using, or returning to the use of, a mood-altering substance.

Are you in sleep debt?

You need sleep, and good-quality sleep at that, and if you don't get enough you are in sleep debt. Sleep debt is simply the amount of sleep you require minus the amount of sleep you're getting. For example, if you require eight hours of sleep and you're getting only five, your sleep debt is three hours.

Signs of sleep debt

The easiest way to know if you are getting enough is to notice simply whether you become sleepy during the day – while driving, watching TV, at meetings or lectures. If so, you probably have a substantial sleep debt or deprivation.

Other signs of sleep debt are frequent blinking, difficulty focusing eyes, heavy eyelids, daytime drowsiness, impatience, irritability, being quick to anger, having difficulty listening to what is said or understanding directions, difficulty remembering or retaining information, making frequent errors or mistakes, depression or being in a bad or negative mood.

To help identify if you are suffering from excessive daytime sleepiness and poor quality of sleep complete the questionnaire below.

QUESTIONNAIRE: excessive daytime sleepiness

(the Epworth Sleepiness Scale)

Rate the chance that you would doze off or fall asleep during the following daytime situations from 0 to 3, as below:

0 means you would never doze off or fall asleep in a given situation.

1 means there is a slight chance that you would doze off or fall asleep.

2 means there is a moderate chance that you would doze off or fall asleep.

3 means there is a high chance that you would doze off or fall asleep.

Situation

1. Sitting and reading.

2. Sitting inactive in a public place (such as a theatre, lecture or meeting).

3. Watching TV.

4. As a passenger in a car for an hour or longer without a break.

5. Lying down to rest in the afternoon.

6. Sitting and talking to someone.

7. In a car, while stopped in traffic.

Total score:

Score

10 or more

You most likely suffer from excessive daytime sleepiness, a strong indication that you are sleep deprived and need to improve the quality and/or duration of your sleep. People who continue to suffer from poor sleep are more prone to depression, anxiety, drug cravings and relapse.

Inadequate sleep and the effects of alcohol and antidepressants

During sleep there is a complex feedback system at work between serotonin and the sleep hormone melatonin (which is made from serotonin) and also other hormones such as cortisol (linked with stress). An imbalance between these often lies behind sleeping problems. Alcohol and antidepressant drugs suppress dream sleep, and when a person stops using them, there is a rebound effect causing disturbed sleep in abstinence.[65]

The healing power of sleep

When you sleep your brain goes through a sequence of stages, each of which has its own benefit. Stage One is a transition state between waking and sleep. During Stage Two and Stage Three the brain waves continue to slow. Stage Four is deep sleep during which the body releases the rejuvenating growth hormone and heals your body. Most people cycle through the four stages of sleep about every 90 minutes throughout the night. If you do not go through all the stages of sleep, you will be deprived of many of the benefits of sleep. Each of the stages is punctuated by dream sleep, and this is a vital stage for repairing our brains especially, as explained below.

Dream sleep: replenishing neurotransmitters

At the end of each sleep cycle there is a period when the eyes move rapidly beneath the lids, called rapid eye movement (REM). Although we may dream during all stages of sleep, dreams occur most frequently in REM sleep, and are usually more vivid and emotional than during other stages. Because dream sleep is so important for our brains, it offers one of the clearest arguments for getting at least seven or eight restful uninterrupted hours of sleep.

During REM sleep the brain replenishes its supply of neurotransmitters – such as noradrenalin, dopamine, GABA and serotonin – crucial for new learning, memory, retention, organisation, reorganisation, mood enhancement, calmness and emotional balance. It's now also well established that dreaming sleep is vital for effective learning.

Dreaming may also be a way of sorting out emotional problems that you haven't dealt with during the day. Dreaming is how we process and help to release unexpressed emotions. If you don't do this, your brain ends up in permanent 'stress' mode – the hallmark of addiction. In fact, REM sleep is rather like running a clean-up programme on your computer. Dream sleep tidies up the fragmented and corrupted files we generated during the day as well as releasing unexpressed emotions. Without it, our mental processes are likely to run slower and less efficiently, to say nothing of the occasional system error and total crashes that we are likely to face.

Dream time may be cut if you are taking antidepressants that boost the hormone serotonin (known as SSRIs, such as Prozac or Seroxat). That's because serotonin levels normally drop right down when we are dreaming.

Vitamins for dream recall

Your ability to recall dreams and whether or not your dreams are in 'black and white' or technicolour is a function of your vitamin B_6 and zinc status. In fact, we often use dreams as a measure of vitamin B_6 and zinc status and recommend vitamin supplements for those in recovery who do not remember their dreams.

Causes of sleep debt

Most researchers now agree that we need around seven to nine hours of largely uninterrupted sleep each night, ideally between 11pm and 7am. As we have stated, use of mood-altering substances affect your sleep, as does quitting the use of those substances. But there are also other causes that contribute to sleep debt and affect your recovery. There are many disorders and conditions that deprive us of sleep, such as insomnia, sleep apnoea, restless-leg syndrome, and bruxism (grinding the teeth while asleep), which can disturb sleep.

Insomnia

The most common of some 84 different sleep disorders, insomnia is defined as:

- Difficulty falling asleep (on average taking more than 30 minutes to fall asleep).

- Waking up frequently during the night and having difficulty getting back to sleep.

- Waking up too early in the morning and being unable to return to sleep.

- Waking up tired or exhausted – which can persist throughout the day, making you feel irritable, anxious or depressed.

Long-term insomnia may be due to 'hyper-arousal'. Insomniacs often have a faster heart rate, higher levels of the stress hormone cortisol and more of the alert beta brainwaves before sleep. Stimulant drugs, including caffeine, can cause this state of hyper-arousal and make it difficult to go to sleep and stay asleep. In response, many people take substances that induce sleep, creating a cycle of taking stimulants to wake up and relaxants to go to sleep.

Lack of deep sleep

The inability to go into, or stay in, deep sleep is a serious problem, because this is the time when cell repair takes place. The consequence of not getting adequate deep sleep is extreme fatigue and physical pain. In fact, the very painful condition of fibromyalgia is associated with lack of deep sleep. The body needs deep sleep to regenerate and that includes regeneration of brain cells damaged by addiction.

Sleeping too much

Some people sleep too much. But, fortunately, the same kind of diet, supplements and lifestyle that help reduce cravings and restore natural energy will help to decrease excessive sleepiness. The most common causes of over-sleeping are deep depression, adrenal exhaustion from too much stress and blood sugar problems (see Chapter 11).

Why sleeping pills are not the cure for sleep problems

If you can't sleep and you go to your doctor, the chances are you will be prescribed sleeping pills, also known as tranquillisers, sedatives or hypnotics. Despite having a long charge sheet of side effects,[66] hypnotic drugs still regularly feature in the top 20 most-prescribed drugs both here and in the USA. Not only that, but they aren't very useful, according to a report in the *British Medical Journal*[67] which concluded that there is plenty of evidence that they cause 'major harm' and that there was 'little evidence of clinically meaningful benefit'.

In fact, many of these drugs may actually suppress REM sleep, prevent deep sleep, reduce available neurotransmitters and block growth hormone release, thereby aggravating low moods. You can see now why deep sleep deprivation, fatigue and sleep medication often develop into a self-perpetuating cycle.

> Taking sleeping pills because of the inability to get restful sleep reduces both REM and deep sleep. This prevents rejuvenation and release of stress. Stress and fatigue increase the desire for sugar, alcohol, stimulants and relaxants, which leads to the inability to get restful sleep . . .

Just how marginally effective sleep medication is was vividly illustrated in a study by the American National Institutes of Health, which found that the newer drugs like Ambien (zolpidem) made volunteers fall asleep only 12.8 minutes faster than when they had taken a fake pill, and sleep for just 11 minutes longer.[68]

Despite this, sales of sleeping pills run at 4.5 billion dollars in the US, because patients are very keen on them and believe they work much better than they actually do. This could be because of one of the side effects, according to the same report: the pills interfere with memory formation so you simply forget all that tossing and turning.

Sleeping drugs can cause addiction

Even when they seem to work and the side effects are mild, there is a grave danger in using any drug for sleep. And that danger is the danger of addiction. If you can't sleep because you have stopped drinking or taking some other mood-altering substance, it will not help you to take something that will create another addiction for you. Why trade one addiction for another? And whether or not a drug is known to be addictive when you take it, the real effects might not be known at the time. As we explained in Chapter 6, most drugs that promote sleep were not thought to be addictive when they came out. And when it was found that they were, they were replaced with a 'non-addictive' one that later turned out to be addictive.

Virtually every sleeping pill targets the neurotransmitter GABA, which promotes sleep by preventing brain cells from firing. You now know natural ways to increase GABA production. So why not do it the natural way – with nutrients?

Using nutrition and supplements to promote sleep

If you don't get enough sleep, it's much harder to quit any addictive substance. Our How to Quit Diet and supplement recommendations in Part 4 will help restore your normal brain chemistry. Even if you've quit an addictive substance, if you haven't restored your brain chemistry to normal, the chances are you'll have sleeping problems. So, what can you do to get a good night's sleep?

You'll almost certainly have raised levels of the stress hormone cortisol, which, along with keeping you aroused at night, also has the effect of lowering production of the growth hormone needed for cell repair. To bring cortisol down you need to introduce fish and fish oil along with vegetables into your daily diet and keep a stable blood sugar level, which means avoiding sugar and refined carbohydrates. How to do this is explained in our How to Quit Diet in Chapter 28.

Raising melatonin – naturally

As we have mentioned several times, the main sleep hormone is melatonin which your body manufactures from serotonin, so although chronically raising levels with medications can cause problems, providing the natural chemicals that make serotonin naturally in the body can raise melatonin without creating excessive levels of serotonin. These raw materials include the amino acid tryptophan (found in milk, as well as chicken, turkey, seeds, nuts and cheese) and 5-HTP.

Several minerals and vitamins are also involved in good sleep. Calcium and magnesium are calming and aid muscle relaxation. Being highly stressed or eating a lot of sugar lowers magnesium levels. Calcium is found in milk, green vegetables and molasses; magnesium in seeds, nuts, green vegetables and seafood. You could supplement with 600mg of calcium and 400mg of magnesium before bed. B vitamins are also involved in handling stress, but, generally, they are best taken earlier in the day, as they can be energising and therefore might keep you awake.

What about taking melatonin supplements?

Produced by the pineal gland, located in the middle of the brain, melatonin regulates the sleep–wake cycle, which is why it seems the ideal sleep aid. Some sleep clinicians recommend 0.5–3mg melatonin under your tongue two hours before bed, but the results from trials have been mixed. However, a recent study found that melatonin significantly improved the quality of sleep, producing alert feelings in the morning, without any side effects and no problems when it was stopped.[69]

CAUTION Melatonin's side effects include nausea, dizziness and loss of libido and its long-term safety has not been determined. Headache and transient depression have been reported. In people who are depressed, melatonin may worsen symptoms. Melatonin is available by prescription only in the UK.

Our Sleep Prescription

Try our Sleep Prescription (see page 397), which contains a combination of 5-HTP or tryptophan, niacinamide (vitamin B_3), magnesium and vitamin B_6 and/or valerian (see page 213).

Or take 3,000–4,000mg tryptophan (only available in 220mg capsules over the counter in the UK or on prescription as Optimax in 1,000mg).

Melatonin is also helpful: take 1–3mg melatonin alone 60–90 minutes before bedtime on an empty stomach with 50/50 unsweetened fruit juice and water.

These options are outlined in detail in Part 4, page 397.

(Please note the caution below.)

Using herbs

Many herbs are said to have sleep-inducing properties. Best known is valerian; others include chamomile, passion flower, lavender, hops and lemon balm. One study of 600mg of valerian, standardised, taken 30 minutes before bedtime for 28 days found it to be as effective as oxazepam, a drug normally used to treat anxiety. Another found that the combination of valerian and lemon balm was as effective as the hypnotic Halcion, but it produced no drowsiness the next day. For more detailed advice contact the National Institute of Medical Herbalists www.nimh. org.uk/index.html.

Another recent development is herbal sources of melatonin. In fact many of the plants with the highest concentrations are in herbal medicine, such as St John's wort, sage and feverfew. Another is the herbal remedy Asphalia, which contains a grass called *Festuca arundinacea*, and which has the highest melatonin content of any plant. So far it has only been tested in one small controlled study, which showed that it improves sleep.

CAUTION Although it's safe to combine behavioural techniques such as sleep hygiene with, say, taking 5-HTP, it's best to avoid taking all of these substances in combination. For example, take either melatonin or 5-HTP or tryptophan, possibly with some valerian, but not all of them together, unless otherwise advised by your health-care practitioner.

Other ways to improve your sleep

The following techniques address ways of thinking and behaving that can affect sleep. If you have an underlying sleep disorder, they probably won't solve your problem, but they may help. If your underlying sleep problem is an addiction, then your first priority should be resolving your addiction issues. These guidelines are only suggestions – see if any work for you.

Cognitive behavioural therapy (CBT)

Long-term sleep problems can be the result of an illness such as diabetes or a painful condition such as arthritis, or from any number of physical problems we have discussed. But sometimes the cause is not physical – or doesn't seem to be. By following our nutrition recommendations for quitting addictive substances naturally you may find your sleep problems simply go away. Stress, anxiety or depression can be emotional or situational as well as physical, and if you are still experiencing problems having followed our nutritional approach you might find psychotherapy helpful. Psychotherapy such as CBT is able to help by encouraging people to acknowledge the stress that is preventing them from sleeping and then helping them develop ways of dealing with it.

This might be by identifying negative or unhelpful thoughts – 'I just can't sleep without my pills' – and changing them. A review in the *Lancet* in 2004 found that various forms of counselling and psychological help are not only the most effective way but also the safest way to tackle chronic insomnia.[70] A more recent study compared CBT with one of the new sleeping pills called zopiclone. While CBT improved the percentage of time spent asleep from 81.4 per cent to 90.1 per cent after six months, zopiclone actually reduced it from 82.3 per cent to 81.9 per cent.[71] In a proper evidence-based system, we'd have most people being referred to counsellors and few being prescribed drugs, instead of the other way round. Your doctor can refer you to a CBT psychotherapist.

Sleep hygiene

Some essentially common-sense advice, rather quaintly known as 'sleep hygiene', forms part of most sleep regimes. The idea is to create regular sleep-promoting habits on the grounds that the less successful you are at getting to sleep, the more you are going to worry about it.

Good sleep hygiene

- Keep the bedroom quiet and dark.

- Wear comfortable clothing to bed.

- Do not have a big meal before bed.

- Keep artificial light to a minimum in the bedroom. (Being exposed to bright light can turn off production of melatonin, which peaks at around 1.00am. Have a light with a low-wattage bulb in the bedroom or hallway in case you need to get up in the night.)

- Exercise regularly, but not after 7pm.

- Avoid coffee after noon and alcohol in the evening.

Good results have been reported for something similar to sleep hygiene known as 'stimulus control therapy', which essentially involves ensuring that the bed is associated only with sleeping. Patients are advised against having naps, to go to bed when sleepy, to get up within 20 minutes if they haven't fallen asleep, to do something relaxing until they feel drowsy and to try again, but to get up again if it fails.

Musical rhythms of sleep

New York psychiatrist Dr Galina Mindlin uses 'brain music' – rhythmic patterns of sounds derived from recordings of patients' own brainwaves – to help them overcome insomnia, anxiety and depression. The recordings sound something like classical piano music and appear to have a calming effect similar to yoga or meditation. A double-blind study by Toronto University found 80 per cent of those getting brain music reported benefits.

We have had excellent results reported by insomniacs with Dr John Levine's CDs, *Silence of Peace* and *Orange Grove Siesta* (available from www.patrickholford.com/CD), played quietly as you go to sleep. Henrietta is a case in point:

Case study HENRIETTA

'After spending years controlling my sleep and alertness during the day with sleeping pills, my body had forgotten how to sleep. The last thing I remember thinking that [first] night, as the didgeridoo kicked in, was, "This CD's rubbish. It doesn't work." I woke up the next morning, after sleeping all the way through with no interruptions.' The didgeridoo begins 20 minutes into the CD. *'Twenty minutes is a dream compared with the two hours of restlessness I usually had before falling asleep.'* Henrietta found that something as simple as listening to alpha-wave-inducing music has helped silence the thoughts that drive her towards addictive substances, which she describes as a 'monkey on her shoulder'.

For further information read John Levine's book, *The Miracle of Alpha Music* (see Further Reading).

Chilling out

Insomniacs may have a hotter core temperature. Scientists at the University of South Australia have reported that the core temperature of normal sleepers dropped about one degree one to five hours before sleep, unlike that of insomniacs. However, naturopaths claim poor sleepers may benefit from a warm bath before bed, citing improved relaxation after a 15–20 minute hot bath, containing one to two cups of Epsom salts (magnesium sulphate). Of course, it could be the magnesium that also helps relaxation. For most people, a bedroom temperature of 20°C (68°F) is associated with the best-quality sleep.

Relaxation exercises

There are many relaxation exercises that you can use to help you go to sleep. Deep relaxation is a way of relaxing the body and mind to reduce stress and produce a sense of well-being. What happens when you relax is the opposite of what is called the 'fight or flight' reaction. When you relax, your muscles become heavy, your body temperature rises, and your breathing and heart rate slow down.

To experience deep relaxation, create a quiet place for yourself. Separate yourself from the world in your quiet place. Lie on your back or sit in a comfortable chair with your feet on the floor. Close your eyes, release distracting thoughts, try to put background noises and sounds out of your thoughts. Breathe deeply and relax your body. You do not *make* your body relax; you *allow* it to relax. You focus your concentration on one thing and allow distractions to drift from your awareness.

Focusing on physical or mental states

With some relaxation methods, the focus is on the physical states you are trying to change (your muscles, body temperature, breathing or heartbeat). With other methods, you do not concentrate on your physical state, but on a colour, a sound, a word or mantra, or a mental image.

Physical If you choose to focus on physical states, begin with your muscles. Allow them to become heavy. Then concentrate on raising your temperature. You can do this by sensing a spot of heat in your forehead or chest and allowing it to flow throughout your body. Then think about your breathing. Let it become slower and slower. Breathe from your abdomen, rather than your chest. Then feel your heartbeat and concentrate on slowing it down.

Mental If you choose to relax by concentrating on something other than your physical state, you can think of a colour. Concentrate on that colour, fill your mind with that colour, become a part of that colour. Or feel yourself in motion, floating, tumbling and rolling. Alternatively, you can repeat a pleasant word over and over to yourself, or imagine yourself in a soothing place, such as a quiet lake or green meadow. These are relaxation exercises you can do by yourself without the aid of a book or a tape, but there are also numerous books and tapes available to guide you through the relaxation process if you prefer. You could also record yourself talking through your relaxation technique and play it when you want to relax. Deep relaxation reduces your stress and helps you feel better. Relaxation exercises can help you manage abstinence symptoms and heal your addicted brain.

SUMMARY

- ▶ Avoid sugar and caffeine and minimise your intake of alcohol. Don't combine alcohol with sleeping pills or anti-anxiety medication.

- ▶ Take our Sleep Prescription (see page 397) one hour before going to bed.

- ▶ Consider taking valerian, hops, passion flower, St John's wort or a 'sleep formula' combining several of them. Choose a standardised extract or tincture and follow the dosage instructions.

continues ▶

▶ Eat more green leafy vegetables, nuts and seeds to ensure you're getting enough magnesium, and consider supplementing 300mg of magnesium in the evening with or without calcium (500mg).

▶ Eat unfried oily fish three times a week and eat nuts and seeds daily.

▶ Find the right kind of psychotherapy, especially cognitive behavioural therapy.

▶ Practise 'sleep hygiene'.

▶ Exercise regularly but not in the evening before sleep.

▶ Listen to alpha-wave-inducing music while in bed and practise relaxation techniques.

14.

SOLVING FOOD ALLERGIES THAT MAKE YOU CRAVE

A fascinating piece of the addiction puzzle is that addicted people and food-allergic people both suffer from many of the same symptoms and medical conditions: ADHD, depression, insomnia, cravings, nervousness and other symptoms that you are familiar with from the Scale of Abstinence Symptoms Severity. Perhaps this is because people who are prone to food allergies are also prone to addiction. Often people crave substances they are allergic to and sometimes addictive substances contain common allergens, for example the milk in your coffee or the yeast in your beer.

What is an allergy?

The immune system, which is the body's defence system, has the ability to produce 'markers' for substances it doesn't like. The classic marker is an antibody called immunoglobulin type E (IgE). These attach to something called 'mast cells'. When the offending food, called an allergen, latches onto its specific IgE antibody, the IgE molecule triggers the mast cell to release gran-

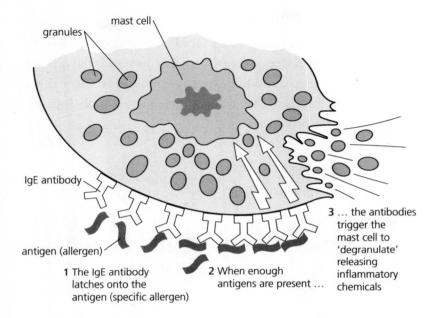

granules

mast cell

IgE antibody

antigen (allergen)

1 The IgE antibody latches onto the antigen (specific allergen)

2 When enough antigens are present …

3 … the antibodies trigger the mast cell to 'degranulate' releasing inflammatory chemicals

How IgE antibodies cause allergic reactions

ules containing histamine and other chemicals that cause the classic symptoms of allergy. These can include skin rashes, hay fever, rhinitis, sinusitis, asthma, eczema, gastrointestinal upsets or swelling in the face or throat. All these reactions are immediate, severe inflammatory reactions to the offending food.

It is easy to tell if you have an IgE-based food allergy. If you develop a rash shortly after eating strawberries, it is fairly safe to assume that you are allergic to strawberries. But, what if the reaction were to come two days later? You probably wouldn't connect the reaction to the strawberries.

Hidden food allergies

Food allergies with delayed reactions are called hidden food allergies, for the obvious reason that it is difficult to connect cause and effect. The emerging view now is that most allergies and intolerances are not IgE based, but involve another marker, known as immunoglobulin type G (IgG). Most food intolerances do not produce immediate symptoms, but have a delayed, accumulative effect, taking anywhere from two hours to three days or longer to show themselves, and are therefore much harder to detect by observation alone.

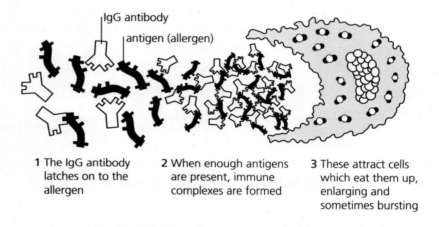

IgG antibody

antigen (allergen)

1 The IgG antibody latches on to the allergen

2 When enough antigens are present, immune complexes are formed

3 These attract cells which eat them up, enlarging and sometimes bursting

How IgG antibodies cause allergic reactions

Allergy and addiction

If you suffer from a hidden food allergy, you are prone to food addiction; that is, you are more likely to become physically addicted to those foods that are causing a delayed allergic reaction.

> Food allergy-induced food addictions in turn play a key role in a predisposition to and perpetuation of alcohol and drug abuse, chronic abstinence symptoms and a tendency to relapse into substance abuse over and over again.

In one study, 96 patients diagnosed as suffering from alcohol dependence and major depressive and psychiatric disorders were compared to 62 healthy volunteers selected from adult hospital staff members for a possible food or chemical intolerance. The results showed that the group of patients diagnosed as depressives had the highest number of allergies: 80 per cent were found to be allergic to barley (which contains gluten) and 100 per cent were allergic to egg white. Over 50 per cent of alcoholics tested were found to be allergic to egg white, milk or gluten grains. Only 9 per cent of the control group were found to suffer from any allergies.[72]

Food addiction

Dr Theron Randolph, the doctor who really put allergies on the map back in the 1960s and 1970s, was the very first to propose that many physical and emotional symptoms and diseases are caused or aggravated by eating certain foods and exposure to environmental chemicals. He observed that food-allergic people frequently develop addictions to the foods they are allergic to. He observed that, at first, many food-allergic people experience a pleasing addictive high, followed eventually by the development of tolerance, and acute withdrawal symptoms when they abruptly stop eating these same foods. He said:

> [Allergic] foods eaten frequently and regularly are rarely ever suspected as [addictive] offenders. Persons addicted to common foods simply use them as often as necessary to keep well. In other words, 'hooked' persons eat or drink their favorite 'pick-me-ups' (food mixtures or primary foods) in order to remain 'picked-up' (stimulated) and postpone or treat their 'hangovers' (or withdrawal effects). If food addictants are . . . eaten regularly, obesity, alcoholism, hyperactivity, insomnia, nervousness, and/or anxiety tend to develop; or persons may become self-centered, excited, aggressive, and agitated . . . These developments, often called the 'onset' of the present illness, usually prompt persons so affected to seek medical help.

When we ask patients to eliminate IgG-allergic foods abruptly from their diets, about one-third experience moderate-to-severe difficulty in getting through the first two or three days of abstinence. They universally complain of strong food cravings for the forbidden foods, and often report a multiplicity of other symptoms as well, including but not limited to, headaches, insomnia, irritability, depression, anxiety, shakiness, inability to concentrate, confusion, mental fogginess and fatigue. If they give in to their cravings and return to the forbidden allergic foods – and, of course, some do – the symptoms abate immediately. These signs and symptoms of withdrawal are not unlike those we observe in alcoholics and chemically dependent clients in recovery.

Allergy or indigestion?

Digestive problems are often the underlying factor that leads to the development of allergies. Many people dealing with addiction have digestive problems that cause allergic reactions, which in turn bring on abstinence symptoms. Many substance abusers and allergy sufferers have been found to have low stomach acid, essential for digesting food proteins. Zinc deficiency is extremely common among allergy sufferers and alcoholics. Zinc is not only needed to digest all protein but it's also essential for the production of stomach acid, which helps digest food. Certain foods are also inherently difficult to digest, the worst being gluten in wheat and casein in dairy products. Wheat and dairy are Britain's top two allergy-provoking foods. Many allergy sufferers and almost all alcoholics may have excessively 'leaky' digestive tracts, allowing undigested proteins to enter the bloodstream through the gut wall and cause reactions.

We recommend alcohol abstinence when you're coming off a food allergen, not only because withdrawal often increases cravings for alcohol but also because alcohol damages the gut, making it more leaky which, in turn, increases your allergic potential.

So, identifying and avoiding what you react to is part of the equation. Excessive stress, consumption of alcohol and excessive caffeine, frequent use of painkillers, deficiency in essential fats or a gastrointestinal infection or infestation such as candidiasis are all possible contributors to leaky gut syndrome (where the gut wall becomes damaged, allowing bacteria and undigested food to escape into the body) that need to be corrected to reduce intolerance to foods. Frequent use of antibiotics, which wipe out gut bacteria, paving the way for candidiasis, therefore also increase the risk of developing food intolerances.

Foods that promote healthy digestion

Improve your digestion by eating plenty of fresh fruit, vegetables, seeds such as pumpkin seeds, and oily fish such as salmon, which contain essential fats and zinc. Take a digestive enzyme supplement, with probiotics (friendly bacteria) for a month, to re-inoculate your digestive tract with good bacteria. And keep alcohol, painkillers and antibiotics to a minimum.

The ADHD–allergy–addiction link

Our work with children has shown that hidden food allergy plays a key role in up to 80 per cent of ADHD patients. Food allergy-induced ADHD is associated with numerous seemingly unrelated symptoms such as food cravings, mood problems, sleep problems, conduct disorders, seizures and digestive problems. These are the same symptoms we often see in people in addiction recovery.

In fact, ADHD occurs in a majority of alcoholics. Significantly more children with ADHD develop problems with alcoholism or drug addiction than do children without ADHD. Many people with ADHD are children of alcoholics, and ADHD is common in the relatives of ADHD children. Why?

One possibility is that there is a genetic predisposition that links ADHD, food allergy and addiction. Another is that common food allergens and addictive substances do something similar to the brain. In Chapter 3 we learned that many people with addictive tendencies have brain chemistry imbalances and crave substances that provide a brain chemical reward by stimulating dopamine, the feel-good brain chemical.

The two most common food allergens, wheat and milk, can be rapidly converted into feel-good substances in the brain.

> If you are suffering from a neurotransmitter imbalance with the symptoms of impulsivity, hyperactivity and lack of concentration, it may be that wheat and dairy, as well as alcohol, caffeine and other drugs, are your way of trying to feel better.

Depression, allergy and addiction

Depression is another commonly shared symptom of both addiction and allergy. Depression that is unresponsive to antidepressant prescription drugs is a common presenting symptom of hidden food allergy, especially in the gluten-sensitive. Some authorities claim that clinical depression is the most common presenting symptom in untreated coeliac disease, which is the most extreme form of allergy related to wheat, barley and rye.[73]

In general, low brain levels of serotonin and/or noradrenalin are the most commonly identified biochemical causes of depression. Low brain levels of these chemicals are found in food-allergic, depressed patients and in recovering alcoholics. For some, simply eliminating food allergens from the diet results in restoration of normal brain chemistry and may result in the relief of depression in chronically depressed recovering alcoholics.

Test for allergies if you are still suffering with symptoms

So many people who have given up their substance of abuse still feel lousy and often substitute other potentially addictive/allergic foods instead. If you have many symptoms on the Scale of Abstinence Symptoms Severity on page 26 our first recommendation would be to get yourself IgG-allergy tested. (See Resources for testing laboratories.)

One of the first nutrition-based recovery programmes in the US was that of Dr Joan Mathews Larson, author of best-selling book *Seven Weeks to Sobriety*. One of the key components of her revolutionary therapy was routine laboratory testing for IgG food allergies. Which are the most common food allergens showing up in recovering alcoholics? You guessed it: wheat and dairy.

What are the warning signs?

If you have a history of infantile colic, frequent ear infections, eczema, asthma, hayfever, seasonal allergies, digestive problems (especially bloating), frequent colds or daily mood swings, or if you function better when you don't eat certain foods, you may have an unidentified food allergy. If you suffer from depression, seizures or osteoporosis that doesn't respond well to therapy, or if you have insulin-dependent diabetes, thyroid disease, balance problems (ataxia), short stature, liver enzyme elevation or anaemia of an unknown cause, recurring canker sores or problem pregnancies, you may be suffering from gluten sensitivity and coeliac disease.

What is your next step?

If you suspect you might have an allergy there are two courses of action. One involves a pin-prick IgG ELISA blood test. This state-of-the-art method of measuring IgG sensitivity will tell you which foods you are currently eating that cause an IgG reaction, and how severe that reaction is. Ideally, it is best to also have an IgE ELISA test too. This information can help your health-care practitioner devise a diet for you that avoids these allergy-provoking foods and replaces them with suitable alternatives.

The other course of action is to strictly avoid the suspected substances for two weeks, then reintroduce them in a controlled way, recording your symptoms. This is best done under the guidance of a nutritional therapist (see Resources to find one near you), which is doubly important if you've ever had a severe reaction, such as asthma or seizures poorly controlled by medication. It is, however, rather hit-and-miss, and is only successful if you both guess correctly what you may be allergic to and are rigorous in your avoidance and reintroduction.

The top food allergies

Wheat Most food allergies develop in reaction to the proteins in food, and particularly foods we eat most frequently. Wheat tops the list, probably because it contains the protein gluten. Gluten sensitivity can produce or aggravate depression, anxiety and headaches, as well as digestive disorders.[74]

(Oats contain much less gluten than wheat, and it is a different kind. For this reason, some people who are wheat intolerant – including most coeliac patients – are not intolerant to oats.[75] However, one study showed that small numbers of people with coeliac disease react to a protein in oats called avenin.[76])

Dairy produce This includes cheese and yogurt. A few people can tolerate goat's or sheep's milk but not cow's milk. Many can't tolerate any of these. Mild allergy symptoms are varied but often include a blocked nose, frequent colds, post-nasal drip, bloating and indigestion, a 'thick' head, fatigue and headaches.

Other foods Oranges, egg white (the yolk rarely provokes an allergic response), other grains apart from wheat, yeast-containing foods, shellfish, nuts, soya and members of the nightshade family: tomatoes, peppers, potatoes and aubergine. Some people also develop allergies to tea, coffee, tobacco and marijuana, whereas alcohol, which irritates the gut wall and makes it more leaky, often increases allergic sensitivity to anything eaten.

What should you do if you are allergic?

The emerging view, shared by an increasing number of allergy specialists, is that food sensitivity is a complicated phenomenon possibly involving poor nutrition, pollution, digestive problems, heavy drinking and overexposure to certain foods. Removing the foods may help you recover, but other factors need to be dealt with in order to have a major impact on long-term food intolerance. Because of the complex factors involved in food allergies and intolerance, it is often best to see a nutritional therapist who can pinpoint the likely culprits from your symptoms and eating patterns, advise you on tests (should they prove necessary), and help you to correct digestive problems that increase your allergic potential.

Foods that evoke an immediate and pronounced IgE-type reaction may need to be avoided for life. The 'memory' of IgE antibodies is certainly long-term, if not for ever. In contrast, the cells that produce IgG antibodies (delayed reaction) have a half-life of six weeks. That means that there are half as many six weeks later. The 'memory' of these antibodies is short term and within three months there is unlikely to be any residual 'memory' of reaction to a food that's been avoided. The exception is coeliac disease, which is a genetic disease reversible only on a permanent wheat-, rye- and barley-free diet.

Foods such as wheat and milk, which are more likely to evoke an allergic response, are probably best avoided or at least minimised as much as possible for those who show allergic tendencies. This is especially true for wheat, since even IgG sensitivity to wheat appears to be a life-long condition, and is possibly genetically predetermined. One way to minimise the impact of a food is to 'rotate' it by eating it only every four or five days. However, if you are truly allergic the only solution is total avoidance.

Chapter 28 in our How to Quit Action Plan includes recipes for your recovery programme and we address the issue of allergies there. Many of the recipes in this book and the guidelines we give you are compatible with a wheat-free and dairy-free diet.

If you'd like to find out more about allergies, read *Hidden Food Allergies* (by Patrick Holford and Dr James Braly).

SUMMARY

▶ If you suspect you have a food allergy, get yourself tested (see page 227). A nutritional therapist can test what you are allergic to and devise a course of action to reduce your allergic potential.

▶ Avoid wheat and dairy products strictly for two weeks and see how you feel. In any case these food groups are best not eaten frequently.

▶ Improve your digestion by eating plenty of fresh fruit, vegetables, seeds and fish, which contain essential fats and zinc.

▶ Take a digestive enzyme supplement, with probiotics (friendly bacteria) for a month, to re-inoculate your digestive tract with good bacteria. Take glutamine daily to accelerate healing of the gut lining. Quercetin is a powerful anti-allergy bioflavonoid.

▶ Keep alcohol, painkillers and antibiotics to a minimum. These damage the digestive tract.

15.

REJUVENATE YOUR LIVER

Forget diamonds. Your liver is your best friend, and knowing how to look after your liver could literally mean the difference between life and death. If you've been drinking too much alcohol or caffeinated drinks, or taking too many drugs (including painkillers) for too long, your liver is likely to have suffered and, as a consequence, may have less ability to detoxify your brain and body from the harmful effects of these substances. At its worst you may increase your risk of liver disease and liver failure.

Liver failure is among the most common causes of premature death – along with cardiovascular disease, diabetes, cancer and prescription medication. It accounts for over 4,000 deaths a year in the UK – that's more than road-traffic accidents – and costs the National Health Service £1.7 billion a year. However, liver dysfunction plays a part in most of these other common diseases as well. In the US obesity has become the most preventable cause of premature death – and a major driver of what's called non-alcoholic fatty liver disease. The thing about the liver is that many people don't know anything is going wrong until it's too late, although now there's a simple liver test you can do which gives you a clear measure of your liver's state of health (more on this in a moment).

What your liver does

The liver is the greatest multi-tasking organ, and as a result its function – or dysfunction – has an incredibly important impact on your health and on the degree of your abstinence symptoms. The following are the liver's main functions:

Breaking down and eliminating toxins The liver is the major organ of detoxification. When it is not working properly, toxins from both inside and outside the body remain in the system and can even cause your immune system to treat some of them as if they were invading organisms. This can lead to many health problems including inflammation, increased likelihood of infections, and food allergies and sensitivities. The breakdown products of alcohol, caffeine, cigarettes and other drugs all tax the liver.

Breaking down and eliminating excess hormones When this function is not working optimally, all kinds of hormonal imbalances can occur.

Balancing blood sugar When our blood sugar levels are high, the hormone insulin triggers the liver to store the excess as glycogen. When blood sugar levels fall, the liver releases glycogen to be broken back down into glucose. If the liver fails in this task, the result is chronic fatigue, sugar cravings, weight gain and, ultimately, diabetes. Blood sugar imbalance leads to cravings for stimulants.

Producing bile This vital substance helps digestion by breaking down fat and removing excess cholesterol. Without it cholesterol levels rise and many digestive disorders can result, including bloating, irritable bowel syndrome (IBS), gall stones, nausea, food allergies and the malabsorption of nutrients, especially the fat-soluble vitamins A, D, E and K.

Storing nutrients The liver stores many essential vitamins and minerals, including iron, copper and vitamins A, B_{12}, D, E and K.

Creating albumin Albumin produced by the liver helps transport nutrients and other chemicals in the blood. For example, it helps carry tryptophan to the brain. When albumin is low – as it often is with liver disease and zinc deficiency – it is associated with an increased risk of premature death from all causes.

Do you need to detox your liver?

Improving your liver-detox potential helps you recover your health and energy quickly, with minimal withdrawal or abstinence symptoms. Complete the questionnaire below to discover whether you need to improve your liver detoxification potential.

QUESTIONNAIRE: check your liver-detox potential

Tick the boxes if your answer is yes to the following questions:

1. Do you often suffer from headaches or migraine? ☐

2. Do you sometimes have watery or itchy eyes, or swollen, red or sticky eyelids? ☐

3. Do you have dark circles under your eyes? ☐

4. Do you sometimes have itchy ears, earache, ear infections, drainage from the ears or ringing in the ears? ☐

5. Do you often suffer from excessive mucus, a stuffy nose or sinus problems? ☐

6. Do you suffer from acne, skin rashes or hives? ☐

7. Do you sweat a lot and have a strong body odour? ☐

8. Do you sometimes have joint or muscle aches or pains? ☐

9. Do you have a sluggish metabolism and find it hard to lose weight, or are you underweight and find it hard to gain weight? ☐

10. Do you often suffer from frequent or urgent urination? ☐

11. Do you suffer from nausea or vomiting? ☐

12. Do you often have a bitter taste in your mouth or a furry tongue? ☐

13. Do you have a strong reaction to alcohol? ☐

14. Do you suffer from bloating? ☐

15. Does coffee leave you feeling jittery or unwell? ☐

Total score: ☐

Score

7 or more
If you answer yes to seven or more questions you need to improve your liver-detox potential.

4–7
If you answer yes to between four and seven questions you are beginning to show signs of poor detoxification and need to improve your liver-detox potential.

Fewer than 4
If you answer yes to fewer than four questions, you are unlikely to have a problem with liver detoxification.

How your liver deteriorates

There are four stages to the decline and fall of your liver:

1. An overload of toxins and a lack of supporting protective nutrients cause certain liver enzyme pathways to become overloaded and consequently to underfunction.

2. Then you start to accumulate fat in the liver, officially called steatosis or fatty liver.

3. Enough of this and you start to get an inflamed liver, called hepatitis.

4. This inflammation damages liver tissue causing fibrosis and cirrhosis, in other words cell death. If you have liver cirrhosis, also read Appendix 3 (which is on our website www.how2quit.co.uk) for strategies on liver regeneration.

Since the liver is the central clearing house of your body (detoxifying toxins, making fat from sugar, sugar from fat, and breaking down proteins, plus thousands of other critical functions) this final stage has many repercussions. Your immune system starts to break down, you lose blood sugar control, excess fats accumulate elsewhere, leading to cardiovascular disease and other diseases.

Check your liver

The easiest way to know where you are in this chain of events is a simple pin-prick blood test, which tests two liver enzymes called AST and ALT. The higher these are, the further along this slippery path you are. Your doctor can run this test or, alternatively, you can do it yourself using a home test kit called Livercheck. The test gives you personalised advice on how to reverse the trend (see Resources for a home test kit). This is a major advance and a test well worth having, especially if you have been struggling with addiction for many years or are a 'vino' drinker – someone who knocks back half a bottle of wine most evenings – or if you have any of the other risk factors shown below. Dr Ravij Jalan from University College London, one of the UK's leading liver experts, says, 'There is no doubt in my mind that it has the potential to save lives. If someone knew they were going to get liver disease, they would do something about it. Checking the health of the liver could prevent them getting to the stage where they are doing themselves real harm.' He reckons that 80 per cent of the deaths caused by liver disease are entirely preventable simply by early screening for liver problems.

What causes liver problems?

Alcohol As you might have guessed, the number-one cause of liver problems is excess alcohol. Over 350,000 people in Britain are admitted to hospital for alcohol-related conditions each year, many of which relate to liver overload. That's a rise of 27 per cent in five years. According to Professor Mark Bellis, director of the Centre for Public Health at Liverpool John Moores University, which compiled the information on alcohol-related admissions from the NHS's Hospital Episodes Survey, 'A lot of attention is paid towards binge drinking in younger people. But large numbers of people of all ages are simply drinking too much.'

Diabesity Diabetes and obesity, which affects close to one in five people over 40, is a major cause of fatty liver. These promote, and are in part caused by insulin resistance, which means you cannot keep your blood sugar levels even. The excess sugar is converted to fat, mainly in the liver, and some of it stays there. There is also evidence that fruit drinks, including naturally sweetened drinks, are a frequent cause of a fatty liver.

Viral hepatitis This infection damages the liver directly. Worldwide, hepatitis and other infections, such as malaria, are a major cause of liver failure. In the Western world hepatitis C infection, mainly from heroin users sharing dirty needles, is a major contributor (see Appendix 3 – which is on our website www.how2quit.co.uk – for a nutritional strategy for hepatitis C).

Drugs As few as 12 paracetamols can kill you – and eight can harm you, especially if you've been drinking as well. A common cause of acute liver failure is paracetamol overdose. Four grams (8 × 500mg tablets) pushes up those liver enzymes AST and ALT.[77] Although paracetamol is the most common drug-induced cause of liver failure, many other drugs are liver-toxic. If you are taking medication, do check it for liver toxicity.

Coeliac disease High blood levels of ALT and AST of unknown origin may be caused by undiagnosed coeliac disease (see Chapter 14 on allergies).

Gut problems There's a direct link between gut health and liver health. When the gut wall becomes more permeable, more un-desirable material enters the blood, which the liver has to clean up. Alcohol, non-steroidal anti-inflammatory (NSAID) pain-killers such as aspirin and ibuprofen, antibiotics and food allergies can all irritate and damage the gut. Glutamine powder (see page 147) last thing at night can help heal the gut, but too much of any amino acid or dietary protein is bad news if you have a very damaged liver, because the liver has to process amino acids. Therefore, glutamine powder should not be taken if there is liver damage.

> The cause of a quarter of all cases of liver failure is unknown, so we have a lot to learn. If your liver is somewhat damaged, combinations of all the above may just tip you over the edge.

How to detoxify your liver and keep it healthy

The good news is that your liver is a highly regenerative organ; and if you can create the biochemical equivalent of a health farm, your liver can regain its ability to detoxify your brain and body in two to three months. Of course, the first step is to avoid the substances that give your liver a hard time. These include:

- **Caffeine and alcohol**

- **All addictive recreational and medicinal drugs** These place an enormous load on the liver, especially painkillers; the average person in the UK takes over 300 of them in a year!

- **High sugar and refined-carb diets** including fruit drinks, sweetened and unsweetened.

- **High-meat diets** Particularly burned meats and processed meats high in preservatives.

- **Deep-fried foods and damaged 'hydrogenated' or 'trans' fats** as found in most margarines, bought biscuits and cakes.

- **Salt**, which is a stomach irritant, linked to gastric cancer and high blood pressure.

- **Processed foods** high in chemical flavour enhancers, such as tartrazine and MSG, or preservatives such as benzoates.

- **Environmental pollutants**, which include cigarette smoke and exhaust fumes.

Combinations of all these are particularly dangerous. For example, drinking large amounts of caffeinated drinks in combination with the painkiller paracetamol triples the production of a potentially fatal toxic by-product called N-acetyl-p-benzoquinoneimine (NAPQI) that can be responsible for liver failure.[78] Combining these with alcohol can be a lethal combination.

The liver-friendly diet

In previous chapters we've suggested the best diet for reducing cravings, which is also the best diet for helping support your liver. This is explained in Chapter 28 and incorporates the following key principles:

- **Low-GL** A high intake of sugar and refined carbohydrates is a major contributor to fatty liver disease.[79] Eating a low–GL diet helps the liver recover.

- **High in antioxidants** All the antioxidant-rich foods in Chapter 12 – including fruits, vegetables, cruciferous vegetables, onions and garlic – help the liver to detoxify.

- **High in essential fats** You need essential fats, especially omega-3, which, together with vitamin E, help regenerate the liver.[80]

- **Low in allergens** Any food allergy taxes your immune system and your liver. If you are allergic to wheat or dairy products and have these foods on a daily basis your liver has to work harder. In Chapter 14 we explained how to identify, avoid and recover from food allergies.

- **High in nutrient-rich wholefoods** Your liver needs the many vitamins and minerals provided in wholefoods; so refined, processed, junk food is out if you want to support your liver.

- **Drink at least 1 litre (1¾ pints) of water every day** Drinking eight glasses of water is the simplest step you can take to help dilute toxins in the blood and support your liver and kidney function.

How your liver detoxifies

If eating the right food is one side of the coin, detoxification is the other. From a chemical perspective, much of what goes on in the body involves substances being broken down, built up and turned from one thing into another. A good 80 per cent of this work in the body involves detoxifying potentially harmful substances. Much of this work is done by the liver, which represents a clearing house able to recognise millions of potentially harmful chemicals and transform them into something harmless or prepare them for elimination. This often means turning a fat-based toxin into something water-soluble that can be eliminated in the urine. The liver is the chemical brain of the body: recycling, regenerating and detoxifying in order to maintain your health.

> The extent to which a substance is bad for you depends as much on your ability to detoxify it as on its inherent toxic properties.

The external toxins (exo-toxins), such as alcohol, caffeine and nicotine, represent just a small part of what the liver has to deal with; many toxins are made within the body from otherwise harmless molecules. Every breath and every action can generate toxins. So, too, can and do the bacteria and yeasts that live inside us. These internally created toxins (endo-toxins) have to be disarmed and eliminated in just the same way that exo-toxins do. If they are not eliminated, the body becomes irritated and inflamed. Antibodies formed to protect us against the harmful effect of these endo-toxins often trigger an autoimmune response, so our body actually starts fighting itself. If toxins can't be broken down, they are stored in the liver and in fat. If you don't burn sugar for energy, for example, the excess is stored as fat.

So, the extent to which a substance is bad for you depends as much on your ability to detoxify it as on its inherent toxic properties. If your ability to detoxify is overloaded, you may have more toxins in your system. And on top of that, other key functions in the liver may be impaired; for example, the liver's ability to activate vitamins and minerals, which it needs to process to become effective, or its ability to burn fat for energy. You may end up with a fatty liver as a result.

Liver detoxification is a two-step dance

The ability of the liver to detoxify has two distinct phases. You can think of Phase 1 as the preparation phase, where toxins are acted on by a series of enzymes (called P450). This phase converts toxins into a form that can be disarmed. Often, however, this process itself can produce unwanted by-products or 'reactive intermediates' such as free radicals that could actually produce even more toxins. To avoid this Phase-1 side effect there is a whole series of nutrients, particularly antioxidants, which you need to support your liver:

Detox nutrients: the Phase-1 heroes

The first phase of liver detoxification (the grey area above the line in the illustration on page 243), which involves the P450 family of enzymes, mainly depends on having a great supply of antioxidant nutrients. These include:

Glutathione and/or N-acetyl cysteine[81] – found in onions and garlic

Coenzyme Q_{10}[82] – found in oily fish, spinach, raw seeds and nuts

Vitamin C[83] – found in broccoli, peppers, citrus fruit and berries

Vitamin E[84] – found in raw seeds, nuts and fish

Selenium[85] – found in raw seeds, nuts and fish

Beta-carotene[86] – found in carrots, peaches, watermelon, sweet potato and butternut squash

Omega-3 fats – found in unfried, oily fish

These antioxidants are team players. You need all of them for your liver-detox potential to be optimum. (See Antioxidants Are

Team Players diagram on page 194, to see how antioxidants work together.) There are also various phytonutrients (substances from plants that have nutritional value) and herbs that can help. These include:

DIM (di-indolylmethane) A substance in cruciferous vegetables such as broccoli that helps detoxify excess oestrogens and hormone-disrupting chemicals such as PCBs and dioxins as well as some herbicides and pesticides.[87]

Bioflavonoids[88] These include **anthocyanidins** in blueberries,[89] **quercetin** in red onions,[90] **polyphenols** in green tea[91] and the standardised herb **milk thistle,** which contains a powerful detoxifying nutrient called **silymarin** that protects liver cells from all kinds of toxins.[92] **Turmeric**, the yellow curry spice, contains curcumins, which are potent antioxidants and increase production of glutathione. Both curcumins and glutathione protect against alcohol-induced oxidation.[93]

There are other herbs that help support liver function. One of the more researched herbal remedies is sho-saiko-to (SST), which is a combination of seven herbs including bupleurum. For more details see Appendix 3, which is on our website www.how2quit.co.uk.

During Phase 2 these reactive intermediates are rendered non-toxic. This happens by enzymes linking the toxin to another molecule that makes it more water-soluble and less toxic. This process is often called 'conjugation' where the toxin is 'married' to a key detoxifying nutrient. For example, the diagram opposite shows you how your body detoxifies paracetamol, aspirin and caffeine. (Nutritional therapists often use a simple urine test that involves you taking a measured amount of caffeine, paracetamol and aspirin, then collect a urine sample to determine how well each of these pathways are working and, consequently, which nutrients you are likely to benefit most from.)

The body processes toxins in the liver using different chemical pathways. The diagram opposite shows examples of what the

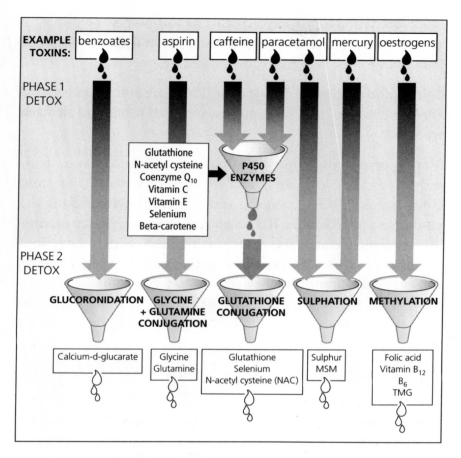

EXAMPLE TOXINS: benzoates | aspirin | caffeine | paracetamol | mercury | oestrogens

PHASE 1 DETOX

Glutathione
N-acetyl cysteine
Coenzyme Q_{10}
Vitamin C
Vitamin E
Selenium
Beta-carotene

P450 ENZYMES

PHASE 2 DETOX

GLUCORONIDATION **GLYCINE + GLUTAMINE CONJUGATION** **GLUTATHIONE CONJUGATION** **SULPHATION** **METHYLATION**

Calcium-d-glucarate | Glycine Glutamine | Glutathione Selenium N-acetyl cysteine (NAC) | Sulphur MSM | Folic acid Vitamin B_{12} B_6 TMG

The key detox nutrients your liver needs

liver does with caffeine, paracetamol (acetaminophen) or aspirin. These different pathways (for example, glutathione conjugation or sulphation), need different nutrients to work properly.

Detox nutrients: the Phase-2 heroes

In Phase 2 the liver detoxifies substances by attaching things on to them so that they are ready to be eliminated from the body in the process called conjugation described above. There are five main ways in which the liver detoxifies:

Glucoronidation is possibly the most important detox pathway of all, dependent on calcium-d-glucarate, which is found in apples, Brussels sprouts, broccoli, cabbage and beansprouts.

Glycine and glutamine conjugation These are amino acids found in root vegetables and beansprouts, sprouted beans and Brussels sprouts.

Glutathione conjugation This pathway depends on a good supply of glutathione, an amino acid complex made from three amino acids (glycine, cysteine and glutamic acid). Onions and garlic are a good source. Root vegetables are also rich in glycine. The mineral selenium also helps glutathione to work. Glutathione can be made in the body from N-acetyl cysteine (NAC); supplementing either improves the liver's capacity to detoxify. Interestingly NAC is given in cases of paracetamol overdose to trigger the liver into detoxifying.

Sulphation depends on the sulphur-containing amino acids, found in onions, garlic and eggs. There's a type of sulphur you can supplement, called MSM, that helps the body to detoxify.

Methylation This is a key detoxifying process described in Chapter 9 that depends on B vitamins, especially folic acid (in greens and beans), vitamins B_{12} (animal source only) and B_6, as well as SAM and TMG, found in root vegetables. Folic acid, SAM and, probably, TMG (by increasing SAM and glutathione levels) help the liver to recover.[94]

Eat your way to a healthy liver

You don't need to know the chemistry but you do need to know that each of these foods, rich in key detox nutrients, are included in our recipes and daily menus in our How to Quit Action Plan, Chapter 28. In addition, we also recommend taking specific detox nutrients to provide additional liver support (see page 394).

Heal your digestive tract – and take a load off your liver

Although your liver does most of the detoxing, effectively filtering and cleansing the blood of toxic material, your digestive tract is the gateway between the food you eat and your bloodstream. It is actually the first line of detoxification. Your digestive tract can be healthy or unhealthy. If it is unhealthy it will become more permeable, which means that larger food particles not on the 'guest list', so to speak, will get into the bloodstream. This is called leaky gut syndrome. Whole food proteins, rather than their constituent amino acids, will gatecrash into your bloodstream and your body's policemen – immune cells and antibodies – will attack, forming what is known as an 'immune complex'. This is then treated by the body as a toxin and forms the basis of most food allergies and sensitivities, which have a detrimental effect on our overall health. So, one immediate way to help detox your body and support your liver is to improve the integrity of your digestive tract.

The G factor: your gut's best friend

Although most of your body's organs are fuelled by glucose, your digestive tract is a different story. It's a vast and highly active interface between your body and the outside world, and it needs a lot of fuel to work properly day in and day out. It runs on an amino acid called glutamine – thus sparing the glucose from your food for your brain, heart and liver. Glutamine also helps you make the calming neurotransmitter GABA and the potent antioxidant glutathione.

Not only does glutamine power your gut, it heals it as well. As your 'inner skin', your gut takes lots of hits: alcohol, NSAID painkillers such as aspirin or ibuprofen, antibiotics, coffee and fried food are some common gastrointestinal irritants.

Many people who use or have quit using an addictive substance suffer from digestive problems and possibly food allergies.

Our top tip (besides avoiding allergenic foods) is to take glutamine every day during the first month of your How to Quit programme, together with digestive enzymes and a probiotic supplement (see Resources). We recommend one heaped teaspoon diluted in a glass of water at least twice daily (that's 8,000mg in total) of glutamine powder taken last thing at night, and again in the morning 30 minutes before breakfast. Under normal circumstances, most of the glutamine in your food gets used up as fuel for your gastro-intestinal tract. However, about 5 per cent of it is used to make glutathione, the liver's most powerful antioxidant. If, however, you have liver disease or poor kidney function, taking in a lot of glutamine is inadvisable – read Appendix 3 (which is on our website www.how2quit.co.uk) on how to regenerate your liver.

Eat to protect your liver

Glutathione boosts your liver and protects every single cell in your body from the dangerous oxidising chemicals: free radicals. As we saw earlier, glutathione is made from three amino acids: glycine, cysteine and glutamic acid or glutamine. Although glutamine is found in protein foods such as beans, fish, chicken and eggs, as well as in vegetables such as cabbage, spinach, beetroot and tomatoes, 95 per cent is destroyed by heating – a good argument for supplementation. Cysteine is a sulphur-containing amino acid found in onions, garlic and eggs. Glycine is found plentifully in root vegetables. By getting more of each of these amino acids, you are providing yourself with the building blocks for glutathione.

Liver detox supplements

You support your liver's ability to detoxify by supplementing the right combination of nutrients. Below, we recommend supplements for you to take only during your withdrawal phase. These are included in your How to Quit Action Plan in Part 4. You don't need to take these for more than 30 to 90 days, unless directed by your health-care practitioner. Once your abstinence symptoms go away and you start the 'maintenance' phase you no longer need these extract nutrients. If your liver function is OK (you've had it tested and there is no raised AST/ALT) but you have some of the symptoms listed on page 233, you could take these for nine days or as long as it takes for most of these symptoms to disappear. (See Part 4 for specific supplementation instructions.)

Our first recommendation is to supplement a combination of digestive enzymes, probiotics and glutamine. Digestive enzymes digest your food, minimising the chances of whole food proteins getting into the blood. Probiotics are essential beneficial bacteria, which also play a part in the digestive process. You need two strains: *Lactobacillus acidophilus* and *Bifidobacteria*. You don't need these every day of your life but a one-month course is a great way to repopulate your gut flora or 'inner garden'. Glutamine is direct fuel for the gut lining. A heaped teaspoon of glutamine powder last thing at night and again in the morning before breakfast will help maintain the integrity of the gut wall, your first line of defence from toxins (but remember that glutamine powder should not be taken if there is severe liver damage, i.e. liver failure and cirrhosis).

Our second recommendation is an all-round antioxidant or liver-support formula (see Resources). Pick a formula that has many of the key liver support nutrients shown in the following list. The ones in bold are the most important, and are needed in substantial quantities, so you may need to take these separately:

Vitamin C

Vitamin E

Coenzyme Q_{10}

Glutathione

N-acetyl cysteine (NAC), * 500mg twice a day

Glycine

Glutamine, ** 1–2 teaspoons (4–8 grams) a day, on an empty stomach

Calcium-D-glucarate

Milk thistle, standardised (silymarin); taking this with phosphatidyl choline helps its absorption by up to 800 per cent

DIM (broccoli extract)

MSM (a form of sulphur)

Trimethyl glycine (TMG), * 1g twice a day. (If you can get it, 400mg of SAM* twice a day is even better.)

Turmeric, high in curcumin, 500mg twice a day. This yellow spice is rarely found in combination formulas.

Bupleurum as found in sho-saiko-to herbal formula (for liver repair, see Appendix 3 on our website www.how2quit.co.uk)

*Although NAC, TMG and SAM may be extremely helpful, these are best given under medical supervision for those with liver damage (see Appendix 3 on the website www.how2quit. co.uk for more details on liver regeneration).

** Those with advanced liver cirrhosis or a history of a risk of liver failure must not take large amounts of glutamine, unless under the supervision of a medical practitioner. All amino acids contain nitrogen, which the liver has to process. In advanced liver damage this puts a strain on the liver.

In addition, you need extra B vitamins and vitamin C, which help methylation, but you'll find these, as well as basic levels of anti-oxidants plus minerals, in a high-potency multivitamin–mineral, recommended as part of the How to Quit supplement programme explained in Part 4, which puts all of these action points into a combined action plan for you to follow.

10 top tips to keep your liver healthy

1. Test your liver function, especially if you drink alcohol on a regular basis or have in the past.

2. Don't have more than one unit of alcohol a day if you're a woman (for example, a small glass of wine), and no more than two units (a large glass of wine) if you are a man; preferably have every third day without alcohol. Drink no alcohol if you have a drinking problem.

3. Drink plenty of water.

4. Eat lots of antioxidant rich fruits and vegetables (see Chapter 12).

5. Eat onions, garlic and eggs – high in sulphur, which is vital for liver function.

6. Eat a low-GL Mediterranean-style diet, limiting sugar and refined carbohydrates and rich in fish, fruits, vegetables, olive oil, whole-grain cereals, legumes, garlic, seeds and nuts (see Chapter 28).

7. Keep your homocysteine low (see page 151) and your SAM high. Methylation is what helps the liver function properly.

8. Keep your gut healthy. If you have digestive problems, explore food allergies (see Chapter 14) and also consider supplementing with glutamine, fish oil and probiotics.

9. Lose weight (if you are overweight) on a low-GL diet (see Chapter 11), plus take exercise.

10. Take supplements that support detoxification.

If you would like to find out more about liver detoxification read *The Holford 9-Day Liver Detox Diet* (by Patrick Holford and Fiona McDonald Joyce).

16.

FIND NEW PLEASURE IN LIFE
BY RAISING ENDORPHINS

When leaving behind the pleasure – perhaps intense pleasure – derived from the 'high' or euphoria of a mood-altering substance, you might feel that life is bland and boring. Whereas eating good-mood foods and taking good-mood supplements will certainly lift your spirit or calm you as need be, you may find yourself yearning for more pleasure and satisfaction in your life. After all, your drug has been a source of intense pleasure. Adjusting to the mundane may be one of the most difficult aspects of quitting.

In Chapter 2 we explained that the most important feel-good chemicals in your brain are endorphins, which promote a feeling of bliss and a sense of euphoria. They are also painkillers, relieving physical and emotional pain. When these are depleted, because of the chemical imbalance in our brain caused by addiction, we can become less able to feel pleasure. This chapter explains how we can raise our endorphins through activities that will bring brightness back into our life. We certainly don't want you to live in joylessness.

Pleasure is learned and, for many in the process of quitting addictive substances, it must be relearned. It is up to you to find what will give your life meaning and purpose: the sources of deep and ongoing joy. But we can suggest some activities that can raise those endorphins so that you can experience some immediate pleasure. This will help lift you out of boredom and provide feelings of satisfaction that may be lacking.

> **A**ctivities that raise your endorphin level are essential for contentment so there is no need to seek pleasure in ways that in the long run take joy from your life.

Exercise

Our number-one suggestion for raising endorphins is exercise. We are not going to discuss the many physical benefits of exercise: weight control, conditioning of heart and lungs, flexibility or building bones and muscles. What we want you to know at this point is that exercise (even moderate walking) produces positive changes in brain chemistry and improves your mood, thereby reducing cravings for *something more* to fill the empty space left when you no longer fill it with an addictive substance. Exercise not only reduces the release of adrenal stress hormones but it also releases growth hormones, increases the supply of blood and oxygen to the brain, and stimulates the release of powerful, mood-elevating endorphins. These chemical messengers create euphoria and pain relief, much stronger than that produced by morphine. These opioids produce the sensation known as 'runner's high'.

Case study OLIVER

'I used to be into all kinds of stimulants, including cocaine. Now I have discovered running, and I have a clear and consistent high. I feel terrific most of the time, without the lows I used to have after coke. I would not trade this feeling for anything.'

Use exercise to beat depression

Oliver is not alone. There have been over a hundred clinical studies examining the link between endorphins and exercise. One of the most interesting compared ten sedentary men with ten men of a similar age who jogged. The sedentary men turned out to be more depressed and had lower levels of endorphins. They also had higher levels of both the stress hormones and the perceived levels of stress in their lives.[95] Other studies have since established that exercise can be as effective as an antidepressant or traditional psychotherapy in treating low moods. Another study found that depressed adults did as well with group-based exercise as those treated with the SSRI antidepressant drug.[96] A third group that performed home-based exercise also improved, though to a slightly lesser degree.

Exercise can help you give up smoking

Taking exercise may also help you give up smoking, at least in the short term. There have been a number of trials which show much better success rates at the end of three months in those who also exercised. (But only one trial showed a significant effect after 12 months.[97] So, while exercise may take the edge off giving up smoking, it alone is not enough. See Chapter 21 for effective methods to stop smoking.)

Exercise will give you a positive mood

According to the US National Center for Health Statistics, frequent exercisers have higher levels of endorphins and demonstrate more positive moods and less anxiety than those who exercise too little or not at all.

> **E**xercise will boost your noradrenalin and serotonin, your feelings of self-confidence and positive thoughts.

What's more, if you exercise in a group this may have added benefits. So there are plenty of good reasons to exercise just to feel good.

We want to encourage you to establish a regular exercise routine, not only so that you will feel good but also to relieve the pain, tiredness, stress, anxiety and other abstinence symptoms you may already be experiencing due to your addictions. The whole purpose of this book is to provide options for increasing pleasure without the need for addictive substances.

The truth is that physical activity can be fun, stimulating and relaxing. A good exercise plan can add pleasure instead of pain to life. The trick is finding a physical activity that is right for you, something you enjoy doing. No one sticks to an exercise programme that is not enjoyable.

Ease your abstinence symptoms through exercise

Many recovering people have found exercise to be extremely helpful in freeing them from the limitations of their abstinence symptoms. We know many recovering addicts who stop in the middle of their day's activities to exercise when they are feeling anxious or when they have difficulty concentrating or remembering. After exercising they feel much better and are more productive (as well as becoming easier to get along with).

The more you move, the better you feel, the more motivated you are to exercise, and the more energy you have.

Case study **DAVID**

'Different forms of exercise have different payoffs for me. I have chosen these forms of exercise to strengthen me since I gave up drugs. Hiking or taking a long vigorous walk gives me time to be completely alone with myself, to meditate, to think more clearly, often working through issues or making short-range plans. I find that a walk enables me to break out of the dull stupor that daily routine can bring.

'Because I automatically feel good while walking, my aware-ness of my surroundings is also sharpened. I then begin to think in a more positive way about myself and my life. I feel more in control of my life. By the end of the walk I am ready to meet new challenges with a new sense of inner strength.

'Tennis relaxes me in another way. It provides strenuous exercise with almost every muscle being used with complete awareness of my physical self. It feels good to reach out and slam the ball, providing a surge of power and energy and anger release. Playing tennis with my partner is also healthy and relax-ing for me. Even though we are competing, it is all in fun. There is laughing, yelling, and just plain "letting go".

'Swimming is my "special" activity. I know of no other recreation that allows me more feelings of surrender. When I let go and be-come part of the water, I seem to flow through it with my worries and tension dissolving. Exercise is a vital part of my programme since giving up drugs and it improves the quality of my life.'

Aerobic exercise

Regular exercise where you use the whole body and keep moving at a steady pace – dancing, jogging, walking, swimming or cycling – is aerobic; it relieves stress and gives you a mood boost. Aerobic exercise increases oxygen intake, and that increases endorphins. Although we do not recommend that you limit yourself to aerobic exercise, we strongly recommend that you do some aerobic activ-ity every day. It is a good idea to have a variety of activities to choose from so that an exercise plan is not dependent on having a partner or the weather.

An excellent form of aerobic exercise is brisk walking, and it is available to almost anybody. It can reduce tension and anxiety immediately. One of the most efficient forms of exercise, it can be done safely throughout your life. Walking is also inexpensive and does not require special equipment, other than good shoes. It offers the extra benefit of giving you time to think and organise your thoughts.

Walking can easily be incorporated into your day. Perhaps you can walk to work or to the bank, post office or to visit a friend. Try taking the stairs instead of the lift. Walk around the station while waiting for your train.

Stretching

Use stretching exercises for warming up and cooling down to make your body more flexible. We recommend that you use them throughout your day to relax your muscles, reduce stiffness and ease any tension. In the next chapter we'll introduce you to some exercises such as yoga and Psychocalisthenics, which incorporate stretching exercises.

Get the most out of exercising

- Whatever form of exercise you choose, going solo is fine and may offer special time alone, but you may also find it's fun if you do some exercises with a friend. Besides the company it provides, having an exercise partner keeps you committed.

- Start your exercise programme gradually, such as with a walk around the block.

- Build up over time to a slow jog, first around the block, or a track, slowly increasing the distance and speed.

- For maximum benefit, build up to a full jog that lasts between 20 and 30 minutes, four to six days a week.

- Jogging, cycling, swimming and calisthenics are all forms of aerobic exercise, which conditions the heart and lungs, and boosts endorphins. Any form of dance is also excellent.

continues ▶

- All exercise takes your mind off your worries: think of the times when you played tag, football, netball or rounders with your friends. Be a kid again!

- Ride your bike or use an exercise bike while watching a DVD, listening to music or reading a book.

- If you do this five days a week, you will feel fabulous, and look good, too.

- Whichever activities you choose, remember the following tips:
  - Wear loose, comfortable clothing and well-fitting running shoes.
  - Warm up before exercise, use a lot of stretches, and cool down afterwards.
  - Do not fall into the 'pain is good' trap. Some muscular soreness or tightness is normal, but pain is a sign that something's wrong. If the pain persists, stop exercising and see your health practitioner.
  - Don't overdo it, especially at the beginning. Rest between exercise sessions. Excessive exercise actually evokes the stress response.
  - Do something you enjoy. The more you enjoy an exercise, the more likely you are to stick with it.

Fun, play and laughter

Having fun is a necessary part of life, but it is often neglected. It is not only a vital part of recovery from any addiction but it is also an essential ingredient of life. Learning to enjoy life naturally may take time and practice if, in the past, fun has occurred unnaturally through mind-altering chemicals. So it will take some time to convince yourself that you do have the ability to have fun and to enjoy and celebrate without altering your mood artificially. Fun and laughter relate directly to the production of endorphins. When you're having fun, your endorphins are raised within minutes and the positive effect can last for hours. First and foremost, fun brings a change of attitude, reaction and perception about yourself, as you slow down and experience your life in the present.

Make play a regular part of your life

We usually think of play as something separate and apart from everyday life; it is the icing on life: as long as we get our work done we can then, and only then, have fun. But life *should* be fun, and fun should be a priority, not something we do when and if we have time. While we are following our recovery plan we can become so serious that we never allow ourselves to lighten up and laugh, but life without fun is like a long dental appointment.

From time to time take breaks that add colour, spontaneity and perhaps some adventure to your life. It could be as adventurous as going on a safari or climbing a mountain, or it might be as simple as spending a day with a child. For others it might be going to an art gallery or the opera.

> The important thing is to do whatever puts excitement and joy back into *your* life.

Learn from children

Do you ever watch children having fun? To them, work and play are the same. Play is their work: they play when they walk or talk, or when they are putting together puzzles. They are constantly using their developing senses to explore this new world and, for the most part, are happy. Don't let society's messages to 'act your age' or 'grow up' or 'stop being foolish' deprive you of the richness of life that play offers.

Play for your health

You may be so programmed to believe that playing is wasting time that you need permission to play. Well, we give you permission. You *must* play for your health, your well-being and freedom from addiction. You will find that you are able to accomplish more if you take time for play than if you neglect it. At work, allow yourself to have outrageous ideas – some of the best innovations start that way.

When you are having fun you will also feel good about yourself. And when you are truly enjoying yourself you will laugh – and that releases endorphins and lightens your heart. After you laugh you will feel better, think better and function better. Humour helps us adapt to change, and giving up an addictive substance requires a lot of change. Why not make it easier on yourself by seeing the humour and learning to laugh at yourself? You then give yourself permission to be imperfect, and when you can find humour in your own imperfections, it is easier to accept imperfections in others.

Research shows that laughter increases creativity and the ability to organise information mentally. Studies also show that humour, laughter or mild elation enables people to remember, make decisions, and work things out better. It seems this feel-good stuff is just what a person with abstinence symptoms needs. Lighten up. Laugh a lot. It can only do you good.

Touching

Touching is pleasurable and so raises endorphins, but it is also a human need. We have tended to become isolated as a society – distanced as families and neighbours, whether because of the increased use of technology, the impersonal workplace or our fear of crime and abuse. Physical contact has suffered as a result. But the skin needs nurturing.

Touching is a great source of pleasure. Even petting animals significantly raises serotonin levels and can help fight depression, as is being shown in an ongoing study in the US.[98]

Many massage and touch therapies are becoming increasingly popular as their benefits become better known. Try Swedish massage, reiki, therapeutic touch, reflexology, rolfing, myofascial release, Rosen therapy or shiatsu.

Enjoying water

There is a natural healing power to water. We use it to hydrate our bodies as well as for cleansing, nutrition, relaxation and recreation. It stimulates, warms, cools, soothes and also fulfils the need for touch.

Showering does more than cleanse, however, it also raises endorphins. Use it to experience the healing power of water. Try standing under a shower and enjoying the feel of the water on your skin. To awaken your senses and increase circulation, alternate hot and cold water or try a shower massager.

Like a shower, a bath can also be used for more than cleansing, as the water can touch you all over. A bath or hot tub can soothe and relax you through its buoyancy, warmth and gentleness. The whirlpool jets in a hot tub can relieve an aching, sore body as well as soothing and relaxing your muscles.

If you swim, you will have complete exercise as well as a sensuous experience – and you can meditate at the same time. If you wear goggles and earplugs, the sound of water gurgling as you swim will help you to relax. Because the water supports every part of your body, this form of exercise can seem effortless – the water supports as it caresses.

Whether you're a swimmer or a fairly brave non-swimmer,

enjoy the buoyancy of the water by submerging yourself and floating to the top. There is nothing quite as luxurious as surrendering to the water by floating on your back, arms to your sides, eyes closed, and the water supporting you. Relax and feel the water surround you.

Music

Some sounds soothe and some invigorate. The sounds of music, waterfalls, rustling leaves, ocean waves or birds singing are usually pleasing and enjoyable. Other sounds are pleasing to some people but not to others, so be selective and choose those sounds that help you to feel more comfortable. These raise your endorphins and can brighten your spirits or calm them down depending on the type of sounds or music you play.

The activities we have discussed in this chapter are a vital part of your How to Quit programme – they will bring you happiness and contentment as you learn to live without your addiction.

SUMMARY

▶ Addiction recovery is more than abstinence, eating correctly and taking supplements; enjoying life is an essential part of giving up and staying clean.

▶ Activities that raise endorphin levels provide enjoyment so that there is less need to seek pleasure in ways that eventually rob you of joy.

▶ Endorphin-raising activities include physical exercise, laughing and having fun, touching and listening to or playing music.

17.

GENERATE VITAL ENERGY: THE CHI FACTOR

For thousands of years oriental traditions and those of India have based medical practices on the importance of vital energy and how it flows through our being. In Chapter 4 we explained how we sometimes use drugs to block out our emotional pain, but in doing so we deplete our vital energy – the 'down' we feel afterwards. To be well again we need to replenish our vital energy, so that we will feel re-energised in mind and body. In this chapter we explain how we can restore our vital energy through the use of exercises such as yoga, t'ai chi, qigong and meditation, as well as the use of complementary therapies such as acupuncture. Acu-detox (ear acupuncture) is also highly effective at reducing withdrawal symptoms.

In China vital energy is called *chi*, in Japan it is called *ki* and Indian traditions refer to the flow of *prana*. The whole basis of hatha yoga is a series of movements and stretches that are designed to generate this vital energy. Meditation techniques also aim to generate an increase in vital energy and a state of mindful awareness, and martial arts, such as t'ai chi and qiqong (pronounced 'chi gung'), focus on generating chi through awareness of your body, breath and movement. The whole basis of the healing treatment, acupuncture, is to create the correct flow and balance of chi. Although no one claims to know exactly how it might work, acupuncture itself – and a form of needleless acupuncture, called auricular therapy – has an excellent anecdotal track record of helping people end their addiction.

> **E**xcess use of addictive substances leads to the loss of vital energy and a greater tendency to get stuck in negative thought and behaviour patterns. By practising meditation, yoga, t'ai chi or other chi-generating exercises, many people find that their desire for addictive substances becomes less.

Even though this chi or vital energy has so far eluded objective scientific measurement, more and more studies are confirming the positive consequences of yoga, meditation, acupuncture and chi-generating exercises.

Psychocalisthenics

One of our favourite exercises, and best ways of generating vital energy, is called Psychocalisthenics® – a precise sequence of 23 exercises that leave you feeling fantastic. Patrick has been using it for 20 years and has found nothing better to keep him trim and feeling great, which is not bad for just 15 minutes a day! Each exercise is driven by the breath and, afterwards, your body feels lighter, freer and thoroughly oxygenated. It's a simple routine, which anyone can do.

Psychocalisthenics is the brainchild of Oscar Ichazo. An expert in martial arts and yoga since 1939, Ichazo developed Psychocalisthenics to be a daily routine that could be done in less than 20 minutes. 'In the same way that we have an everyday need for food and nourishment, we have to promote the circulation of our vital energy as an everyday business,' says Ichazo. At first glance it looks like a powerful kind of aerobic yoga.

Whereas most exercise routines simply treat the body as a physical machine that needs to be worked to stay fit, Psychocalisthenics is designed to generate both physical fitness and vital energy by bringing mind and body into balance. The key lies in the precise breathing pattern that accompanies each physical exercise. According to Jane Alexander of the *Daily Mail*, 'Psychocalisthenics is exercise, pared to perfection. I wasn't sweating buckets as I would after an aerobics class. But I had exercised far more muscles. I was clear-headed and bright rather than wiped out.'

The best way to learn Psychocalisthenics is to do a short course. You can also teach yourself from a book and CD, but it is best to learn it 'live' (see www.patrickholford.com/psychocalisthenics for trainings). One of the things we like most about Psychocalisthenics is that you don't have to go anywhere, wear special clothes or buy any equipment. Once you've learned the routine you can do it in under 20 minutes in your own home, accompanied by the CD with its 'talk through' music track. It takes half a day to learn and will leave you feeling blissful and energised.

The science of yoga

One consistent finding in studies on yoga is that it lowers levels of the hormone cortisol, which is associated with stress and anxiety, and it raises levels of GABA, the relaxing neurotransmitter, helping to induce a natural state of relaxed alertness.

One such study, at Boston University, measured GABA activity in the brain using an advanced magnetic resonance technique developed at Harvard Medical School. They compared eight people before, during and after an hour of yoga, versus 11 people who read a book instead. The yoga practitioners had a 27 per cent increase in GABA levels,[99] associated with inducing a deep state of relaxation.

Other studies have measured numerous health benefits, including lowered cortisol levels, in controlled trials on yoga, meditation and yogic-breathing techniques, with participants reporting reduced anxiety, stress and depression compared with those in the control groups.[100]

> **A**lthough there are few trials directly on the benefits of yoga in relation to abstinence, it has certainly been our experience that people who take up a regular practice in one of these energy-generating exercises are less likely to relapse.

Meditation

There have been a number of studies looking at the effects of meditation, including a meta-analysis of 19 studies (with 4,524 participants) on the effects of Transcendental Meditation (TM) on the use of alcohol, cigarettes and illicit drugs.[101] It showed that the effect from the TM technique was substantially greater than from relaxation programmes or preventive education programmes. A number of studies have reported finding a positive correlation between TM technique and various health benefits, including reduction of insomnia,[102] decreased cigarette smoking,[103] decreased alcohol use[104] and decreased anxiety.[105]

The technique comprises 'mindfulness' which, through meditation, develops an awareness of emotions and physical feelings and then guides people to make creative choices about how to respond to them. Other meditation techniques based on developing mindfulness have also been shown to help. Dr Paramabandhu Groves, a consultant psychiatrist at the Alcohol

Advisory Service in London, has successfully run workshops with people with addictions using a combination of a Buddhist-style mindfulness meditation together with cognitive behavioural therapy (CBT). He ran a pilot study in which 15 people with alcohol problems undertook mindfulness-based cognitive therapy (MBCT). Each member was given a CD and asked to practise at home. One reported that it gave him a spiritual practice he found lacking in other recovery methods; others said it had given them a more immediate and conscious awareness of how they felt at a given moment. Most said they found it helped them in their battle against alcohol and reported that it gave them the tools to challenge the negative thoughts that drove them to drink. 'It emphasizes critical awareness, rather than concentration,' said Dr Groves, who went on to say:

> In meditation the mind keeps wandering off, so you note where the mind has gone and then you come back to the body sensation. When you do this, you begin to notice where the habitual patterns are, and this gives you the ability to stay with negative thoughts. Once you stay with these negative thoughts, you can diffuse them and take the power out of them.

By doing this, said Dr Groves, the vicious cycle of addiction can be broken. Negative thoughts, particularly linked to an external trigger, such as a row with a partner, can trigger a relapse and lead to substance use. 'Mindfulness can break this link,' says Dr Groves. His clients are taught how to recognise and resist negative thoughts by observing themselves non-judgementally and learning to accept their emotions.

T'ai chi – movement in meditation – and qigong

The martial art t'ai chi chuan is another vitality-generating physical exercise. Originating in China, its aim is to allow the chi, or vital energy, to flow unhindered through the body. T'ai chi involves learning a series of precise movements that flow into each other, and through them you learn how to relax certain muscles rather than tensing them, which helps to reduce the background tension we all hold within our bodies. The movements also help to open up the joints, allowing the chi to flow unhindered. T'ai chi is therefore about developing a harmony with the self through posture and a strength through yielding. Once the sequence is learned by attending classes with a qualified teacher, t'ai chi can be practised at home.

Another chi-generating set of exercises from China is qigong. This comprises a series of positions practised in a similar way to meditation, with a specific pattern of breathing (see Diakath breathing below).

Finding peace through deep relaxation

Although there is much we don't know about how yoga, meditation and chi-generating exercises work, it is clear that they help many people access a state of deep relaxation, leading to a more mindful state of awareness that allows for the opportunity to examine one's thoughts and feelings, rather than being a slave to negative patterns that lead to addictive behaviours.

For this reason we recommend establishing a regular practice of yoga, t'ai chi, qigong, Psychocalisthenics and/or meditation as a key to successful recovery from addiction. (Details on organisations offering trainings and classes in these practices are given in the Resources section.)

Using Diakath breathing

An example of the kind of mindful breathing exercises that accompany yoga, t'ai chi and qigong is Diakath breathing, which is an essential part of Psychocalisthenics, the exercise system designed to generate vital energy. It's also excellent if you are experiencing abstinence symptoms, as it helps to balance both your mind and body.

This breathing exercise (reproduced with the kind permission of the Arica Institute, a school for self-knowledge) connects the *kath* point – the body's centre of equilibrium – with the diaphragm muscle, so that deep breathing becomes natural and effortless. You can practise this exercise at any time, while sitting, standing or lying down, and for as long as you like. You can also do it unobtrusively during moments of stress. It is an excellent natural relaxant and energy booster, helping you to feel more connected and in tune.

The diaphragm is a dome-shaped muscle attached to the bottom of the rib cage. The *kath* is not an anatomical point like the navel, but is an energy point located in the lower belly, about three finger-widths below the navel (see diagram on page 268). When you remember this point, you become aware of your entire body.

You can do this anywhere, standing or sitting, but ideally find somewhere quiet first thing in the morning and practise before breakfast for a few minutes.

EXERCISE: Diakath breathing

1. Sit comfortably, in a quiet place with your spine straight.

2. Focus your attention in your *kath* point.

3. Let your belly expand from the *kath* point as you inhale slowly, deeply and effortlessly. Feel your diaphragm being pulled down towards the *kath* point as your lungs fill with air from the bottom to the top. On the exhale, relax both your belly and your diaphragm, emptying your lungs from top to bottom.

4. Repeat at your own pace.

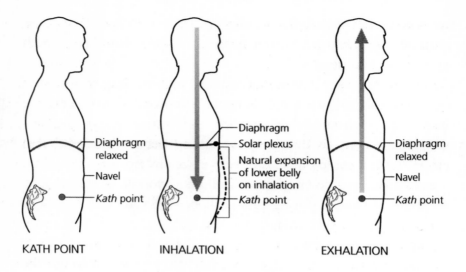

KATH POINT Diaphragm relaxed — Navel — *Kath* point

INHALATION Diaphragm — Solar plexus — Natural expansion of lower belly on inhalation — *Kath* point

EXHALATION Diaphragm relaxed — Navel — *Kath* point

Diakath breathing

Whenever you are stressed throughout the day, check your breathing. Practise Diakath breathing for nine breaths. This is great to use before an important meeting, or when something has upset you.

(© 2002 Oscar Ichazo. Diakath breathing is the service mark and Kath the trademark of Oscar Ichazo. Used by permission.)

Acupuncture

The system of complementary medicine known as acupuncture dates back thousands of years – many experts estimate at least five thousand years. Yet, in the Western world, it has only recently begun to be recognised as a valid form of treatment for a variety of health conditions. Although there is still scepticism among medical practitioners, there is strong evidence that it works, especially in the alleviation of pain: it has been used successfully as anaesthesia for animals – and placebos don't work with animals.

Traditionally, acupuncture healers seek to restore the balance of two complementary energy forces (yin and yang) that travel through the body by way of channels called meridians. These energy forces must be in balance for our vital life functions – including physical, emotional, mental and spiritual states – to operate correctly. The meridians surface at various locations – called acupuncture points – on the body. Acupuncture involves stimulation of these points on the skin with ultra-fine needles that are manipulated manually, and sometimes electrically.

Balance and the relief of pain

The ancient explanation for the effectiveness of acupuncture is that when conditions interfere with the energy flow through the meridians, toxins build up in the body and block body systems from functioning optimally. Stimulating the acupuncture points releases the flow, and balance is restored. Western scientists suggest a different or an additional explanation for the effectiveness of this ancient procedure: it mobilises endorphins in the reward system of the brain. As we have stated previously, the endorphins reduce pain even more effectively than drugs and without the side effects.

Specialists in pain management often use acupuncture. If you are recovering and abstaining from mood-altering substances, such as painkillers, acupuncture may be a good alternative for pain relief. People who suffer from back pain, bursitis, osteo-arthritis and headaches can benefit from using acupuncture.

Acu-detox (ear acupuncture)

About 2,500 years ago it was discovered that there were points in the ear that, when manipulated with needles, could relieve the discomfort of withdrawal from opium. In more recent times Dr H.L. Wen successfully applied electrical stimulation to needles inserted in the ear to relieve opiate withdrawal symptoms. Over several years Michael Smith, a physician at Lincoln Hospital in Bronx, New York, and his associates, refined the system to use just five ear points that are manipulated with needles. Currently this procedure has been used in the United States in numerous settings including drug treatment programmes, jails and prisons.[106]

When acu-detox is used with inpatients, the severity of their withdrawal symptoms has been reduced and seizures have been controlled. It is, however, limited to detox from opiate-type drugs such as heroin, methadone and barbiturates as well as alcohol, but has not been found to be helpful in detox from stimulant drugs such as cocaine. Also, it is a detox tool – therefore used for a brief period of time – not a tool for ongoing recovery.

Needle-less auricular therapy (auriculotherapy)

Although the term auriculotherapy is sometimes used to refer to any type of ear therapy, including ear acupuncture, we use it here to describe a needle-less procedure that utilises four cranial nerves and three cervical ganglia within the ear, not acupuncture points. It uses a microcurrent device to diagnose and treat these nerves, which are a direct port of entry to the brain and spinal cord.

Auriculotherapy is used to identify the location and measurement of an abnormal nerve point and then to treat that point with a micro-amp current at a specific frequency depending on where the point is located. The practitioner uses a hand-held device to locate abnormal points of increased skin conductivity on the ear and then to treat those identified points. Once the points have been located, the microcurrent device is used to stimulate the nerve to decrease skin conductivity at that location. The less conductive the skin, the healthier it is.

An advantage of auriculotherapy over some therapies for addiction is that it enables the release of the *specific* neurotransmitters that may be in short supply in the individual receiving it.

Auriculotherapy has been found to be safe and effective. There are hundreds of conditions that can be treated, but there are two for which it is most successful: pain management and addictive disorders. Its effects for pain management are almost instantaneous; however, the benefits for addiction take longer: about ten treatments of 15 minutes each. (For addiction recovery there is no quick fix.)[107]

Cranial electrical stimulation

As we have pointed out, research has demonstrated that the brain makes use of electrical activity; therefore, we can affect mental functions by affecting the brain's electrical activity. Cranial electrical stimulation (CES) provides a gentle electrical current that stimulates the production of brain chemicals, which then increase a feeling of well-being. The electrical stimulation is passed through two electrodes usually positioned behind the ear, or clipped to the upper portion of the ear lobe (although some clinicians apply the electrodes to the head and the wrist). Normally, CES is used once or twice daily for 30 minutes per session. Improvement is achieved over a period of two to three weeks. It might then be used occasionally as needed to maintain the achieved level of improvements. The CES unit is pocket-sized so that it can easily be carried from place to place.

During CES, an electric current promotes an increase in endorphins, serotonin and dopamine, and a decrease in the level of cortisol, the stress hormone. While using CES and for some time after, users are usually in an alert, yet relaxed state. And the improved brain chemical levels and the decreased stress hormone can have long-lasting effects.

Studies have shown that such low-voltage electrical stimulation of the brain is therapeutically beneficial in the treatment of such conditions as depression, substance-use disorder, withdrawal symptoms and insomnia.[108] There have been no major complications or negative effects associated with CES. A few users feel mild discomfort while using CES but suffer no long-term difficulties.[109]

Although the exercises and therapies we have mentioned above may seem unusual to you, many people have benefited hugely from them. We wholeheartedly recommend you try perhaps just one. We feel sure you will be pleasantly surprised at the peace of mind and body they can bring, and it will help you on your road to recovery using our How to Quit programme.

SUMMARY

▶ Take up yoga, Psychocalisthenics, t'ai chi, qigong or some form of mindful meditation, both to help generate a state of relaxed alertness, and also to give you the ability to observe your thoughts and feelings and become more able to turn away from negative patterns of addictive behaviour.

▶ Consider acupuncture, acu-detox, auricular therapy or cranial electrical stimulation (CES) to help you detox and to reduce abstinence symptoms.

18.

GET THE PAST OUT OF
YOUR FUTURE

As we have seen, quitting your addictive substance is not only a matter of what you eat and what supplements you take, it is also about what you do for your emotional, social and spiritual well-being. But – you might be thinking – haven't we been telling you that addiction is a physical condition? Yes, we have. And yes it is. Addiction itself is what happens in your *body* as a result of your use of a mood-altering substance.

But *recovering* from addiction requires emotional, social and spiritual healing as well as physical healing. It is more than changing what you do or don't put into your body. It's about changing how you think and feel, changing how you view yourself and relate to others, and changing what you value.

> In order to get the past out of your future, you have to change how you respond in the present.

Healing emotional pain is as important to your ability to maintain your commitment to be free of addiction as healing your body. You may have begun using a substance in the first place to relieve emotional pain, as we explained in Chapter 4. Or you may be experiencing emotional pain that has developed as a result of your addiction. Or your emotional pain may be due to the loss of giving up what you have used for so long to feel good.

Self-medicating to relieve your pain

Life can be emotionally painful for someone at risk of becoming addicted, regardless of whether that pain is caused by genetic reward deficiency or just the circumstances of living. As we pointed out in Chapter 3, there is pain associated with reward deficiency long before a person finds a substance that works to relieve it.

Children with genetic reward deficiency often have problems in childhood. They may have ADHD or at least some of the same symptoms: inability to concentrate, impulsivity, hyperactivity, difficulty organising and prioritising, difficulty staying on task, difficulty remembering or an inability to wait. As a result of these symptoms they may become underachievers, develop social problems and have low self-esteem. Painful school experiences and social interactions, feeling the disappointment of parents and teachers, never knowing quite what is expected of them – all contribute to a sense of self as being defective. This forms an underlying core of emotional pain that grows more intense over time.

If this has happened to you, you have probably internalised the messages you perceive coming from your world as: (1) not being good enough; (2) not being smart enough; or (3) not being loveable enough. And you have built a sense of self as being bad, incompetent or unlovable. We call these your shameful self-perceptions.

Perhaps it was not your reward deficiency that became the source of unresolved pain for you, but someone else's. Many people who are addicted grew up in families where there was addiction. Was one of your parents an alcoholic? Or perhaps it was not a substance that created a problem but a behaviour like gambling, overworking or risk taking. Children who grow up in a family where there is addiction or compulsive behaviour of any kind don't develop a sense of what is 'normal'. So when they are unable to adjust to the inconsistencies and unpredictability of their lives, they come to believe that there is something wrong with them.

And again, this results in a mistaken sense of self as being defective with the shameful self-perception of being not smart enough, not good enough, not loveable enough.

Of course, there are many other circumstances that become a source of pain that can lead you to use a mood-altering substance for relief and eventually addiction. Maybe you have experienced some stressful situation or trauma that was so painful that you welcome whatever would blot out that trauma. In any case, use of a mood-altering substance becomes a form of self-medication. It *works*. And it becomes a welcome friend. Whatever the circumstance that led to addiction, the pain of it will still be there when a person stops using the pain-relieving substance. So, in addition to the physical discomfort of withdrawal, there is the emotional discomfort that has been covered up for years by addiction.

Getting long-term pain out of your future

An important part of healing from a painful childhood is changing your 'shameful' perception of yourself. By changing the internal messages you give yourself on a daily basis you can transform the way you see yourself. You can interrupt the 'shame' messages you give yourself and replace them with more accurate messages that say, 'I am a good, competent, loveable person.' When you hear yourself say to yourself, 'I am never good enough,' stop and give yourself credit for the good things you do and the good person you are. When you hear yourself saying, 'I am so stupid; I never do anything right,' remind yourself of what an accomplishment it is that you are doing what it takes to stop your addiction.

Take it one step at a time

Painful memories that were avoided by addiction and carried into recovery won't go away just because you take amino acid supplements and eat oily fish to heal your brain, or eat fruit and vegetable to support your liver. But having a healthy body and brain will make it easier for you to confront the pain of the past. So we recommend that you give yourself time to get physically and mentally fit before seriously tackling your emotional health.

When you feel ready to face the issues that you have used your addiction to avoid, *find a professional person to help you*. If you try to tackle these issues alone, you may find facing your painful memories may lead you back into your addiction. Find someone who will lead you *gently* through this emotional healing process. And be patient with yourself as you heal. (See Resources for details on finding a suitable therapist.)

Retreats and workshops

There are transformational retreats and workshops that can help you move beyond the past. One of the best is an intensive one-week residential course called the Hoffman Process. The Hoffman Process helps those who have given up their addiction but who have not filled the spiritual void that made them reach out for a substance or activity in the first place. The Process allows us to heal the addictive nature of our personality by concentrating on a forgiving and loving relationship with ourselves and an acceptance that we are good enough as we are. It crosses the fine line between psychology (healing the psyche) and spirituality: getting back in touch with our bigger self or soul. Since 1967, more than 50,000 people, worldwide, have used the techniques of Hoffman to achieve personal strength, clarity and inner peace. They have also felt the benefits of developing loving relationships with family members and being able to communicate more effectively at home and at work. (See Resources for contact details.)

The shame and guilt of addiction

Regardless of what may have contributed to your becoming addicted in the first place, addiction creates its own pain. Shame and guilt are the companions of addiction. There is the shame of doing over and over again what you have repeatedly told yourself you will never do again. And there is the guilt you feel for disappointing people who care about you for what you have done to lose their trust. The need to keep using an addictive substance has probably caused you to do things that have violated your own values. Have you ever lied about your smoking or drinking? Have you ever hidden alcohol or cigarettes or biscuits so that no one would know how much you were consuming? If you place a high value on being honest and trustworthy, guilt is the outcome for violating those values.

Case study **GRANT**

Grant's father was an alcoholic who left the family when Grant was very young. Over the years they had little contact and eventually none at all. As Grant grew older he sometimes thought about his father and wondered where he was and what might have become of him. But not for long, because he believed that certainly his father didn't think about him. Years went by and Grant became a successful person in his chosen profession and gained prominence from his many accomplishments. He thought little about his father. Then came word from officials in another city that his father had died and had left Grant's name as next of kin. When he arrived at the place his father had called home, Grant found very little to give him any feeling of connection to the person who had lived in this one room with little furniture and little to indicate he had actually had a life beyond his addiction. Then Grant found this man's wallet – an item where most of us keep evidence of what is of value to us. There was no money and nothing of much worth. But imagine Grant's surprise and surge of emotion when he found prominently displayed in the wallet of this 'stranger' a picture of himself as a baby. In tears, Grant realised that addiction had not robbed his father of the value he had for family. It had only robbed him of his ability to live in harmony with that value.

Certainly this is an extreme story, and perhaps you are thinking that your addiction would not cause you to abandon your family. But the story clearly illustrates the extent to which addiction can cause us to violate our own value system. And the greatest burden of guilt comes from living out of harmony with what we value.

Using the 12 Steps of Alcoholics Anonymous for any addiction

One of the best tools we know for resolving shame and guilt is the 12 Steps of mutual help, a programme based on one used by Alcoholics Anonymous. It is interesting that in all of the steps, alcohol (or whatever substance or behaviour your particular group addresses) is only mentioned once and that is in the first step. So the focus is not on the substance but on doing what it takes to live emotionally and spiritually free. Alcoholics Anonymous is a spiritual programme but not a religion. The 'God' referred to in the 12 Steps is a god of your personal understanding; it is defined by each individual, and a higher power can be whatever you find that gives you strength and hope.

The first three steps help you take an honest look at your

situation, acknowledge that what you have been doing is not working for you, and accept the fact that you need help from a power greater than you, whatever that means for you.

Step 1: *We admitted we were powerless over alcohol, that our lives had become unmanageable.*

Step 2: *We came to believe that a power greater than ourselves could restore us to sanity.*

Step 3: *We made a decision to turn our will and our lives over to the care of God as we understood Him.*

The next four steps ask you to take an honest look *inside* yourself and your 'defects of character', those traits that keep you from living in harmony with your values:

Step 4: *We made a searching and fearless moral inventory of ourselves.*

Step 5: *We admitted to God, to ourselves, and to another human being the exact nature of our wrongs.*

Step 6: *We were entirely ready to have God remove these defects of character.*

Step 7: *We humbly asked Him to remove our shortcomings.*

The next two steps ask you to look *outside* yourself at the harm you have done and to what has become part of the burden of guilt that may have contributed to your addiction or resulted from it:

Step 8: *We made a list of all persons we had harmed and became willing to make amends to them all.*

Step 9: *We made direct amends to such people wherever possible, except when to do so would injure them or others.*

The last three steps are sometimes called the 'spiritual' steps because they ask you to continue to look honestly at yourself but along with that to move beyond the guilt and shame to build an uplifting life – a life with meaning and purpose:

Step 10: *We continued to take a personal inventory and when we were wrong promptly admitted it.*

Step 11: *We sought through prayer and meditation to improve our conscious contact with God, as we understood Him, praying only for knowledge of His will for us and the power to carry that out.*

Step 12: *Having had a spiritual awakening as the result of these steps, we tried to carry this message [of hope] to alcoholics, and to practise these principles in all our affairs.*

Grieving the loss of what you are giving up

Let's be honest, if the mood-altering substance you use wasn't giving you pleasure or relieving your pain, you wouldn't need it. Giving it up would be a piece of cake. (Pardon the metaphor if your feel-good substance is sugar.) Of course, part of why it is hard to give it up is that using it relieves the pain of physical dependence.

But isn't it more than that? Hasn't the substance you use become your friend? A friend that you have depended on when you felt you couldn't depend on anything or anyone else? A friend that could do something for you that you couldn't find anywhere else – a friend that you looked forward to spending time with? Hey, that's quite a friend. It's normal to feel an emotional bond to such a friend and to feel a sense of loss when you don't have that friend any more.

Grieving the loss of your friend means

- Acknowledging the profound nature of the loss for you.

- Letting yourself feel the sadness of what you are losing.

- Adjusting to life without your feel-good substance.

- And then taking the emotional energy you have been investing in the past and investing it in what lies ahead.

- Only then does it become part of your past and not part of your future.

The healing power of the serenity prayer

You may find it helpful to say the serenity prayer:

God grant me serenity to accept the things I cannot change, courage to change the things I can, and the wisdom to know the difference.

Wisdom for healing lies in the words of the serenity prayer. To move beyond the pain, shame and guilt of the past it is necessary to identify what you have the power to change and what you can't do anything about. The real trick is learning which things are which. As long as you are expending your energy trying to change what you are powerless over, you are not expending it on what you can change. And the cycle of failure, shame and guilt goes on and on. You can fret about the past, but you can't change it. You can only change the present and with that change the future.

Finding serenity from freedom to change

Recognising that there are things you cannot change frees you to take responsibility for what you can and should change. Now that you know ways to overcome addiction you can free yourself from its bonds. You are free to change.

And with that freedom comes serenity. Serenity doesn't mean you don't have any unpleasant feelings. It means you accept life as it is without expending excessive energy fighting against what you can't change. It does not mean that you do not get angry or afraid. Serenity means accepting and acknowledging *all* of your feelings. Serenity is acceptance that your feelings are valid so you don't have to be ashamed or feel guilty about them.

Serenity is also knowing that what you feel and what you do about your feelings are not the same thing. You can be afraid and not run from what you are afraid of. You can be angry and not become violent. You can be sad and not give up on life. You can learn ways to express your feelings that are appropriate and healing.

Living in the present

Perhaps the real secret of serenity is in living in the present – being present in the moment. There is little serenity in replaying what has already happened or waiting for some time in the future to enjoy life. If you are living for tomorrow you are missing out on today. Serenity increases as the experience of being present and comfortable in the moment increases.

'One day at a time' is a slogan learned in AA that is helpful in recovery because it teaches one to focus on the present. Sometimes it can be broken down to 'one moment at a time'. Now is all you have. The past is history. You cannot change it. The future is a mystery. You cannot experience it. *The present is where life is lived.* It's a gift. That's why it's called the present. Enjoy it for what it is and leave the past behind.

SUMMARY

▶ Recovery from addiction requires more than physical wellness; it also requires emotional, social and spiritual wellness.

▶ Healing emotional pain from the past is possible with counselling and/or a mutual help programme such as Alcoholics Anonymous.

▶ Grieving the losses that accompany giving up an addictive lifestyle require acknowledging the losses and adjusting to life without what you have given up.

Finding serenity in recovery requires:

▶ Accepting what you cannot change.

▶ Finding the courage to change what you can.

▶ Learning to tell which things are which.

PART 3

HOW TO QUIT *YOUR* ADDICTION

When you become aware that the symptoms or pain you associate with using a substance – including the likely consequences if you continue to use it – are more severe than the symptoms of giving it up, you are ready to quit. However, the idea of stopping usually brings with it a sense of dread, based on three fundamental fears: (1) the fear of facing the stresses, hassles, trials and tribulations of life without the substance; (2) the fear of simply living without the pleasure these substances can bring; and (3) the fear of physical withdrawal.

Now that you understand how the addicted brain tricks you into thinking you are always in need of something, and have learned the fundamental keys to living life free from the desire for addictive substances, in this part you will learn what you need to do to quit your particular addictions with minimal abstinence symptoms, and with rapid recovery of your innate capacity for feeling good without needing anything extra. This is the beginning of your How to Quit programme.

Share your commitment to quit with someone you trust. Let them know what you are doing and check in with them along the journey.

Each chapter in this part describes a strategy for quitting one of the major addictive substances. It should be used alongside our How to Quit Action Plan in Part 4, which includes our How to Quit Diet and our tailor-made prescriptions for addictions and abstinence symptoms.

19.

CAFFEINE: HOW TO INCREASE YOUR ENERGY WITHOUT IT

Every addictive substance has benefits, and caffeine is no exception. Otherwise, we would not be drinking an estimated 300 million cups of tea and coffee every day in Britain! That's the equivalent of over 100,000 cups in your lifetime! When you first started drinking coffee (or tea or other caffeinated drinks) you no doubt got a buzz – an increase in energy, clarity, motivation and mood. It also helps you recover in the morning if you've had too much alcohol the night before or you have taken drugs. It can even reduce your appetite and stop you gaining weight. Perhaps these are some of the reasons you kept drinking it.

So, why do you want to give it up? Is it because it doesn't give you a buzz any more? Or do you need to drink more and more to get the same effect? Or have you noticed that you feel tired, stressed or don't sleep well and think coffee or caffeine is the cause? Perhaps you've read that caffeine raises blood pressure[1] and increases the risk of heart disease,[2] as well as raising homocysteine,[3] although, surprisingly, it appears to lower diabetes risk.[4]

Whatever the reason, our purpose is to help you stop being dependent on caffeine so that you will feel good, normal or less bad, and be able to quit without experiencing terrible withdrawal symptoms. To do this we need to recap what caffeine does in the brain to understand the basis for how to undo it.

What caffeine does

Caffeine raises the stress hormones cortisol and adrenalin, as well as dopamine, the feel-good neurotransmitter from which adrenalin is made. It also depresses the action of adenosine, a chemical that helps switch off excess adrenalin, thus calming you down, and insulin, which is the hormone that controls your blood sugar.[5] This can lead, in turn, to either more caffeine cravings or sugar cravings. (Read Chapter 5 for more on the stress-sugar-cigarette-stimulant trap.) It only takes one or two cups of coffee for you to start to become addicted to it. Some people are addicted to just one cup of coffee. The national daily average is about 280mg – the equivalent of about one to two mugs of coffee or three to five cans of a soft caffeinated drink.

How you might feel when you quit

If you quit caffeine without correcting the biochemical imbalance it creates in your brain and body's chemistry, you are likely to experience the following symptoms:

- Headaches

- Fatigue or drowsiness

- Flat mood, including depression and irritability

- Difficulty concentrating

- Flu-like symptoms of nausea, vomiting and muscle pain or stiffness

It takes about 15 hours for caffeine to leave the system, so these symptoms usually start within 12 to 24 hours, hit peak intensity around day two, and last for anything between two and nine days. Half the number of people who give it up get headaches, and about one in nine feel so bad they can't function well enough to work. That's what happens if you go cold turkey with no nutritional support.

Do you need to quit completely?

This is a difficult question and one that only you can answer. Our advice is to quit completely, following all our diet and supplement guidelines, for at least 30 days. If you feel fantastic, you have your answer. If you choose to consume caffeine in moderation bear in mind that tea, and especially green tea, is not so bad for you. Unlike coffee, for most people it doesn't raise the stress hormone cortisol. In fact it reduces it. This alone suggests coffee is much worse for you, and that tea might even be beneficial in moderation. Green tea can boost glutathione levels[6] and both black and green tea are quite high in antioxidants. The L-theanine content in both green and black tea may also act as a relaxant. In fact, in one study drinking tea was shown to lower the stress hormone cortisol and to help people relax.[7] A fallback position could be two medium-strength cups of black tea, or up to three cups of green tea from the same tea bag. This is how the Chinese and Japanese drink their tea: they put some leaves in the pot, drink their tea, then, later in the day, add more water to the pot, but not more leaves. Decaffeinated tea or coffee is, of course, better, but watch out because this still keeps you hooked into the taste and the ritual of coffee or tea.

Caffeine-free alternatives

Nowadays there are many caffeine-free drinks available for you to choose from. Most people like red bush (rooibos) tea, which can be drunk with milk and tastes closest to the real thing, but has no caffeine and is high in antioxidants. There are also sweet fruit and herbal teas. Try Yogi teas such as Cinnamon Spice, or peppermint or rosehip tea. As we saw in Chapter 5, of the caffeine-containing teas, green tea is the least bad, and has some positive benefits, but don't have more than three cups a day.

▶ HOW TO QUIT caffeine

Use the following guidelines alongside our How to Quit Action Plan in Part 4.

1. A week before you start to reduce or quit caffeine follow our How to Quit Diet in Chapter 28, paying special attention to the three low-GL rules: eat low-GL foods, eat protein with carbohydrates, and graze (eat little and often) rather than gorge – it's also important to start your day with a low-GL breakfast.

2. A week before you give it up, start taking the Basic Supplements recommended for everybody on page 388.

3. Give caffeine up slowly. Set yourself the target of getting down to one regular coffee (100mg), one cup of black tea, one high-strength caffeinated drink (80mg), or two regular caffeinated drinks (for example 40mg × 2), before quitting completely. Do this by cutting your daily intake by a third each day until you reach a daily intake of no more than the equivalent of 100mg. For example, if you have three coffees a day, have two tomorrow, and one the next day, then quit completely.

4. On the day before you give it up, also start taking the Stimulant Prescription (page 403). This includes extra dosages of

the amino acid tyrosine to support your own ability to make dopamine and adrenalin, as well as extra chromium to help increase your sensitivity to insulin, plus adaptogens such as standardised ginseng, which help with fatigue.[8]

5. For the first week after quitting have two cups of green tea a day.

6. You may feel sleepy for the first few days. Let yourself sleep. There's a good chance that you're an adrenalin addict and are simply in sleep deficit (see page 204). Let yourself recover. That's why it's best to quit when you don't have too much going on, or during a holiday. Let yourself unwind.

7. If you do get a terrible headache, take 3g vitamin C every hour for several hours and drink lots of water.

8. If you feel really edgy or irritable take chromium 200mcg up to a maximum of three a day.

9. If you feel really depressed take SAM 400mg, or alternatively 1,000mg of tyrosine on an empty stomach. Break open the tyrosine capsule and swill it around your mouth and under your tongue before swallowing to help it to be absorbed quickly.

10. Drink at least 1 litre (1¾ pints), preferably 2 litres (3½pints), of water a day for the first week after quitting.

Using the 12 Keys to Unaddicting Your Brain

The most important keys from Part 2 for you are:

- Rebalance Your Brain with Amino Acids (Chapter 7) – this is because specific amino acids, especially tyrosine, help stimulate the brain naturally once you've removed your daily fix of caffeine.

- Raise Your Methyl IQ with Vitamins and Minerals (Chapter 9) – this is because caffeine messes up methylation, and specific B vitamins help improve your concentration without the need for caffeine.

- Balance Your Blood Sugar to Gain Energy and Reduce Cravings (Chapter 11) – caffeine messes up your blood sugar balance and this chapter explains how to restore it.

- How to Get a Good Night's Sleep (Chapter 13), if you don't sleep well – learning how to get a good night's sleep is going to stop you craving caffeine.

- Find New Pleasure in Life by Raising Endorphins (Chapter 16) – by exercising regularly your energy level will go up, reducing your 'need' for stimulants.

- Generate Vital Energy: The Chi Factor (Chapter 17) – by learning how to do this you'll find a natural, clean energy that is much nicer than the effects of caffeine.

What to expect 30 days later

It takes, on average, about 30 days to recover and normalise your brain's chemistry and blood sugar balance. Of course, this depends greatly on whether caffeine is your only vice. If you've been using a variety of addictive substances for years, our advice would be to stick to this kind of recovery programme for at least 90 days.

Otherwise, provided your Scale of Abstinence Symptoms Severity score has dropped by two-thirds (see Chart Your Progress on page 385), stop the Stimulant Prescription, but keep taking the Basic Supplements.

20.

SUGAR: HOW TO LOSE YOUR SWEET TOOTH

Everyone likes sugar, and the more you have the more you want. You get used to higher and higher levels of sweetness so that after a while the desire for sweet foods can literally take over. Richard is a case in point. He was averaging over 100 teaspoons a day – drinking a 2 litre (3½ pint) bottle of cola every day, containing 45 teaspoons, plus chocolate, biscuits, sweets and sugar in drinks and on cereal. Often, if you are eating excess sugar you will also suffer from hyperactivity, impulsive behaviour and poor concentration. Too much sugar leads to blood sugar peaks and troughs. The troughs make you tired, so if you have a sugar habit you will probably also go for caffeinated drinks and other stimulants to counter the sugar blues. Sugar, just like cocaine and heroin, stimulates dopamine and endorphins, leading to reward deficiency.[9]

Dr Candace Pert, Research Professor in the Department of Physiology and Biophysics at Georgetown University Medical Center in Washington DC, says: 'I consider sugar to be a drug, a highly purified plant product that can become addictive. Relying on an artificial form of glucose – sugar – to give us a quick pick-me-up is analogous to, if not as dangerous as, shooting heroin.'[10]

What is more, whether you have a serious sugar problem or a mild one, just substituting foods or drinks with artificial sweeteners doesn't reset your sweet tooth. As with any addiction it takes time and good nutrition to get your brain's chemistry back into balance.

What sugar does

Of course, with too much sugar comes other problems such as weight gain, depression, craving for alcohol and drugs, diabetes, heart disease, kidney problems, thrush, failing eyesight and numbness in the fingers and toes. You might have decided to curb your sweet tooth because of one of these problems or just because you recognise that you have become addicted.

How you might feel when you quit

If you just quit all sugar and sweet foods completely, with none of the nutritional support we recommend, you will simply crave it. You may feel more tired and low, lacking in motivation. It takes about a week for these symptoms to recede to an extent. It takes a week for your blood sugar levels to adjust to the lack of a constant, daily fix.

How supplements will help

On the other hand, if you also take the amino acid, vitamin and mineral supplements that we recommend, the results are very different. This is because a lot of people crave sugar due to an underlying serotonin deficiency. By supplementing the right amino acids to correct this (mainly tryptophan and/or 5-HTP) sugar cravings often reduce substantially and, with that, excessive weight gain.

A good example of this is a study involving a group of carbohydrate bingers. Those who were put on a low-carb diet and also took the amino acid supplements for 90 days lost an average of 12.2kg (1 stone 13lb/27lb) and only 18 per cent relapsed. They were compared to a group not taking the supplement that lost an average of 4.5kg (10lb) and had a relapse rate of 82 per cent.[11]

In another study, published in 1997, two groups of dieters were monitored for two years after they had completed a medically monitored fast, involving liquid meals, which had resulted in significant weight loss. Following completion of the 'fast', one of the two groups took a formulation of nutrients each day and the other group did not. And this is what happened. At the end of two years the group that took the amino acid formulation showed the following: a twofold decrease in percentage overweight for both males and females (meaning that whatever percentage each person was overweight before, that percentage had de-creased twice as much in the supplement group as in the other group), a 70 per cent reduction in cravings for women and a 63 per cent reduction for men, a 66 per cent decrease in binge eating for women and a 41 per cent decrease for men, and only 15 per cent of the weight lost was regained. In the group without the supplements, 41.7 per cent of weight lost was regained.

Richard Wurtman, a professor of brain and cognitive science at the Massachusetts Institute of Technology in Cambridge, believes that some people crave carbohydrates not because they lack willpower but because of an imbalance in serotonin. This theory is supported by evidence that obese people and people who crave carbohydrates often have lower serotonin levels than do lean people or people who prefer protein-rich snacks. Their extra-low serotonin levels leave them feeling anxious, irritable and craving a serotonin 'fix'. The reason why sugar works is that sugar causes a release of insulin, and insulin carries tryptophan in the blood into the brain, where it can be converted into serotonin. This is probably why you crave sugar when you're feeling low, and feel better for it, and why we give upset children something sweet and they perk up.

Chromium, which helps insulin to work, also substantially reduces craving, as well as improving mood. It halves cravings in eight weeks and improves mood in people prone to depression in two out of three who supplement 600mcg a day.[12]

Do you need to quit completely?

Sugar itself is not bad – it just becomes so when you have too much. It is also refined and thus devoid of the nutrients, especially B vitamins, vitamin C and chromium, needed to turn it into energy.

Having said that, to break the habit, it is best to set yourself a clear line: nothing with added sugar. There are many names for sugar, including:

Glucose (syrup)

Dextrose

Malt

Honey

Sucrose

Fructose

These are best avoided, although fructose has half the effect on your blood sugar as sucrose, which has almost half of the effect of glucose. So, fructose is the lesser of these evils.

This also means avoiding chocolate, which is high in sugar. However, the occasional bit of dark chocolate (with 70 per cent cocoa solids and low in sugar) is no big deal – as long as you don't eat a bar a day.

Instead, eat whole fruits, which provide fructose and nutrients. The best fruits are apples, pears, berries, cherries, plums and peaches. Oranges aren't bad, but watch out for guzzling loads of juice. As a rule of thumb, don't have more than the juice of one orange per day or an equivalent amount of apple juice. Dilute this with one-third water. Then, after the first week, start diluting half and half with water. Have a maximum of two such juices a day.

Sugar-free alternatives

One of the best natural sugars is xylose, also called xylitol. About two-thirds of the natural sugar in berries, cherries and plums is xylose, which tastes sweet but doesn't raise your blood sugar level. Nine teaspoons of xylitol has the same effect on your blood sugar level as one teaspoon of sugar or honey. Nowadays, you can buy it easily in supermarkets, health-food shops and by mail order (see Resources). It tastes just like sugar and the only thing it won't do is caramelise. So you won't be able to make crème brûlée with it.

Because xylitol attracts water in the gut, if you have too much you get looser bowels, which, although not harmful, is quite a good indicator to have less xylitol. It is also positively good for your teeth. You might have seen the ads on TV for xylitol mouth-wash or chewing gum. This is because xylitol stops bacteria sticking to the teeth.

▶ HOW TO QUIT sugar

Use the following guidelines alongside our How to Quit Action Plan in Part 4.

1. One week before you begin to quit, take the Basic Supplements (page 388), plus the Mood Prescription (page 416), which includes tryptophan and/or 5-HTP for promoting serotonin, as well as chromium for supporting blood sugar balance.

2. Set yourself reasonable targets based on halving your sugar intake each week until you have none. For example, if you normally have two sugars in your tea, have one in the first week, and half a teaspoonful in the second week.

3. Switch to xylitol so that you don't have the blood sugar rush.

4. Have half a teaspoon of cinnamon in a drink, on your cereal or on a light dessert. You can also get supplements of cinnamon, in which case take these with the chromium supplement in the Mood Prescription.

5. If you are craving sugar, first have a large glass of water, then a piece of fruit with some nuts or seeds (eating protein with carbohydrate keeps your blood sugar level even).

6. Always eat breakfast. You are aiming for three meals and two snacks a day. By eating little and often you help support your blood sugar balance.

7. Minimise caffeine and alcohol, as these both affect your blood sugar.

8. Follow our How to Quit Diet in Chapter 28, Part 4.

Using the 12 Keys to Unaddicting Your Brain

The most important keys from Part 2 for you are:

- Rebalance Your Brain with Amino Acids (Chapter 7) – this is because specific amino acids, especially tryptophan, help restore the underlying serotonin deficiency that leads to carbohydrate craving.

- Balance your Blood Sugar to Gain Energy and Reduce Cravings (Chapter 11) – this gives you the understanding necessary to become a master of controlling your sugar balance, energy, weight and cravings.

What to expect 30 days later

After 30 days your cravings for carbs will be much reduced and probably your need for extra chromium will be too. So, cut back to one 200mcg tablet with breakfast, but do keep taking the Basic Supplements. If you find this doesn't work as well as the two you were taking as part of the Mood Prescription, there's no harm in continuing. Perhaps try taking 2 × 200mcg.

21.

NICOTINE: HOW TO CUT YOUR CRAVINGS

Once you've started smoking it's very hard to quit. You probably smoke because it wakes you up in the morning, calms you down when you're stressed, helps you concentrate, helps you chill out after a meal, or even gives you something to do with your hands or something to put in your mouth, or to suppress your appetite. Any drug that offers you all this is attractive, right? So why do you want to quit?

Perhaps you're fed up with having to go outside to smoke or the social pressure on you to quit. Perhaps you're afraid of cancer, or perhaps you've been getting infections and finding them hard to shift. You may simply be fed up with 'needing' a cigarette and the withdrawal effects you get when you haven't had one, or how you smell, your dry-cleaning bill, and how much you spend on cigarettes.

The first thing we want to say is: you can quit. This statement might seem counterintuitive if you've tried and failed, or can't imagine ever stopping. And there's no doubt that nicotine is addictive stuff. In fact, it's more addictive than heroin.

What nicotine does

Nicotine produces a stimulating effect even in small doses, and in large amounts acts as a sedative. This is its attraction: on the one hand, it can give you a lift; on the other, it can calm you down. Before a meal it can stop you feeling hungry; after a meal it can stop you from feeling drowsy. These effects are mainly down to nicotine's action on adrenal hormones and blood sugar balance.

Biochemically there's a very close link between nicotine addiction and alcohol addiction. If you stop one, but not the other, the underlying biochemical imbalance doesn't change. You need to quit *both* otherwise you will keep craving. This may sound almost impossible, but you will find, with the back-up of our nutritional approach, that this will not be as hard as you imagine. However, you may choose to stop one for two weeks to get over the worst of the withdrawal effects before you stop the other.

Over 90 per cent of people who smoke 40 a day plus have an underlying alcohol dependency. If this applies to you, have a look at Chapter 22 on alcohol and how to lose your craving.

How you might feel when you quit

If all you do is quit nicotine without correcting the biochemical imbalance it creates in your brain and body's chemistry, the chances are you'll be climbing the walls – feeling agitated, irritable, moody, hungry, spacey and desperate for a cigarette and the whole ritual of smoking. You are likely to feel that you can't relax and chill out without a smoke.

Many people feel nauseous, have headaches and flu-like symptoms, feel lethargic, depressed, have blood sugar lows where they crave something sweet and, consequently, gain weight.

For many people these symptoms last a week. The bad news is that, for some people, these symptoms are still there weeks, and even months, later. The good news is that this need not happen if you get your brain chemistry back into balance with our nutrition programme.

Do you need to quit completely?

The simple answer is yes. Of course, there are people who just have the odd cigarette, but these people usually aren't going to get addicted anyway. The chances are you aren't one of these people or you wouldn't be reading this. Our advice is to quit completely.

Although you might find it useful to wean yourself off cigarettes and on to nicotine patches for a while, this is only a stepping-stone to quitting completely.

▶ HOW TO QUIT nicotine

Use the following guidelines alongside our How to Quit Action Plan in Part 4.

1. Before you even begin to try to give up cigarettes, we recommend you take the Basic Supplements (page 388) and the Stimulant Prescription (page 403) and follow the How to Quit diet strictly for one month. At the end of this period you should no longer be consuming any other stimulants (such as tea, coffee and chocolate) or sugar. Instead you'll be eating small, frequent meals, with an emphasis on foods containing slow-releasing carbohydrates combined with foods rich in proteins. Your background blood sugar balance will be much better, which means you'll experience less withdrawal symptoms on quitting.

2. Break all the associated habits. The average smoker is addicted not only to nicotine, but also to smoking when tired, hungry or upset, on waking, after a meal, with a drink, and so on. Before you actually give up smoking altogether, it's best to break these mental associations.

3. At first don't attempt to change your smoking habits. Just keep a diary for a week, writing down every situation in which you smoke, how you feel before, and how you feel after smoking. You can copy the example on the following page seven times to record your one-week smoking diary. When the week is up, add up how many cigarettes you smoke in each situation. Your list might look something like this:

With a hot drink: 16

After a meal: 6

With alcohol: 4

Difficult situation: 4

After sex: 3

4. Now set yourself weekly targets. For the first week, smoke as much as you like whenever you like but not when you drink a hot drink. For the next week, smoke as much as you like whenever you like but not when you drink a hot drink or within 30 minutes of finishing a meal. Continue like this until, when you smoke, all you do is smoke, without the associated habits. Having said that, set yourself a maximum of six weeks to complete this phase. This will be tremendously helpful for you when you quit. Most people start again because someone phones them with a problem, a work colleague brings in a coffee, offers them a cigarette . . . and before you know it they're smoking.

5. Put your cigarette butts in a big glass jar with a sealing lid. Fill it half with water. Keep this in clear view in your living room. You will begin to associate cigarettes with the nasty stuff in your jar.

6. Now it's time to reduce your nicotine load gradually. Week by week, switch to a cigarette brand that contains less nicotine, until what you smoke contains no more than 2mg per cigarette. Now reduce the number of cigarettes you are

Smoking diary		
Day _____ Time Situation	Feeling Before	Feeling After
9 am: with coffee	tired	awake

smoking until you smoke no more than five cigarettes a day, each with a nicotine content of 2mg or less. If you wish, stop smoking and replace it with nicotine gum as an intermediate step. (Nicotine gum comes in two strengths: 4mg and 2mg.)

7. You want to be down to a maximum of 10mg of nicotine a day before quitting – that is, five pieces of 2mg nicotine gum, or five 2mg nicotine cigarettes.

8. For the first week of quitting also take an extra 8g of vitamin C (there are two tablets in the Basic Supplements, so this gives you 10g in total). Buy some magnesium ascorbate powder (this is a form of vitamin C). Magnesium is a calming mineral. Put 8g worth of it in a bottle of half water and half juice. Drink it throughout the day. It is likely you will get slightly looser bowels.

9. Also take chromium 200mcg: one with breakfast and one with lunch. This helps stabilise your blood sugar level.

10. Take 50mg of niacin (nicotinic acid) twice a day. (You'll probably need to buy a 100mg niacin tablet and break it in half.) You will experience a blushing sensation when first taking niacin. This is harmless and usually occurs 15 to 30 minutes after taking it, and lasts for about 15 minutes (so don't take it at work). The blushing is less likely to occur if you take niacin with a meal, and will diminish and, in most cases, stop completely after a week if you keep taking it. The reason for taking this is that both nicotine and niacin occupy the same receptors in the brain – so giving yourself more niacin is likely to reduce your cravings.[13]

11. Eat an alkaline-forming diet: one that is high in fruit, vege-tables and seeds. (It's better to have a more alkaline-forming diet than one that is acid forming.) Also, make sure you are supplementing a total of 850mg of magnesium and calcium combined. A good multivitamin will provide 200mg calcium and 150mg magnesium, and there will be at least 500mg in

the magnesium ascorbate powder noted above. These alkaline minerals will have an alkalising effect on your body. Whenever you feel the need for nicotine, first drink a glass of water and eat an apple or a pear. This will raise your low blood sugar level, which is often the factor that triggers such a craving.

12. Improve your breathing. Your lungs are damaged by smoking and it's really important to do something that stimulates breathing and their recovery. At least, go for a brisk walk every day, ideally in clean air or in the park. Any exercise that focuses on the breath, such as some forms of yoga and Psychocalisthenics, is ideal. This is a great time to sign up at your local gym or to start jogging, cycling or swimming.

13. If you have difficulty sleeping, or are irritable or depressed, supplement 200mg of 5-HTP. This is an amino acid that the body converts into serotonin, an important brain chemical that controls mood. Nicotine withdrawal tends to lower serotonin levels. The supplement 5-HTP is best absorbed if you take it away from protein foods and with carbohydrate foods, so either take it on an empty stomach, or with a piece of fruit. And because serotonin levels rise at night, promoting a good night's sleep, the best time to take your 5-HTP is one hour before bed.

14. Another useful aid during the first month is sugar-free liquorice, which promotes the action of adrenal hormones. Since nicotine acts as an adrenal stimulant, additional adrenal support can be helpful during the withdrawal phase. Liquorice is either available as a supplement or as a bar, but make sure you are getting the real thing. As far as supplements are concerned, the amount to take is 1–2g powdered root, or 2–4ml fluid extract, three times a day. Check the manufacturers' instructions, as potencies can vary.

CAUTION Liquorice should be avoided by people with high blood pressure.

Detox your body to reduce cravings

One factor that helps to reduce cravings is boosting the body's ability to detoxify and eliminate nicotine. There are five things you can do to speed up this process: exercise, sweating, drinking plenty of water and supplementing vitamin C and niacin. Put these all together, and you've got a winning formula for rapid detoxification. If you have access to a sauna or steam room, here's what to do (most gyms have one or the other).

1. Take 1g of vitamin C and 100mg of niacin (if you do this you don't need to take the extra niacin outlined on page 305).

2. Go for a run or undertake any cardiovascular exercise that raises your pulse rate and stimulates circulation.

3. Once you start blushing as a consequence of the niacin, enter the sauna or steam room. The sauna should never be at a temperature above 27°C (80°F).

4. Take 1 litre (1¾ pints) water into the steam room with you and drink it at regular intervals.

5. Do this for half an hour every day. This routine is *not* recommended for those with a history of cardiovascular disease. Although no danger is anticipated or reported, the combination of exercise, niacin and saunas is a substantial stimulation to circulation and detoxification.

Using the 12 Keys to Unaddicting Your Brain

The most important keys from Part 2 for you are:

- Rebalance Your Brain with Amino Acids (Chapter 7) – read this chapter to understand why you need specific amino acids to use your brain's natural ability to wake up and relax without nicotine.

- Raise Your Methyl IQ with Vitamins and Minerals (Chapter 9) – check your homocysteine level to find out your ideal level of B vitamins. Smoking definitely raises it.

- Balance Your Blood Sugar to Gain Energy and Reduce Cravings (Chapter 11) – your blood sugar balance will be out, so read up on how to eat to keep your blood sugar in check. This will prevent rebound overeating.

- Repair Your Brain with Antioxidants (Chapter 12) – this will help you understand why you need to up your antioxidants to undo the damage from smoking.

- Find New Pleasure in Life by Raising Endorphins (Chapter 16) – exercise really helps to get your lungs back to shape (but start gently).

What to expect 30 days later

It takes, on average, about 30 days to recover and normalise your brain's chemistry and blood sugar balance. Of course, this depends greatly on whether nicotine is your only vice. If you've been using a variety of addictive substances for years, our advice would be to stick to this kind of recovery programme for at least 90 days.

Otherwise, provided your Scale of Abstinence Symptoms Severity score has dropped by two-thirds (see Chart Your Progress on page 385), stop the Stimulant Prescription, but keep taking the Basic Supplements. By now you'll know the effects of the other temporary supplements – niacin, chromium and 5-HTP. Reduce or stop these according to your need.

22.

ALCOHOL: HOW TO LOSE YOUR CRAVINGS

You probably started drinking alcohol for some of the same reasons millions of other people do. Your friends drank; it was a rite of passage; it was the social thing to do. However, if you are reading this chapter, it's very likely that alcohol is now causing you problems or you are recovering from alcoholism and still finding it tough going.

What's your problem?

Of course, not everyone who considers themselves to have a 'drink problem', or even everyone who needs to quit, is an alcoholic. There are many different ways that alcohol problems are classified. But the most helpful is probably to divide problem drinkers into two categories – those who abuse alcohol and those who are alcohol dependent.

Alcohol abuse

An alcohol abuser is someone who drinks irresponsibly and continues to do so despite harmful consequences but who does not have the symptoms of alcohol dependence, such as increased tolerance, withdrawal symptoms and loss of control (see opposite). In other words, an alcohol abuser drinks for psychological or social reasons, for fun or just to get drunk. An abuser can stop drinking for any length of time without experiencing withdrawal symptoms. A person who is not physically dependent on alcohol, but who drinks and drives is abusing alcohol. College students who don't drink at all during the week but who get together and drink for the sole purpose of becoming intoxicated are drinking irresponsibly (abusers) but in most cases are not alcohol dependent.

Even for alcohol abusers, however, there are serious consequences of drinking to excess. Alcohol abuse can damage relationships, affect performance at work, lead to problems with the police – and it can damage your body and brain. The body does not distinguish between alcohol consumption by an abuser and consumption by a person who is addicted. So an abuser is also susceptible to damage to the liver, digestive tract, heart and brain. There is also a problem that is sometimes referred to as 'psychological dependence', which makes giving up alcohol very difficult. If you use alcohol to relieve emotional pain and you come to rely on it to do that for you, you will experience a kind of emotional withdrawal when the pain returns after you quit drinking. Perhaps, for example, you don't know how to be sociable without drinking. This can cause pain and even craving when you try to interact with people or have a good time without alcohol. Obviously the score on the Scale of Abstinence Symptoms Severity for an abuser who is quitting is lower than for someone who is physically dependent, but the abuser will still have many of the symptoms and can use it to gauge when they can move into the maintenance phase (see Chart Your Progress on page 385).

Alcohol dependence

An alcohol-dependent person drinks in response to the physiological compulsion to do so. There are three very straightforward criteria for alcohol dependence:

1. **Tolerance** The physical ability to drink large amounts of alcohol without showing signs of intoxication and eventually the need to drink greater amounts of alcohol to feel the same effects.

2. **Withdrawal** Symptoms such as nausea, sweating, shakiness and anxiety occur when regular alcohol use is stopped.

3. **Loss of control** The inability to limit your drinking on any given occasion.

You might not be experiencing symptoms of alcohol addiction but you could still be on your way to becoming dependent. Even if your problem seems to be one of abuse at the present, we would advise you to evaluate your drinking to determine your risk of becoming dependent, because it is difficult to distinguish abuse from early stage dependence. Here are some warning signs that indicate you may be at risk of developing alcoholism.

- The main sign that you may be at risk of dependence before you develop noticeable symptoms is that your drinking seems to you and to others to be beneficial rather than harmful.

- You may experience fewer problems than others while drinking the same quantities and with the same frequency. If you can drink more than your peers without becoming intoxicated, you may be in the early stage of alcoholism.

- While alcohol has a sedating effect on most people, those at risk of alcohol addiction often have a period of stimulation when they feel more alert and may actually function better when they drink. This period of stimulation might last past the point at which drinking companions have stopped drinking, gone to sleep or passed out. But beware: this 'magic' period can come to a halt quite rapidly and you then find yourself drunk.

- For a while the period of stimulation may increase, but eventually you will find that you can drink less and less before losing control. Symptoms of addiction may then become noticeable. Once this occurs, you can't go back, no matter what you do – you can never go back to the 'magic' days when alcohol was your friend instead of your foe.

- Even if you don't see the pattern of risk that we have described here, you should be aware that anyone who drinks hard enough and long enough can become addicted. And if this seems to be your pattern, you are to be commended for doing something about it now before it becomes a much more serious problem.

CAUTION If you are addicted to alcohol, we do not recommend that you quit drinking on your own. Withdrawal from alcohol can be serious and even life-threatening. The detoxification process should be medically supervised. So if you are alcohol dependent, seek help from your doctor in the first instance and then you can follow our programme (see page 316).

The stages of alcohol dependence

The criteria for alcohol dependence outlined on page 311 reflect the progression of alcohol dependence through the following three stages:

The first stage is that period of time when you can drink large quantities of alcohol without becoming intoxicated. This is a period when you appear to be less likely to have a drinking problem than either a 'vino' (someone who drinks half a bottle of wine most evenings) or an alcohol abuser. While drinking you are more sociable and more comfortable than when not drinking. It is difficult at this stage to recognise that alcohol might be a problem because you can 'hold your liquor' better than people who are drinking with you. The body, however, is changing and adapting to the regular ingestion of large quantities of alcohol. Tolerance is developing even without outward signs.

In the middle stage tolerance becomes dependence; want becomes need. As the cells of the brain change to tolerate large quantities of alcohol, so need increases. As this happens, the person has less and less control over drinking and drinking behaviour. There is increasing loss of control over frequency of drinking, over behaviour while drinking and over the ability to stop drinking.

The chronic stage of alcohol dependence is marked by deterioration. The main deterioration is physical; all body systems can be affected. Complications such as liver damage, malnutrition and severe brain impairment occur. The tolerance for alcohol is nearly non-existent. The loss of control becomes more and more dramatic, ending in more and more serious consequences. Psychological and social disruptions become severe, and life becomes unmanageable. At this point your alcoholism is recognisable.

Do you need to quit completely?

If you are an alcohol abuser it is very possible that you can learn to drink in moderation. If you believe you are an abuser and not alcohol dependent, you will probably want to try this approach. Here is our advice. Follow the recommendations given below for alcohol abusers, for at least 30 days, including abstaining from alcohol. Ideally make a decision to quit for 90 days. Then drink no more than one drink a day, if you are a woman, or two drinks a day, if you are a man. If you are able to do this without losing control or drinking irresponsibly, you are probably not alcohol dependent. If you are able to do this and feel comfortable without gradually increasing the amount you drink, you are probably an abuser and have now learned to drink responsibly. But if this was very difficult for you, if you had strong cravings or a feeling of compulsion to drink more, you should be very cautious. At any time that you find yourself repeatedly drinking beyond one or two drinks a day, then you should consider the possibility that you are already dependent and need to stop completely.

If you are alcohol dependent, our answer is yes, you need to stop completely. Although some people will tell you that it is possible to learn to drink in moderation despite a history of addictive drinking, we have not seen evidence of this in 25 years of experience. We strongly advise against attempting it. Some people become sensitised to alcohol and the slightest intake triggers relapse.

▶ **HOW TO QUIT** recommendations for alcohol abusers

Use the following guidelines alongside our How to Quit Action Plan in Part 4.

1. One week before starting to quit, take the Basic Supplements (page 388) and the Alcohol Prescription (page 406) as described in Part 4. The Alcohol Prescription includes trypto-

phan or 5-HTP, GABA or glutamine and taurine: the nutrients needed to calm your hyperactive nervous system.

2. Most people who abuse alcohol are sleep-deprived. Use the Sleep Prescription (page 397) to increase serotonin and melatonin levels and induce deep, regenerative sleep.

3. Follow our low-GL diet (see Chapter 11), being sure to include unfried oily fish three times a week, olive oil, garlic, nuts, beans and lentils, and whole grains.

4. Many of those with a high alcohol intake are deficient in omega-3 fatty acids. Supplement 2g fish oil daily with meals.

5. To help eliminate cravings and improve your mood take 500mg D-phenylalanine twice daily on an empty stomach.

6. In the case of alcohol liver damage take liver regenerative nutrients as described in Appendix 3 (which is on our website www.how2quit.co.uk). If you have liver damage, regardless of the cause, you should take liver regenerative nutrients.

7. Test for hidden (IgG) food allergies and eliminate allergic foods for three months (dairy and wheat products are the most common allergens found in alcoholics, so it's also probably worth checking if you are an alcohol abuser).

Using the 12 Keys to Unaddicting Your Brain

The most important keys from Part 2 for you are:

- Rebalance Your Brain with Amino Acids (Chapter 7) – fundamentally, excessive alcohol intake creates GABA, serotonin, endorphin and dopamine deficiencies. This chapter is therefore very important to help you understand why you need amino acids to heal your brain.

- Balance Your Blood Sugar to Gain Energy and Reduce Cravings (Chapter 11) – most heavy drinkers have blood sugar problems and strong sugar cravings. This chapter will help you keep your blood sugar level.

- How to Get a Good Night's Sleep (Chapter 13) – alcohol disturbs sleep therefore you are very likely to be sleep deprived and REM-sleep deprived. This chapter will give you guidelines on getting a good night's sleep.

- Rejuvenate Your Liver (Chapter 15) – by improving your liver's ability to detoxify and regenerate, you can heal your liver of the damage caused by alcohol.

- Get the Past Out of Your Future (Chapter 18) – alcohol is often used as a means of avoiding life issues (particularly in alcoholics) and many people gain enormous benefit from help in unravelling these.

- Find New Pleasure in Life by Raising Endorphins (Chapter 16) – by exercising regularly, your energy level will go up, thereby reducing your 'need' for alcohol.

▶ HOW TO QUIT alcoholism

1. As we pointed out in the warning on page 312, if you are addicted to alcohol, you should not quit drinking on your own. Withdrawal from alcohol can be serious and even life-threatening. The detoxification process should be medically supervised so seek help from your doctor in the first instance and then you can follow our programme. The usual method of detoxing from alcohol is to use a longer acting sedative drug in decreasing doses to reduce discomfort and the risk of seizures and/or death.

2. After medical detox, intravenous (IV) nutrient therapy to relieve alcoholic abstinence symptoms is extremely effective (see Chapter 30). In fact, we have found it more successful when used with alcohol addiction than with any other addiction. At present it is not widely available in the UK (though this situation should soon improve) but if you can access this therapy, we highly recommend it.

3. We recommend you attend an addiction treatment centre, inpatient or outpatient, whichever is appropriate for you. In addiction treatment you will receive education about alcoholism and recovery, and addiction-specific counselling.

4. Become part of an Alcoholics Anonymous group where you can meet other recovering alcoholics, who will give you support and encouragement.

In addition to these recommendations you should also follow all those that apply to alcohol abusers – see pages 314–16.

How you might feel when you quit

When an alcoholic chooses to abstain, early withdrawal symptoms can become severe and can last up to ten days. Symptoms include tremors, loss of appetite, sweating, nausea and vomiting, agitation, low stress tolerance, hyperactivity of the nervous system, confusion, hallucinations, disorientation, seizures, delirium and in rare instances death.

Once the symptoms of acute withdrawal subside, other abstinence symptoms begin to emerge and persist into long-term recovery. The most pronounced abstinence symptoms for alcoholism are hypersensitivity, confusion, difficulty concentrating, memory problems, sleep problems, depression and anxiety.

What to expect 30 days later

It takes, on average, about 30 days to recover and normalise your brain's chemistry. Of course, this depends greatly on whether alcohol is your only addiction – whether you are an abuser or alcohol dependent – as well as the severity of your addiction if you are dependent. If you've been using a variety of addictive substances for years, our advice would be to stick to this kind of recovery programme for at least 90 days.

Otherwise, provided your Scale of Abstinence Symptoms Severity score has dropped by two-thirds (see Chart Your Progress on page 385), stop the Alcohol and Sleep Prescriptions but continue taking the Basic Supplements.

23.

SLEEPING PILLS AND BENZODIAZEPINES: HOW TO SLEEP WELL WITHOUT THEM

Tranquillisers and sleeping pills are some of the most widely prescribed drugs, and are often given to people to help them cope with the withdrawal symptoms they are suffering after they have quit other substances. Unfortunately, these too create dependency and can be exceptionally difficult to get off, as we explained in Chapter 6. Before we start talking about sleeping pills and benzodiazepines (called benzos), perhaps we should tell you what we mean when we use these terms. Sleeping pills, as you would expect, are any prescription medication intended to help you go to sleep or stay asleep. Benzos are sleeping pills. But that is not their only use. They are also prescribed for anxiety. The most commonly prescribed of these drugs are diazepam, lorazepam, temazepam, zopiclone and zolpidem. Of these lorazepam and temazepam are the more addictive, because they are shorter acting than diazepam. So, in this chapter we are talking about a variety of kinds of drugs with a wide range of addictiveness and severity of withdrawal. Although these drugs need to be tapered off very slowly with medical supervision, the nutritional support recommended in this chapter and our How to Quit Action Plan can greatly reduce your abstinence symptoms and improve your chances of success.

Did you start taking a benzo drug or a prescription sleeping pill or tranquilliser because you couldn't sleep, or because of extreme anxiety, or both? Did you intend to take them for a short period of time until your anxiety or inability to sleep subsided but found it too difficult to stop taking them? It might be that you were prescribed them because of anxiety you were having when you quit another addictive substance.

Despite having a long charge sheet of side effects,[14] these drugs still regularly feature in the top 20 most-prescribed drugs both in the UK and the US. Not only that, but they aren't very useful according to a report in the *British Medical Journal*,[15] which concluded that there is plenty of evidence that they cause 'major harm' and that there was 'little evidence of clinically meaningful benefit'.

What benzos and sleeping pills do

Benzodiazepines work by attaching to the GABA receptor site like neurotransmitters and can have an effect on the brain similar to the brain's own neurotransmitters. However, when benzos are used to take the place of GABA for an extended period of time, the body begins to reduce production of GABA. This can create a GABA deficiency in the brain. The function of GABA includes calming the brain and reducing stress, tension and anxiety.

Some of the benzodiazepines are among the most addictive of all substances. In our experience, they are the most difficult to get off once addicted.

CAUTION Benzodiazepines are so addictive and the withdrawal so severe that you should ***never*** under any circumstances quit taking them abruptly ('cold turkey'), because this can be life threatening.

This caution is essential for the benzos. Seizures are not uncommon. You should *always* be under medical supervision and taper them off very gradually, over months (see Resources for CITA charts, which tell you exactly how to do this for each drug).

How you might feel when you quit

If you reduce your medication too fast, you will feel confused, depressed, anxious, panicky and lacking in coordination, and be unable to remember things; you will experience an extreme inability to sleep and, consequently, daytime drowsiness. Another problem is ataxia: a loss of balance, and internal and external tremors and shakiness. For many people these symptoms may last for years.

Even the Zs, such as zolpidem or Zimovane, can be very addictive for some. For these sensitive people, taking the tablets for as little as two weeks leads to tolerance, so that they need more. The experience of needing more to get the same effect, hence experiencing more anxiety and less ability to sleep, and almost immediate withdrawal symptoms, is a strong motivator to get out of this vicious cycle. But being motivated to quit and successfully quitting are not the same thing.

The non-benzos are not quite so bad, but you still need nutritional support, as Pauline found out:

Case study PAULINE

Pauline was prescribed Zimovane, but managed to come off it with a carefully balanced nutritional plan. As she explains: 'After a very bad viral infection my doctor put me on Zimovane because I needed to sleep. I remained on it. I tried so many times to come off it and failed. Once I didn't take any for three days, couldn't sleep and drove into the back of a car! I decided I wanted to come off it and followed your advice. I took a supplement containing 5-HTP, B vitamins and magnesium, plus some valerian and soon

I was off Zimovane. To this day I still take these nutrients and I feel great. Goodbye Zimovane!'

Bear in mind that it is quite common, as you quit benzos and Zs drugs, to have panic attacks in which you think a symptom of anxiety, such as a raised heartbeat, is a heart attack. Your panicky mind thinks of the most catastrophic interpretation of what you are feeling which, of course, feeds back into the anxiety you are feeling. The amino acid glycine, put under the tongue, is often the best remedy for reducing panic attacks (see page 324).

Do you need to quit completely?

If you are addicted to any of these medications, you will not be able to take them in small amounts for very long. You have probably already found that they lose their effectiveness and you need to take more and more to get the intended effect. The only solution to this problem is to stop taking them and find other remedies for your sleeplessness and anxiety. If you can keep the amount you take to a low dose and not increase it over time, you may not need to quit completely. But these drugs are so addictive that we believe you should try safer options to get the effects that these powerful and addictive drugs are used for.

▶ HOW TO QUIT sleeping pills and benzodiazepines

You need to have proper medically supervised slow drug withdrawal, but your symptoms will be greatly reduced by following our How to Quit Action Plan. Usually this gradual tapering of the more addictive and potentially dangerous benzos such as Xanax involves gradually replacing them with a less addictive and longer acting benzodiazepine such as Valium and then slowly reducing the Valium over a period of two to six months. If you are addicted to Valium, this is usually tapered off, again over a period of months. It is very important that you do this with the supervision of a doctor well experienced in taking people off benzodiazepines.

WARNING Many doctors are experienced in prescribing benzos, but not taking people off them. Tapering off these drugs is so important that it is perfectly acceptable to ask your doctor to take you off gradually over a period of months. If he or she is not experienced in doing this, ask if they would refer you to someone who is, or contact CITA (see Resources) who specialise in helping people to come off these drugs.

Use the following guidelines alongside our How to Quit Action Plan in Part 4.

1. One week before beginning to reduce your dosage, take the Basic Supplements (page 388).

2. Take the Chill-out Prescription (page 420). This provides vital nutrients for you, including GABA, which is depleted in the brain by benzodiazepines. GABA is available over the counter in the US, but in the UK you will need a prescription. An alternative to GABA is taurine, which encourages the brain to make GABA. Start with 1g, which will probably mean 2 × 500mg of taurine, increasing to 1g three times daily if needed for anxiety, tension or sleep. Some people respond well to glutamine, the precursor of GABA. All these nutrients are part of, and clearly explained in the Chill-out Prescription. The prescription also includes niacin, thought to have a similar relaxing effect, and magnesium. Niacinamide (a form of niacin that does not make you flush or blush) has a benzodiazepine-like effect in large doses, but is not addictive.[16]

3. Be kind to yourself. Don't do anything or take on anything that is stressful for you because, as you detox, your ability to deal with stress anxiety is vastly compromised. Create a low-key and stress-free life, pampering yourself as much as you can through the detox phase.

3. Glycine is another calming amino acid and neurotransmitter. If you feel a panic attack coming on, take glycine under the tongue. Break two to four capsules of glycine 500mg and swill it under your tongue for at least one minute before swallowing with water. You can do this three to five times with five-minute intervals if you continue to panic. Don't exceed 10g of glycine a day.

4. If you have trouble falling asleep, consider taking the well-known anxiety-relieving sleep aid, standardised valerian, but only under medical supervision. As we've said, valerian is a great help in the process of withdrawal. A GABA enhancer, it will have similar actions to benzos, but is much gentler and doesn't have the same addictive potential. The same is true for kava, although this has now been voluntarily withdrawn from the UK market pending investigation into its safety. The idea is that you gradually reduce the benzo dose while increasing valerian, but it's best to seek professional help from a qualified nutritional therapist while doing this.

CAUTION Since benzodiazepines, alcohol and valerian all enhance GABA, the combination of the herb with benzo drugs or alcohol can make the drug's effects more potent. For this reason, valerian should be viewed in the same way as any medicine and taken in carefully scheduled doses as part of the medically super-vised withdrawal programme. In other words, you should not just add them in yourself. It is also helpful to add supplements that support the liver's ability to detoxify these drugs, such as stan-dardised milk thistle (*Silybum marianum*), 120mg three times a day. This liver-enhancing herb helps to speed up the metabolism of benzos while protecting the liver. Generally, as we gradually decrease the benzo dose, we gradually increase the amount of valerian, replacing the drug with the herb. Since valerian is not addictive and does not build tolerance, the person doesn't have to be weaned off it later. The effective dose range for standardised valerian is 280mg two to three times daily. You must take it for at least eight weeks to get maximum benefits.

You need to support your liver. Since the liver is responsible for breaking down these drugs, improving your liver function helps you detoxify the drug (see Chapter 15).

Using the 12 Keys to Unaddicting Your Brain

The most important keys from Part 2 for you are:

- Rebalance Your Brain with Amino Acids (Chapter 7) – fundamentally, sleeping-pill or tranquilliser addiction creates GABA deficiency or inefficiency, hence the most vital step is restoring your ability to make GABA and have it work effectively for you.

- Rebuild Your Brain with Essential Fats (Chapter 10) – here you'll find advice to help your brain recover more quickly.

- How to Get a Good Night's Sleep (Chapter 13) – the best cure for anxiety is a good night's sleep, and this chapter contains gems to help you achieve this.

- Rejuvenate Your Liver (Chapter 15) – by improving your liver's ability to detoxify and regenerate you can get over dependency to these drugs faster.

What to expect 30 days later

If you do all this and feel fine 30 days later, or have a two-thirds drop in your key abstinence symptoms (see Chart Your Progress on page 385), well done! You can stop the Chill-out Prescription. However, with benzo withdrawal, this is unfortunately rare. It is more likely that you'll need these supplemental nutrients for a good three months, if not six. As far as benzos are concerned get ready for the long haul.

24.

ANTIDEPRESSANTS:
HOW TO BOOST YOUR MOOD
WITHOUT DRUGS

Antidepressants are routinely prescribed to people suffering from depression, even though they can be highly addictive and have a long list of unpleasant side effects, as we explained in Chapter 6. Withdrawal symptoms can be so bad that sufferers become caught in a trap of dependency and discomfort. Although you must taper off these drugs with the help of a medical practitioner, this chapter explains how our How to Quit Action Plan will help you to succeed while minimising your abstinence symptoms.

Why did you begin taking antidepressants? Perhaps it was because of a life situation, such as a loss of some kind, and you thought that taking antidepressants would be temporary until you were feeling better. Unfortunately, many people then find they can't stop taking them without experiencing withdrawal symptoms or abstinence symptoms.

Perhaps you began taking antidepressants because you were diagnosed as being clinically depressed. However, even though they worked for you at first, eventually they lost their effectiveness and you found yourself not only depressed but also addicted.

It may be that depression was an abstinence symptom that you experienced as a result of getting off another addictive substance, and not knowing this you sought medical help and were prescribed an antidepressant. Now you've traded one addiction for another.

The trouble is that most antidepressant drugs create their own problems. They carry a potential increased risk of suicide, an increased risk of cardiovascular disease, and an increased risk of bone loss and bone fractures. There is also an increased risk of bleeding in your gut (by up to 600 per cent) if the antidepressant is taken with painkillers.

Long term, they are really not that effective.

Antidepressants don't work 30 to 40 per cent of the time, and when they do work, on average, there is only about a 50 per cent reduction in the depression. One study found that 60 per cent of people who continued to take them for two years had a return of their depression while on the drug, compared to only 8 per cent who stopped the drug.[17] Cognitive behaviour therapy (CBT) worked much better. So, why take the risks associated with antidepressants?

Perhaps your desire to quit using an antidepressant is due to these concerns or perhaps you have experienced side effects.

What antidepressants do

Up to a quarter of the people taking antidepressants experience side effects, the milder ones including nausea, vomiting, malaise, dizziness and headaches or migraines. Prozac, the original market leader and prescribed to more than 38 million people worldwide, has 45 listed side effects – and more: if you're under the age of 25, there is the increased risk of suicide, as we have seen, and there can also be severe withdrawal problems, in particular with SSRI antidepressants.

How you might feel when you quit

The most common withdrawal symptoms are balance problems, flu-like symptoms, blurred vision, irritability, tingling sensations, uncontrollable crying, diarrhoea, vivid dreams, nervousness and sleeping problems. Some people continue to experience these symptoms for up to a month. Without any nutritional support the depression that was the reason for starting antidepressants in the first place is likely to return along with other long-term abstinence symptoms. This can be avoided with the correct nutritional support.

Do you need to quit completely?

In the long run, yes – particularly for those who find the drugs lose their effectiveness and they need to take more and more to get the intended effect. The only solution to this is to find other remedies for your depression and associated symptoms. Those who can keep the amount they take to a low dose and not increase it over time may not need to quit completely. However, we believe you should try natural ways to get the effects – without the side effects – that these drugs are used for.

▶ HOW TO QUIT antidepressants

Much of what we recommend in our How to Quit Action Plan you can do for yourself or with the guidance and support of a nutritional therapist. However, the process of weaning yourself off antidepressants is something you must do with the support and guidance of your doctor. Ask your doctor to wean you off gradually.

Use the following guidelines alongside our How to Quit Action Plan in Part 4.

1. A week before you begin reducing your antidepressant, start taking the Basic Supplements (page 388).

2. Take the Mood Prescription. This will provide a variety of important nutrients, including B vitamins and essential fats. To boost your intake of essential fats further, eat oily fish three times a week. For some people, fish oil can be miraculous. Alice is a case in point.

Case study **ALICE**

Thirty-year-old Alice had a long history of irritability, anxiety, depression, sleep problems and multiple drug abuse. She entered the clinic on an SSRI antidepressant, Ambien, for sleep, and a tranquilliser, neither of which were helping her much. She was tested for essential fat status using red blood cell membranes, which showed profound omega-3 fat deficiency. In her case she had six days of IV nutrient therapy (see Chapter 30) followed by a low-GL Mediterranean-style diet, supplements, including fish oil and flaxseed oil, and the Sleep Prescription (page 397). She was able to give up all medication and was sleeping well, depression- and anxiety-free after only 28 days. (Incidentally, she had been following a strict low-fat diet before coming for therapy. Low-fat diets among people already omega-3 deficient are dangerous diets to follow.)

3. The Mood Prescription offers the choice of supplementing tryptophan or 5-HTP, however, we recommend that 5-HTP not be taken in significant amounts (above 50mg) if you are on an antidepressant. 5-HTP helps the body make serotonin whereas SSRI antidepressants stop it being broken down. If your doctor is willing to wean you off antidepressants, it helps if you are weaned onto 5-HTP at the same time, gradually building the daily amount up to a maximum of 300mg, but no more than 100mg before you are completely off the

antidepressant. In our experience, this minimises and short-
ens the withdrawal effects that many people experience
when coming off antidepressants. Alternatively, don't take
any 5-HTP until you have stopped the antidepressant drug
completely. Then take 200mg a day. Two of the hardest to
come off are the SSRI, Seroxat, and the new SNRI drug,
Efexor. The withdrawal symptoms are longer lasting and the
drugs are best tapered off gradually over at least three
months. Other antidepressants, such as Lustral (Sertraline)
and Prozac, can be tapered off over a week or two.

4. Make sure you are on a low-GL diet by following our How
   to Quit Diet strictly.

5. The mineral chromium, which is included in the Mood Prescription, helps relieve depression in those with carb cravings
   who are suffering with excessive sleepiness and grogginess at
   the same time.

6. Faulty methylation (the process that makes the brain's neurotransmitters from amino acids) is very strongly linked with
   depression. Do check your blood homocysteine level, which
   can be done using a home test kit (see Resources). The Mood
   Prescription will help bring your level down in the likely
   event that it is high but you should also eat more greens,
   beans, nuts and seeds, as these are rich sources of folate.

7. Exercise is a proven mood booster (see Chapter 16) and
   recent research suggests it can even stimulate the building of
   new brain cells.[18] Sunlight and vitamin D, which is made
   from cholesterol in the skin in the sun, makes a big difference.
   So exercise outdoors regularly and make sure your multivitamin gives you at least 15mcg of vitamin D. If not, and if
   you are prone to depression in the winter, supplement up to
   50mcg a day.

8. Counselling also works, so make sure you have the support of a good counsellor as you come off antidepressants. Often depression is really about unexpressed anger and childhood trauma.

9. Sometimes depression is a symptom of an unidentified food allergy, wheat gluten being one of the most common offending foods. You can test yourself with a home-test kit (see Resources).

10. Sometimes depression is a symptom of an underactive thyroid. Discuss with your doctor a trial period of a low level of thyroxine if you have the following symptoms: you are still exhausted all the time, have a problem with dry skin, constipation and sensitivity to cold, and are also unable to lose weight, even if your blood test is apparently normal, although at the low end of the scale.

11. Some herbs work well for some people. The most popular is standardised St John's wort. When taken alone, it is safe and has few side effects. However, it should not be taken in conjunction with prescription antidepressants.

12. Some people report great results with the herb *Rhodiola rosea*.[19] Try 200 to 300mg twice daily, one early in the morning and the other early in the afternoon, of a standardised extract of 3 per cent rosavins and 0.8–1 per cent salidroside with meals. *Rhodiola rosea* should be taken early in the day because it may interfere with sleep if taken late in the day. If you become overly active, jittery or agitated, then a smaller dose with very gradual increases might be needed. It shouldn't be taken if you are restless, agitated or overly tense, nervous or excited.

Using the 12 Keys to Unaddicting Your Brain

The most important keys from Part 2 for you are:

- Rebalance Your Brain with Amino Acids (Chapter 7) – a lack of serotonin makes you feel depressed, irritable and agitated, whereas a lack of tyrosine gives you low motivation as well as depression. This chapter explains how getting the correct amino acids can get you functioning again.

- Raise Your Methyl IQ with Vitamins and Minerals (Chapter 9) – it's important to understand the role that high homocysteine plays in depression. This chapter provides that knowledge.

- Rebuild Your Brain with Essential Fats (Chapter 10) – if you generally don't eat oily fish or seeds, or have been on a low-fat diet, there's a very good chance that you are essential-fat deficient and will experience a considerable boost from fish plus supplemental fish oils.

- Balance Your Blood Sugar to Gain Energy and Reduce Cravings (Chapter 11) – don't underestimate the power of keeping your blood sugar even. You'll find lots of tips and guidance on this important factor in maintaining equilibrium throughout the day.

What to expect 30 days later

There's a good chance, once you've followed all these factors, that you won't be feeling depressed after 30 days. Most of these nutritional approaches work within days, not months. If your Scale of Abstinence Symptoms Severity score has dropped by two-thirds you could stop the Mood Prescription and continue with the Basic Supplements. We are all different; in this first month you may have found out what works best for you. If so, stick with it.

25.

CANNABIS: HOW TO TUNE IN AND CHILL OUT WITHOUT IT

Cannabis is the most widely used illicit drug in the UK and US. In Ireland, one in ten teenagers surveyed recently were using marijuana daily. This included teenagers as young as 14.

It is one of the more controversial substances in the addiction list. Not all authorities agree that it is addictive, although most do, especially with heavy daily use. Many people smoke it occasionally without any evidence of addiction but, for some, it becomes a daily necessity.

What cannabis does

The effects are quite different from one person to another. You may have started using and continued to use because, like some people with ADHD-type symptoms, you have found that a joint helps quiet the hypersensitivity to sights, sounds and stress that we spoke about on page 22 and helps you to chill out or sleep. Perhaps it helps you relax and sleep.

Over time you might have noticed a decrease in your memory and a loss of drive or motivation in life. You might have become more anxious and occasionally paranoid. You may have noticed that it triggers a lowering of your mood, even depression. You might have heard about the potential brain damage from continued use. Chronic coughing and recurring lung infections may have become more frequent and severe if you are a heavy user. You may have become addicted, especially if you smoke the extra-strong hybrid, skunk, which is many times stronger than regular cannabis.

How you might feel when you quit

An increasing number of studies have surfaced, indicating that some marijuana users experience withdrawal effects when they try to quit, and that these effects should be considered by clinicians treating people with problems related to heavy marijuana use.[20]

Recently, and for the first time, tobacco and marijuana withdrawal syndromes have been compared. A group of researchers at Johns Hopkins University reported that withdrawal from the use of marijuana is similar to what is experienced by people when they quit smoking cigarettes. Abstinence from each of these two drugs appears to cause several common symptoms, such as irritability, anger and trouble sleeping – based on self-reporting in a recent study of 12 heavy users of both marijuana and cigarettes. Overall, withdrawal severity scores associated with marijuana alone and tobacco alone were of similar frequency and intensity. Sleep disturbance seemed to be more pronounced during marijuana abstinence, whereas some of the general mood effects (anxiety and anger) seemed to be greater during tobacco abstinence.

If you just quit without nutritional support you may feel sleepy, unmotivated, a bit down and irritable and possibly have difficulty sleeping. Some people report feeling anxious, others feel more anger and aggression. However, if you smoke joints, the chances are you have become addicted to nicotine and/or alcohol as well. So, some of your withdrawal effects may be due to smoking or drinking less. They tend to be short-lived and may last up to a week. However, in those with lingering brain chemistry imbalances, the withdrawal and abstinence symptoms last much longer.

Exactly why cannabis has its effects and withdrawal symptoms is complex. It affects, and generally depletes, acetylcholine, the memory neurotransmitter. It also affects dopamine and nora-drenalin, which are motivating and make you feel good.

Do you really need to quit completely?

Probably yes, in any event for 90 days. Only that way will you experience the benefits of restoring your brain's chemistry. If you have other addictions, and have resolved all of them, then occasionally (no more than a couple of times a month) you may want to have neat cannabis, no tobacco. There's no clear evidence of harm. However, you run the danger of getting hooked on tobacco again, and whatever else might go with cannabis use. It's also illegal.

▶ **HOW TO QUIT** cannabis

Use the following guidelines alongside our How to Quit Action Plan in Part 4.

1. One week before you quit, start taking the Basic Supplements (page 388).

2. Don't quit cannabis and cigarettes at the same time. Quit one and then quit the other. See Chapter 21 for how to quit cigarettes.

3. Take the Mood Prescription (page 416). Amongst other things this contains essential fats, especially omega-3, essential for normal mood, motivation and memory.

4. Most of the withdrawal symptoms from cannabis have to do with neurotransmitter depletion and imbalance. Since acetylcholine is affected you need more phospholipids, especially phosphatidylcholine. The Basic Supplements (page 388), provide some phospholipids, but we also recommend you have either 2 teaspoonfuls of lecithin or two 1,200mg capsules of lecithin each day for a month and include an egg yolk in your daily diet.

5. If you do feel dopey, tired and unmotivated after quitting, we recommend the Stimulant Prescription (page 403). Among other key nutrients, this contains tyrosine (the amino acid precursor of dopamine and noradrenalin).

6. If your main symptoms after quitting are anxiety or irritability and an inability to sleep you may benefit from more 5-HTP or tryptophan (see the Sleep Prescription on page 397 for details). If you suffer from overactivity, restlessness, poor concentration and impulsivity, take 10mg NADH, 1g of fish oil twice a day, eat unfried oily fish three times a week, and consider hidden (IgG) food allergy testing (see Chapter 14).

7. Cannabis affects your blood sugar balance – hence feeling hungry ('the munchies'). Therefore, it is vital for you to become a master of keeping your blood sugar level even by following our low-GL How to Quit Diet.

8. As you are smoking less, it's important to stimulate your lungs with some clean air, as well as getting some endorphin-boosting, cortisol-reducing exercise. So, go for walks or jogs outside, gradually building up your endurance.

Using the 12 Keys to Unaddicting Your Brain

The most important keys from Part 2 for you are:

- Rebalance Your Brain with Amino Acids (Chapter 7) – here you will find out how your symptoms are all to do with dopamine and opioid shut-down and which specific amino acids will get your brain back on track.

- Rebuild Your Brain with Essential Fats (Chapter 10) – by optimising your intake of the brain's essential fats you can help to undo the damage and get your memory and concentration back.

- Balance Your Blood Sugar to Gain Energy and Reduce Cravings (Chapter 11) – by learning how to eat to keep your blood sugar, and your energy level even, you'll have less cravings for cannabis.

What to expect 30 days later

It takes, on average, about 30 days to recover and normalise your brain's chemistry and blood sugar balance. If you've been using a variety of addictive substances for years, our advice would be to stick to this kind of recovery programme for at least 90 days.

Otherwise, provided your Scale of Abstinence Symptoms Severity score has dropped by two-thirds (see Chart Your Progress on page 385), stop the Prescriptions, but keep taking the Basic Supplements. By now you'll know the effects of the other temporary supplements such as 5-HTP. Reduce or stop these according to your need.

26.

COCAINE, AMPHETAMINES AND OTHER STIMULANTS: KICK-START YOUR BRAIN WITHOUT DRUGS

Whether you currently use cocaine or have used it in the past but still don't feel great, our How to Quit programme can really help you feel good without the need for alternative stimulants, including caffeine and cigarettes. Being one of the most potent stimulants, cocaine takes its toll on your brain's chemical balance. Simply quitting doesn't get you back to feeling normal. Many people start using a stimulant like cocaine or amphetamines to get high with friends. You might have found that it made you more alert and gave you more energy while giving you more of a buzz out of life. Perhaps you used it as an antidote to boredom. Did that high energy, euphoria and stimulation keep you going, at your peak – a high flyer at work and play? You probably loved that full-on engagement. You felt more fearless and 'happy'. You could go for days without much hunger or sleep.

Perhaps you preferred crack cocaine to snorting cocaine, or started freebasing (smoking cocaine). Crack or freebasing provides a blast of euphoria in about five seconds, because the cocaine is absorbed immediately into the bloodstream. The rush is more intense, but the effects do not last as long. For many people this quick high is near impossible to resist.

Is your stimulant of choice an amphetamine (dexedrine, methamphetamine, Ritalin)? Amphetamines have actions similar to cocaine but with longer acting effects. Both amphetamines and cocaine stimulate the central nervous system. Cocaine is an ingredient from a plant (coca), whereas amphetamines are synthetic (made from other chemicals). Methamphetamines can also come intravenously and in a smokable form known as ice or crack.

Most worrying is the escalation in prescriptions of stimulant drugs such as Ritalin, which can also be abused for their stimulant effect. Another common recreational substance of abuse is Ecstasy or MDMA (methylenedioxy-N-methylamphetamine). Ecstasy is chemically related to amphetamines but has different effects on brain chemistry. It produces a dreamy euphoria with an anti-fatigue effect and users take it to enhance the sensation of music and to produce excessive energy. Ecstasy can be very dangerous when used in high doses (which it usually is when used by young people in large group settings).

What amphetamines and other stimulants do

Whatever your stimulant of choice, the chances are you have very quickly found your life spiralling out of control. In addition to the risk and consequences of taking an illegal substance, there has probably been a breakdown of your working life, relationships and finances, or your physical health. You'll have quickly noticed that the high wasn't nearly as high as it used to be and you're extremely agitated if you don't get your fix. You've probably become depressed, irritable and prone to bursts of anger. Having got more and more tired you may be finding it difficult to sleep through the night, or you oversleep – often with unpleasant dreams – which make you even more exhausted. You might have got to the point where your use is more about ending withdrawal symptoms than actually giving you pleasure. Since these stimulant drugs suppress appetite you may have lost weight, have become malnourished and damaged your health.

How you might feel when you quit

If you decide to quit with no nutritional support to restore your brain's chemistry, you are likely to experience depression, extreme agitation, sleeplessness or oversleeping, mood swings, anxiety, uncontrollable appetite, paranoia, exhaustion and the inability to think or act fast. You've gone from the fast lane to the slow lane. Your mood may also become flat where nothing feels pleasurable. This is called anhedonia and is a classic sign of dopamine depletion.

It takes about a week for acute withdrawal symptoms to pass, as the brain 'up-regulates' to make more and become more sensitive to dopamine. But without restoring brain function with optimum nutrition, you are likely to continue suffering from chronic abstinence symptoms, making you feel s**t while abstaining and making you prone to relapse.

New research also shows that there's another neurotransmitter called glutamate that, when depleted, increases the desire for cocaine. By supplementing N-acetyl cysteine (also known as NAC), which is an amino acid, brain glutamate levels increase and the desire for cocaine decreases.[21]

Do you need to quit completely?

Yes. Stimulants are very addictive and best avoided completely if you've ever had any addictive tendencies. Many people make the mistake of quitting for a few weeks then think they've cracked it.

▶ **HOW TO QUIT** cocaine, amphetamines and other stimulants

If you have a serious addiction to cocaine or amphetamines, we recommend that you get professional treatment as an inpatient, or at the very least, outpatient treatment where you will get help from people who understand addiction. In a treatment setting you will get education about your addiction and addiction-specific counselling.

Once you have quit completely (at this stage there is no such thing as occasional use), you need to change your friends and your circumstances. Some people join Cocaine Anonymous (CA) and meet other people committed to staying clean. As they say in CA, you need new playgrounds and playmates. You need to make a break from the kind of situations where you'll be offered a 'line'.

Use the following guidelines alongside our How to Quit Action Plan in Part 4.

1. Start taking the Basic Supplements (page 388) a week before you quit.

2. Follow our How to Quit Diet. You will have neglected your health and your diet, since these drugs are powerful appetite suppressants. Your health now needs attention, so it's time to have a crash course in healthy eating. This will quickly make you feel better and stronger.

3. The chances are if you use cocaine or crack, you smoke cigarettes, another dopamine-elevating stimulant and, ultimately, this is important to quit too. But, for now, at the very least, do not increase the amount you smoke and, ideally, keep it below ten a day. For the same reasons, you're probably a coffee drinker. Similarly, don't increase your caffeine intake and ideally keep to a maximum of two cups a day. After 30 days, work towards stopping coffee (Chapter 19) and then cigarettes when you are ready (Chapter 21).

4. Take 10–20g of oral vitamin C daily in divided doses (or up to 'bowel tolerance': the point where you get loose bowels) as a powder in water diluted one-third with juice. Take this for at least one month until you are through the worst of your withdrawal symptoms.

5. Take the Stimulant Prescription (page 403), which provides tyrosine, adaptogenic herbs and B vitamins, including pantothenic acid (vitamin B_5), needed for the adrenal glands. Also supplement N-acetyl cysteine (NAC) 500mg, three times a day during the first month of quitting.

6. If you are unable to relax or sleep, take the Sleep Prescription (page 397). If you can get it, take 1,000mg of GABA in the evening to help you relax.

Using IV

If you are able to access it, IV nutrient therapy makes the biggest and quickest difference. Withdrawal and abstinence symptoms go away rapidly, often after the first one or two IV sessions. IV therapy is discussed in Chapter 30.

Using the 12 Keys to Unaddicting Your Brain

The most important keys from Part 2 for you are:

- Rebalance Your Brain with Amino Acids (Chapter 7) – you are experiencing neurotransmitter deficiency and this chapter helps you understand your symptoms and why specific amino acids can help you recover quickly.

- How to Get a Good Night's Sleep (Chapter 13) – sleep is a great healer and the chances are you will be chronically sleep-deficient. In this chapter you'll learn how to sleep well.

- Balance Your Blood Sugar to Gain Energy and Reduce Cravings (Chapter 11) – energy comes from a stable blood sugar level and, feeling tired, you might find yourself craving sweet foods and drinks. This is just using sugar as a fix. Instead, find out how to up your energy naturally.

- Raise Your Methyl IQ with Vitamins and Minerals (Chapter 9) – this chapter tells you how to check your homocysteine level and why supplementing the key methyl nutrients (B_6, B_{12}, folic acid, TMG and zinc) improves your 'methyl IQ', and helps make neurotransmitters.

- Rebuild Your Brain with Essential Fats (Chapter 10) – the chances are your diet has been deficient, so guaranteeing a daily intake of the brain's essential fats will help you recover your natural energy and concentration.

- Generate Vital Energy: The Chi Factor (Chapter 17) – by learning how to do this you'll find a natural, clean energy that is much more centering than stimulants.

What to expect 30 days later

It takes, on average, about 30 days to recover and normalise your brain's chemistry and your blood sugar balance. Of course, this depends greatly on your previous level and length of abuse and whether you are still using caffeine or cigarettes. If you've been using a variety of addictive substances for years, our advice would be to stick to this kind of recovery programme for at least 90 days.

Otherwise, provided your Scale of Abstinence Symptoms Severity score has dropped by two-thirds (see Chart Your Progress on page 385), stop the Stimulant Prescription and extra GABA as needed, but keep taking the Basic Supplements. If you still feel tired, add 1g of tyrosine on an empty stomach.

27.

HEROIN AND PAINKILLERS (OPIOIDS): HOW TO ZONE IN INSTEAD OF OUT

Almost the opposite of cocaine, the attraction of heroin is to be completely relaxed, a total chill out. After an injection of heroin, the user has a 'rush' of intense euphoria, followed by alternately wakeful and drowsy states. Mental functioning becomes clouded due to the depression of the central nervous system. Heroin is used to relieve psychological and physical pain, to get away from the world and all its problems and to feel completely cocooned. It can be injected, smoked or sniffed/snorted. Injection is the most common and efficient means of getting the effects.

Whether you first took heroin to see what it was like – and loved it – or started using it to numb out and escape from painful circumstances in your life, it's hard to quit once you're addicted. Heroin is a highly addictive drug. Withdrawal symptoms can appear if heroin has been used continually for as little as three days and is then stopped abruptly. Apart from the risk of getting into trouble due to the illegality, you may have found that your health has gone downhill, as have your relationships, your career and your bank account. The potential consequences of heroin dependency – HIV/AIDS, hepatitis B and C, sexually transmitted diseases (STDs), pneumonia, tuberculosis, crime, violence, imprisonment, as well as disruptions in family, education and career – are devastating. On top of that, the more you have the more you need – and the less the pay-off; it's just not like it used to be. Our How to Quit Action Plan can help you to give up your dependency.

What heroin and other opioids do

Heroin is one drug in a group called opioids, derived from opiates (morphine and codeine). Heroin is a semi-synthetic opioid. Synthetic opioids are painkillers, such as oxycodone (OxyContin), hydrocodone (Vicodin) and meperidine (Demerol). Methadone is another synthetic opioid often used as a legal substitute for heroin that is as addictive as heroin. All opioids are addictive. The effects on your brain chemistry are relatively similar, resulting in low levels of dopamine and endorphins, resulting in pain and extreme discomfort on withdrawal.

How you might feel when you quit

If you just quit heroin or any other opioid abruptly ('cold turkey'), within six to 24 hours the withdrawal begins. The symptoms are often excruciating, including anxiety, depression, muscle cramping in the legs, insomnia, cold sweats, chills, severe muscle and bone aches, nausea and vomiting, diarrhoea, goose bumps and fever. Many users also complain of a painful condition, the so-called 'itchy blood', which often results in compulsive scratching that causes bruising and sometimes ruptures the skin, leaving scabs. These symptoms can be so intense that the desire to start using again is hard to resist. At its worst you feel like you're dying.

These withdrawal symptoms persist in the acute phase for up to 24 hours, although you will probably continue to feel abstinence symptoms for a month or longer. With withdrawal from methadone, the abstinence symptoms might continue for longer.

Do you need to quit completely?

Yes, if you are addicted. There is no social use.

▶ **HOW TO QUIT** heroin and painkillers (opioids)

Firstly, don't do it alone. You need professional support. Our recommendation is that you check into a good treatment clinic where you will be medically detoxed. As well as quitting you need to change your friends and your circumstances. Some people join Narcotics Anonymous (NA) and meet other people committed to staying clean. As they say in NA, you need new playgrounds and playmates. You need to make a break from the kind of situations where you'll be offered heroin.

With medical supervision, the nutritional support recommended in this chapter can greatly reduce your abstinence symptoms and improve your chances of success.

Use the following guidelines alongside our How to Quit Action Plan in Part 4.

1. One week in advance begin taking the Basic Supplements (page 388).

2. It is certain that your digestive system will be damaged, since heroin shuts down digestion, so you need a digestive-system tune up. As a consequence you'll be low in essential fats. Eating oily fish, seeds and supplements of omega-3 can help to heal the damage.[22] Read Chapter 8 and follow the Digestion Prescription (page 393) of our How to Quit Action Plan.

3. In terms of specific supplements, you need the Opiate Prescription (page 411). This contains D-phenylalanine, which is the amino acid that helps restore your brain's normal production of endorphins and enkephalins. It also contains natural relaxants (GABA or taurine/glutamine), magnesium and tryptophan or 5-HTP. If you want to enhance detoxification

and further lift your mood take NAC 500mg twice a day and turmeric 500mg twice a day with meals.

4. Two nutrients included in the Opiate Prescription are niacin (vitamin B_3) and vitamin C. You need these in very large amounts for a small period of time (see box below).

Wonderful vitamin C

Back in 1977 Dr Alfred Libby and Irwin Stone pioneered a detoxifying treatment for drug addicts using megadoses of vitamin C.[23] In one study involving 30 heroin addicts, they gave 30–85g a day and reported a 100 per cent success rate. Dr Abram Hoffer reported similar results in one week with ten heroin addicts using 50g of vitamin C combined with high-dose niacin. The Opiate Prescription contains high levels of vitamin C and niacin.

Using the 12 Keys to Unaddicting Your Brain

The most important keys from Part 2 for you are:

- Rebalance Your Brain with Amino Acids (Chapter 7) – here you will find out how your symptoms are all connected with dopamine and opioid shut-down and which specific amino acids will get your brain back on track.

- A Healthy Brain Needs a Healthy Gut (Chapter 8) – by restoring your gut's ability to digest and absorb, your improved diet and supplements will have a more positive effect.

- Rebuild Your Brain with Essential Fats (Chapter 10) – by optimising your intake of the brain's essential fats you can help to undo the damage.

- How to Get a Good Night's Sleep (Chapter 13) – sleep is a great healer, and learning how to sleep and to chill out without drugs is a key step to recovery.

___ **Using IV** _____

In an ideal world, every heroin addict who wants it would be able
to undergo six to ten days of IV nutrient therapy (see Chapter 30)
at a treatment clinic. The benefit of IV nutrient therapy is that it
speeds up recovery. However we still see great results in people
following our nutritional approach with the appropriate
supplements and diet.

- Get the Past Out of Your Future (Chapter 18) – although this
  might not be something you are immediately keen to be
  involved in, once you get your head clear and your health and
  strength back, there are likely to be issues in your life, and your
  past, that you've been avoiding. You are going to need some
  help unravelling these.

What to expect 30 days later

It takes, on average, about 30 days to recover and normalise
your brain's chemistry and blood sugar balance. Of course, this
depends greatly on your previous level and length of abuse and
whether you are still using alcohol as a downer or cigarettes. If
you've been using a variety of addictive substances for years, our
advice would be to stick to this kind of recovery programme for
at least 90 days.

Otherwise, provided your Scale of Abstinence Symptoms
Severity score has dropped by two-thirds (see Chart Your
Progress on page 385), stop the Opiate Prescription, but keep
taking the Basic Supplements.

PART 4

YOUR HOW TO QUIT ACTION PLAN: A 12-WEEK PROGRAMME

Knowing what to do and doing it are two different things. This action part of the programme lets you know exactly how to quit and recover your health and happiness with minimum abstinence symptoms. We provide a precise diet for you to follow or, if you prefer, you can use the guidelines to work out your own personal eating programme. You'll find guidance on supplements, all the prescriptions referred to in Part 2 and 3 and how you can chart your progress.

The vast majority of people will recover from their addiction within 12 weeks, although those with a minor addiction may take just four weeks, and some addictions, from which you need to taper gradually, may take longer. We explain how you can then decide whether you are ready to move on to the maintenance programme to continue with your recovery. As each person is different, the maintenance phase will begin at different times for everybody. We also look at repeated IV nutrient therapy, which is particularly suited to those with serious long-term addictions.

Of course there is much more to recovery than what you put into your body. With this in mind we also suggest some simple lifestyle changes that will help, as well as how to find the help and support you need to become free from addiction.

If you have not already read the relevant chapter in Part 3 that explains about your own addiction, do that before following the recommendations here.

28.

THE HOW TO QUIT DIET

In Part 2 we introduced you to the key principles of our How to Quit Diet. These key principles will create a diet for you that:

- Gives you high-quality protein three times a day (three 20g servings ideally).

- Keeps your blood sugar level even (low GL).

- Provides essential fats and phospholipids, including fish and eggs.

- Encourages you to include foods rich in cold-pressed omega-3 and 6 essential fats, such as raw nuts and seeds, as well as oils such as flax, walnut, pumpkin, sesame and sunflower, plus extra-virgin olive oil for salads and olive oil or coconut oil for cooking.

- Avoids all damaged and processed fats, including trans fats and deep-fried food. (Fats become oxidised, or damaged, by high heat; trans fats are found in many shop-bought convenience foods).

- Provides lots of antioxidants from fresh fruit and vegetables.

- Requires you to drink eight glasses of water a day.

It is not, however, a deprivation diet. We do not ask you to restrict your calories, only to eat nutrient-rich unprocessed foods. You will not go hungry or lack delicious, tasty and satisfying meals and snacks. There are two ways to do it: by following our menus, or by following our principles and creating your own diet. Whatever you decide, read this chapter so that you understand the principles behind the recipes – you can then invent your own recipes and menus.

One-week How to Quit menu plan

Opposite is a list of seven breakfasts, lunches and dinners to make up a complete week (which you can repeat as necessary). The recipes for these meals are given on pages 357–74. Every day you need to choose one of each, or stick to this One-week Menu Plan as we have arranged it. The lunches and dinners are interchangeable. You must, however, have unfried, preservative-free oily fish three times a week (these recipes have a fish symbol next to them).

All the recipes come from the *Holford Low-GL Diet*. You will also find lots of other delicious recipes there, as well as in the *Holford Low-GL Cookbook*, *Optimum Nutrition Cookbook* and *Food GLorious Food* (by Patrick Holford and Fiona McDonald Joyce).

Watch out for allergens

Please note that if you have tested allergic to a food, such as wheat or milk, you must avoid these foods strictly for three months. In the recipes that follow simply use soya milk or soya yogurt instead of cow's milk, if you are allergic, and oatcakes instead of bread if you're allergic to wheat. The cookbooks mentioned above give plenty of allergen-free recipes, and ways to adapt them to be allergen-free.

> **B**reakfast is your most important meal of the day.

Breakfasts

Boiled Egg on Wholegrain Rye Toast

Low-GL Muesli

Scots Porridge

Fruit Yogurt or Yogurt Shake

Smoked Salmon with Scrambled Egg on Toast

Get Up & Go with fresh fruit (berries are best)

Wholegrain Rye Toast with Nut Butter

Lunches

Sardines on Toast

Beany Vegetable Soup

Rice, Tuna and Petits Pois Salad

Green Bean, Olive and Roasted Pepper Salad

Hot-smoked Fish with Avocado

Low-GL Sandwich (with a choice of fillings)

Low-GL Baked Potato or Sweet Potato

Dinners

Spiced Turkey Meatballs

Fajitas

Pasta with Pumpkin Seed Pesto

Chilli

Sticky Mustard Salmon Fillets

Thai Green Curry

Sweet Potato and Red Onion Tortilla

Snacks

In the same way as it is vital that you eat breakfast every day, it is also vital that you have two snacks: one mid-morning and one mid-afternoon. In this way you are eating 'little and often'. Grazing in this way, rather than gorging, is much better for keeping your blood sugar level even and cravings under control.

The snack rules

- Always combine protein with carbohydrate. See chart opposite.

- Have at least one whole, fresh fruit snack a day.

- Have a tablespoonful of Essential Seed Mix (page 357) on your wholegrain cereal each day or a small handful of raw seeds and nuts, either on your cereal or as part of a snack.

Drinks

The single most important drink is water. You need to drink eight glasses of water a day, ideally filtered or mineral water, but tap water is not bad.

You can have your water as herbal teas, or even green tea, but there is a limit. Whatever substance you are giving up, you will gain the best health, and freedom from disease, if you also give up caffeine. Having said this, we'll be kind. You can have:

- Either one cup of black tea a day;

- Or three cups of green tea a day, using the same tea bag;

- Or two cups of decaf tea a day;

This is because there is evidence that tea lowers the adrenal hormone cortisol, and helps you to relax,[1] whereas coffee raises it.

SNACK COMBOS

Below are ten snack combos for you to choose from.

Protein	Carbohydrate
1 small handful of mixed unsalted nuts (about 8 nuts) such as almonds, walnuts, cashew nuts, macadamia, Brazil nuts	1 whole apple or pear or 2 satsumas
1 tbsp nut or seed butter (no-added-sugar peanut or cashew, or tahini spread)	1 thin slice wholegrain rye bread or 100% wholegrain bread
50g (1¾oz) feta or goat's cheese	3 rough oatcakes
150g (5½oz/½ small pot) low-fat cottage cheese	1 corn on the cob
1 handful mixed raw seeds (sunflower, pumpkin, sesame, linseed/flax seeds)	2 plums or 1 nectarine/peach
½ × 200g (7oz) tub hummus	carrot and celery crudités
150g (5½oz/1 small pot) natural yogurt	½ × 300g (11oz) pack of berries (strawberries, blueberries, raspberries, blackberries)
½ × 125g (4½oz) can of tuna with salsa	1 wholewheat tortilla
1 tbsp of pumpkin seeds ½ grilled free-range or organic chicken breast fillet (no skin)	6 small pieces of dark chocolate (70% cocoa solids, very small bar)
½ × 125g (4½oz) can oily fish (mackerel, sardines, herring, salmon)	3 rough oatcakes

Otherwise it is herbal teas or coffee alternatives. Try any of the following:

Red bush tea

Peppermint tea

Other herb and fruit teas

Caro Extra or Bambu (instant-coffee alternatives)

Teecino (requires a cafetière)

Drinks to avoid

Do NOT drink any of the following:

- Pre-made teas (which contain lots of refined sugar).

- High-caffeine sports drinks – excess caffeine interferes with deep, restful sleep and therefore with recovery).

- Undiluted or sweetened fruit juices – pure fruit juice diluted with at least 50 per cent water is OK. However, you must limit diluted fruit juice to no more than one or two 225ml (8fl oz) glasses daily. Fruit juices in excess are high in sugar, which is linked to a fatty liver and obesity.

- Fizzy drinks, whether with sugar or without, other than mineral water (these drinks often contain caffeine, phosphoric acid, aspartame, and/or refined sugars).

- Caffeinated coffee (excess caffeine interferes with deep, restful sleep and with recovery).

- Flavoured water drinks (even with Splenda).

- 'Alcohol-free' beer.

- Aspartame-containing drinks – these contain aspartic acid, which, in excess, is bad news for brain nerves.

THE HOW TO QUIT Diet recipes

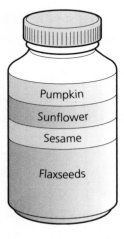 This symbol means an oily fish recipe

Essential Seed Mix

Seeds are incredibly rich in essential fats, minerals, vitamin E, protein and fibre. You need a tablespoon a day for 100 per cent health. Here's the magic formula:

1. Take a glass jar that has a sealing lid and half-fill with flax seeds (also called linseed), then fill the other half with an equal mixture of sesame, sunflower and pumpkin seeds. Shake to mix together.

2. Keep the jar sealed and in the fridge to minimise damage from light, heat and oxygen.

3. Put a handful of mixed seeds in a coffee grinder or nut mill, grind up and put a tablespoon on your cereal each day. Store the remainder in the fridge and use over the next few days.

Pumpkin

Sunflower

Sesame

Flaxseeds

BREAKFASTS

Boiled Egg on Wholegrain Rye Toast

This simple breakfast makes a wholesome start to the day.

SERVES 1
1 large free-range egg
wholegrain rye toast, lightly buttered

Pour boiling water into a small pan and add the egg. Boil the egg to taste (4–5 minutes for soft-boiled). Serve with very lightly buttered wholegrain rye toast.

Low-GL Muesli

You can make this delicious muesli yourself. Experiment with fruit combinations. It tastes best when the oats or rye are soaked overnight in enough water to cover the ingredients.

SERVES 1
50g (1¾oz) soft porridge oat flakes or quinoa flakes
45g oat bran
1 tbsp ground seeds (see page 357 for the Essential Seed Mix)
as many berries as you like (strawberries, raspberries, blueberries)
2 tbsp natural yogurt

Put the flakes, oat bran and seeds into a bowl and pour over cold water to cover. Stir, then cover and leave overnight. Serve with the berries and yogurt

Scots Porridge

On a cold winter's day nothing is more warming than porridge. Oats are full of fibre and complex carbohydrates and make a sustaining breakfast.

SERVES 1

300ml (10fl oz) water

300ml (10fl oz) skimmed cow's milk or unsweetened soya milk

60g (2¼oz) porridge oats

2 tsp mixture of ground flax and pumpkin seeds

1 tsp agave syrup

1 tsp cinnamon (optional)

1 Put the water and half the milk in a pan and sprinkle in the oats. Bring to the boil and simmer for 3–5 minutes, stirring all the time.

2 Serve with the remaining milk, the seeds, agave syrup and cinnamon, if you like.

Fruit Yogurt or Yogurt Shake

Low-fat, live, natural yogurt is a first-class food, unlike its commercial counterpart, in which most bacteria have been destroyed to give the product a longer shelf life. Live yogurt is packed with friendly bacteria that have a spring-cleaning effect on your digestive system, helping prevent allergies and infections, as well as being a good source of protein. Add any fruit in season.

SERVES 1

280g (10oz) very low-fat live natural yogurt

1 tsp agave syrup

1 serving of fruit, such as 1 small or ½ large banana, 1 apple, 1 pear, 1 kiwi fruit, a handful or small punnet of berries

2 tsp ground flax and pumpkin seeds

Combine all the ingredients or, if you prefer, make a smoothie by processing the mix in a blender.

Smoked Salmon with Scrambled Egg on Toast 🐟

Eggs, as part of a balanced diet, are a good source of protein and fat and add variety. If you don't like smoked salmon have 2 eggs instead, but make sure you get your three portions of oily fish per week.

SERVES 1

1 large free-range egg
a dash of skimmed cow's milk or unsweetened soya milk
1 tbsp chopped fresh parsley
small knob of butter
1 thin slice of wholegrain rye toast
75g (2¾oz) preservative-free smoked salmon

1 Break the egg into a bowl, add the milk and parsley, and beat with a fork.
2 Melt the butter in a small pan over a medium heat. Pour in the egg mixture and cook slowly, stirring constantly with a wooden spoon until the eggs form soft curds.
3 Serve on the toast and top with the smoked salmon.

Wholegrain Rye Toast with Nut Butter

Nuts are a great source of essential fats, protein and minerals. Choose the unsweetened, unsalted varieties of nut butter (available in good health-food shops or supermarkets). Wholegrain rye toast with nut butter is the perfect combination of slow-releasing carbohydrate and protein to give you energy to start the day and keep you feeling full.

SERVES 1

1–2 slices of thin, wholegrain rye bread
1 tbsp unsalted, unsweetened nut butter

Toast the bread and spread with the nut butter.

Get Up & Go

Nourishing Get Up & Go is a powdered breakfast drink, which is blended with skimmed milk or soya milk and banana or berries. Nutritionally speaking, it is the ultimate breakfast: each serving gives you more fibre than a bowl of porridge, more protein than an egg, more iron than a cooked breakfast and more vitamins and minerals than a whole packet of cornflakes. In fact, every serving of Get Up & Go gives you at least 100 per cent of every vitamin and mineral and a lot more of some key nutrients. It is widely available in health-food shops. Remember to make whole fruit, rather than juices, your primary source of nutrition. As a general rule, chew your fruit – don't drink it.

SERVES 1
300ml (10fl oz) skimmed milk or unsweetened soya milk
1 portion of fruit, such as 1 small or ½ larger banana, 1 pear or 2
   heaped tbsp berries
1 serving Get Up & Go powder

Blend the milk with the fruit and Get Up & Go powder. Serve.

LUNCHES

Sardines on Toast 🐟

This may take you back to your childhood. Sardines are endowed with lashings of omega-3 fats, and make a fast and delicious meal served this way. Just add a big green salad with red onions and extra-virgin olive oil.

SERVES 1
3 slices wholegrain rye bread
1 tbsp olive oil
2 tomatoes, sliced
170g (6oz) sardines in brine, drained
ground black pepper

Toast the bread and drizzle with olive oil. Put the tomato slices and sardines on the toast and season with black pepper.

Beany Vegetable Soup

This one-pot winter warmer is crammed full of fibre and is just right to take in a vacuum flask to work.

SERVES 6
2 red onions, chopped
450g (1lb) mixed root vegetables, such as carrot, swede and parsnip, peeled and chopped into bite-sized chunks
3 celery sticks, finely chopped
3 leeks, sliced
850ml (1½ pints) vegetable stock
2 × 400g (14oz) cans mixed pulses (or your choice of beans, such as kidney, chickpea, borlotti, butter or flageolet), drained and rinsed
fresh flat-leaf parsley, roughly chopped
Solo salt alternative and ground black pepper

1 Put the onions, root vegetables, celery, leeks, stock and seasoning in a large pan and stir. Cover and bring to the boil,
   then reduce the heat and simmer for 20 minutes.
2 Stir in the mixed pulses, then cover and simmer, stirring occasionally, for 5–10 minutes or until the vegetables are tender
   and beans are heated through.
3 Add the parsley, then check the seasoning before serving.

Rice, Tuna and Petits Pois Salad

This is unbelievably tasty – much more interesting than bog-
standard tuna mayo. Peas are delicious raw, and of course they
retain more vitamins this way.

SERVES 1
100g (3½oz) brown basmati rice
100g (3½oz) tuna in brine, drained and flaked
1 tsp sesame oil
2 tsp tamari or soy sauce
2 tsp lemon juice
1 tbsp fresh, raw petits pois (use frozen cooked if you cannot find
   fresh)
1 carrot, cut into julienne (finely sliced lengthways)
1 spring onion, finely sliced
ground black pepper

1 Rinse the rice and boil in plenty of water for 15 minutes or
   according to the pack instructions. Drain, then spread the
   cooked rice over a plate to cool a little while you prepare the
   remaining ingredients.
2 Combine the rice with the remaining ingredients, tossing
   thoroughly to mix all the flavours.

Green Bean, Olive and Roasted Pepper Salad

A Spanish-style salad that tastes good stuffed in a wholemeal pitta bread.

SERVES 1

2 medium eggs
200g (7oz) French beans, trimmed
1 tsp red wine vinegar
1 tbsp extra-virgin olive oil
1 small red onion, finely chopped
2 roasted red peppers, finely chopped
a handful of stoned black olives, halved
Solo salt alternative and ground black pepper

1 Put the eggs into a pan of boiling water, bring back to the boil and cook for 8 minutes until just hard-boiled. Drain the water and cool the eggs quickly under cold water. Shell and slice.
2 Steam the beans until al dente (tender with a bite), then rinse under cold running water to keep the deep green colour. Dry on kitchen paper and put in a bowl.
3 Whisk the vinegar into the oil and season, then toss over the beans.
4 Stir in the red onion, red peppers and olives, then gently scatter the egg over the top. Serve.

Hot-smoked Fish with Avocado

The avocado provides healthy monounsaturated fat, while the fish gives plenty of omega-3 oils.

SERVES 1

2 fillets hot-smoked preservative-free salmon or trout
5cm (2in) piece of cucumber, cut into bite-sized pieces
½ ripe medium-sized avocado
juice of 1 lemon

1–2 tsp chopped fresh dill or chives
1–2 tsp chopped fresh flat-leaf parsley
Solo salt alternative and ground black pepper

1 Skin the fish and remove any bones, then flake into chunks. Place in a salad bowl with the cucumber.
2 Cut the avocado into bite-sized pieces. Add to the bowl with the lemon and herbs.
3 Season and gently mix together. Serve.

Cook's tip

Leave the stone in the leftover half of avocado and drizzle the flesh with lemon juice to prevent discoloration, then cover and place in the fridge for future use.

Low-GL Sandwiches

When it's lunchtime and you're starving, sometimes only a sandwich will do. Top two slices of wholegrain rye bread or fill a wholemeal pitta pocket with any one of the following combinations.

SERVES 1
- 150g (5½oz) cottage cheese, with cucumber slices and chopped fresh chives
- 150g (5½oz) hummus and lettuce
- 1 small, roasted or grilled chicken breast (skin removed) and 1 sliced tomato
- 1 small preservative-free smoked trout or salmon fillet with a smear of low-fat cream cheese or Pumpkin Seed Pesto (page 374) and watercress
- 60g (2¼oz) canned salmon or tuna in brine, with cucumber and cress
- egg 'mayonnaise' (made with 2 hard-boiled eggs, 1 tbsp cottage cheese, 1 chopped spring onion and Solo salt alternative and ground black pepper)

Low-GL Baked Potato or Sweet Potato with Filling

Many diets give the humble spud short shrift, but a baked potato can be a great base for a satisfying lunch. It's also available at many city sandwich shops in case you've forgotten to bring anything to work with you. All you need to remember is to choose a small potato so that you don't overdo the carbs. Do eat the skins – they're full of fibre. Have them with any of the fillings below and a large salad. A (small) sweet potato makes a delicious change.

SERVES 1

1 small baking potato or sweet potato

Scrub the skin, then prick all over with a fork. Bake at 220°C/ 425°F/Gas 7 for 50–60 minutes or until done but still firm inside. Serve with one of the following fillings:

- 60g (2¼oz) drained tuna in brine blended with 1 tsp cottage cheese or natural yogurt

- 150g (5½oz) low-fat cottage cheese with chives and spring onions

- 150g (5½oz) hummus with a sliced tomato

- 200g (7oz) baked beans, heated until warmed through

- 1 small, roasted or grilled chicken breast (no skin) tossed in 1 tbsp yogurt dressing (blended with paprika, ground black pepper and chopped fresh chives, basil or parsley)

- 2 tsp Pumpkin Seed Pesto (page 374) with 60g (2¼oz) cottage cheese and chopped fresh chives

THE HOW TO QUIT DIET   **367**

DINNERS

Spiced Turkey Meatballs

These patties are a leaner alternative to beef meatballs and have a spicy kick. They go down well with teenagers and are brilliant for barbecues. (If you do barbecue them, avoid charring or blackening the meat.) Serve with baked beans and grilled mushrooms and tomatoes, or wholegrain spaghetti (see Cook's Tip).

SERVES 4
1 tbsp extra-virgin olive oil
2 large garlic cloves, crushed
1 large green chilli, seeded and finely chopped
a large pinch of ground cumin
400g (14oz) lean minced turkey
Solo salt alternative and ground black pepper

1 Put the oil in a pan and gently fry the garlic, chilli and cumin for 2 minutes, then leave to cool slightly.
2 Add the minced turkey, season and mix thoroughly. Shape the mixture into four patties.
3 Grill for 10 minutes or until cooked thoroughly, turning halfway through.

Cook's Tip
If serving with spaghetti, place lightly grilled courgette pieces on the top before adding the meatballs: slice the courgettes lengthways and drizzle with a little oil and Solo salt alternative, then lightly grill, turning halfway through.

Fajitas

Here's a low-fat take on this ever-popular Tex-Mex dish. Double or triple the recipe to make a fun family supper, or a great informal meal for friends. Substitute a can of black-eyed beans if you do not eat meat (see Cook's Tip).

SERVES 2

1 tbsp extra-virgin olive oil

2 red onions, sliced

1 garlic clove, crushed

1 red and 1 yellow pepper, seeded and sliced lengthways

⅔ tbsp Old El Paso Fajita Seasoning

2 chicken breast fillets, skinned and cut into slices

2 tortilla wraps

FOR THE TOMATO SALSA

2 plum tomatoes, chopped

2 spring onions, finely chopped

1 garlic clove, crushed

2 tbsp chopped fresh coriander

1 tbsp lime juice

1 tbsp extra-virgin olive oil

pinch of Solo salt alternative

ground black pepper

1 Put the oil in a pan over a low heat. Add the onions, garlic and peppers. Cover and cook, stirring occasionally, for 5–10 minutes or until tender.

2 Rub the seasoning into the chicken and cook under a medium-hot grill.

3 Mix the chicken into the vegetables.

4 To make the salsa, stir the ingredients together in a large bowl. Divide the salsa between the tortillas and add the chicken and vegetable mixture, then roll up.

Cook's Tip

If you are using black-eyed beans, add the fajita seasoning to the vegetables and cook for a further few minutes. Drain and rinse the beans, then stir into the vegetables. Heat through, then remove from the heat and serve.

Pasta with Pumpkin Seed Pesto

Sometimes at the end of a long day it is all you can do to boil the kettle for some pasta. Luckily, this dish is pretty instant, if you keep some Pumpkin Seed Pesto in the fridge. Serve with a tomato and red onion salad.

SERVES 2

2 tsp pumpkin seeds
170g (6oz) or ⅓ regular pack wholewheat or buckwheat pasta
½ quantity Pumpkin Seed Pesto (page 374)
a handful of fresh basil leaves
ground black pepper

1 Put the pumpkin seeds into a small, dry pan and toast over a medium-high heat for 3 minutes or until golden brown. Set aside. Cook the pasta according to the pack instructions, then drain well and return to the pan.
2 Stir the pesto into the pasta and divide between two plates.
3 Top with the basil, pumpkin seeds and black pepper. Serve.

Chilli

This wonderful dish – just right for a crisp autumn evening – has fooled many a hardy meat eater. You can prepare this in double quantities and freeze it. It works well with brown basmati rice, on a small baked potato or in a toasted tortilla wrap.

SERVES 1

1 tbsp extra-virgin olive oil

1 small onion, sliced

2 garlic cloves, crushed

½ green pepper, seeded and sliced

½ tsp chilli powder

1 tsp paprika

1 tsp ground cumin

1 tsp ground coriander

60g (2¼oz) dried soya mince (pre-soaked) or 170g (6oz) Quorn mince

200g (7oz) canned tomatoes, chopped

1 tbsp tomato purée

110g (3¾oz) canned kidney beans, drained and rinsed

250ml (8¾fl oz) vegetable bouillon

1 Put the oil in a pan over a low heat. Add the onion, garlic and pepper and stir in the chilli powder, paprika, cumin and coriander. Cover with a lid and cook, stirring occasionally, for 5–10 minutes or until tender.

2 Add the pre-soaked soya mince or Quorn mince and stir for 2 minutes.

3 Add the tomatoes, tomato purée, kidney beans and bouillon. Mix well and leave to simmer for at least 30 minutes, stirring occasionally to prevent it from sticking or burning. If the mixture becomes too thick, add a little water.

Sticky Mustard Salmon Fillets 🐟

Salmon not only provides plenty of protein but it is also a rich source of essential fats. Try to go for wild salmon, as it's a healthier option than farmed fish. Serve with steam-fried spinach and red or yellow peppers, and 3 small boiled baby new potatoes per person or brown basmati rice (65g raw weight per person).

SERVES 2
juice and grated zest of ½ orange
1 tsp wholegrain mustard
1 tsp clear honey
2 skinless, boneless preservative-free salmon fillets

1 Put the orange juice and zest into a bowl and whisk in the mustard and honey. Put the salmon in an ovenproof dish and pour over this marinade. Leave the salmon to marinate in the fridge for 30 minutes–1 hour. Meanwhile, preheat the oven to 180°C/350°F/Gas 4.

2 Bake the salmon for 20–25 minutes and serve.

Cook's Tip
This marinade also works very well with tofu slices.

Steam-frying

A healthy way to cook vegetables either as part of a dish or as an accompaniment is by steam-frying. Add about 2 tbsp of liquid (such as water, vegetable stock or a watered-down sauce) to a wok or large frying pan – use one with a lid. When the liquid is boiling, add your vegetables, stir-fry for about 1 minute then place the lid on the pan to allow the ingredients to steam inside. Turn down the heat after a couple of minutes and steam until the vegetables are al dente (tender with a bite) – you can always add a splash more water if the pan dries out.

Thai Green Curry

The aromatic blend of spices and creamy coconut milk in this dish suits a number of protein-rich foods, so you can adapt this recipe to use chicken, tofu chunks or prawns. Green curry paste, fish sauce and kaffir lime leaves are now widely available in most supermarkets. If you can't find the last two, the curry will still be delicious. Serve with brown basmati rice (65g/2½oz) raw weight per person).

SERVES 2

1 tbsp extra-virgin olive oil

1 red onion, chopped

2 garlic cloves, crushed

3 heaped tsp Thai green curry paste

2 small chicken breast fillets or 600g (1lb 5oz) firm tofu, cubed, or
    350g (12oz) cooked, peeled prawns

3 tsp fish sauce

400ml (14fl oz) can coconut milk

2 kaffir lime leaves

2 small courgettes, chopped

a handful of fresh basil leaves

1 Put the olive oil into a pan over a low heat. Add the onion, garlic and curry paste. Cover the pan and cook, stirring occasionally, for 2 minutes.

2 Add the chicken or tofu. Cover and fry for a further 5 minutes.

3 Add the fish sauce, coconut milk and kaffir lime leaves. Stir well, cover and leave to simmer for 30 minutes, adding a little water if necessary.

4 About 10 minutes before serving, add the courgettes and continue simmering. Add the prawns, if using, and the basil leaves 2 minutes before the end of cooking. Serve.

Cook's Tip

If you are cooking the dish for vegetarians, use tofu and omit the fish sauce. Add 1 tbsp tamari or a dash of Solo salt alternative instead.

Sweet Potato and Red Onion Tortilla

This tasty Spanish-style tortilla is an interesting variation on the traditional tortilla, using sweet potatoes, with a lower GL score, instead of potatoes. Cut into wedges and serve with a side salad or steamed broccoli.

SERVES 2
1 large sweet potato, peeled and sliced horizontally into thin circles
1 tbsp extra-virgin olive oil
2 large red onions, chopped
2 garlic cloves, crushed
4 medium eggs
Solo salt alternative and ground black pepper

1 Steam the sweet potato for 5–10 minutes or until tender.
2 Heat half the olive oil in a pan over a low heat. Add the onion and garlic, then cover and cook, stirring occasionally, for 12–15 minutes or until soft. Remove from the pan and set aside.
3 In a large bowl beat the eggs, then stir in the sweet potato and half the cooked onion. Season generously with Solo and black pepper.
4 Heat the remaining oil in a shallow non-stick frying pan until hot, then add the remaining cooled onion. Pour in the egg mixture and cook over a very low heat for 6 minutes or until the bottom is golden and the mixture looks set. Using a spatula, flip the tortilla over and cook the other side for 1–2 minutes.

Pumpkin Seed Pesto

This useful pesto keeps in the fridge for 2–3 days and can be stirred through soup or pasta, or added to bean salads. It makes a pleasant change from the usual variety made with basil and pine nuts.

SERVES 4

60g (2¼oz) raw pumpkin seeds
60g (2¼oz) fresh flat-leaf parsley leaves
60g (2¼oz) fresh basil leaves
2 garlic cloves, crushed
1 tsp Solo salt alternative
2 tsp lemon juice
60g (2¼oz) grated Parmesan cheese
90ml (3fl oz) pumpkin seed oil (roasted if possible)

1 Place the pumpkin seeds in a blender or food processor and add the herbs, garlic, Solo, lemon juice and Parmesan. Blitz until the mixture is blended but retains some texture.
2 Add the pumpkin seed oil and mix until the pesto is an even consistency.

Cook's Tip

If you can't find pumpkin seed oil use the same quantity of pumpkin seed butter and omit the pumpkin seeds (available from Health Products for Life – see Resources).

Do-it-yourself How to Quit Diet

If you want to create the diet yourself, you need to pick foods that will fall into the following categories.

Protein foods

Choose foods that give you quality protein three times a day, this means:

- Always have seeds or nuts on your wholegrain cereal, or add 1 tablespoonful of the Essential Seed Mix (page 357), or have eggs or a kipper for breakfast.

- Have a serving of unfried fish, meat, eggs, lentils or beans as part of lunch or dinner. Your protein serving should be about the size of the palm of your hand, being a quarter of what's on your plate. Choose lean, preferably organic, meat from fit, healthy, preferably wild or organic animals, not processed, chemically treated, preservative-laden meats from intensively reared, fat, unhealthy animals. You become what you eat.

- Have some raw nuts or seeds at least once a day as part of a snack.

Eat low-GL for even blood sugar

Choose foods that will keep your blood sugar level even; in other words low-GL foods. This means:

- Always eat carbohydrate foods with protein foods.

- Have two low-GL snacks a day; for example, an apple or berries with raw almonds or pumpkin seeds (see Snack Combos on page 355).

- Have half of your main meal plate as vegetables, one-quarter as protein (such as fish, meat or tofu), and one-quarter as low-GL carbs (such as brown rice, wholewheat pasta, boiled potatoes, beans or lentils). See the 'ideal dinner plate' on page 185.

Also read Chapter 11 for more guidance on low-GL eating.

Choose the right carbohydrates and avoid the wrong ones

Use these two lists when shopping, to ensure you buy the healthy carbohydrate options.

WHICH FOODS TO CHOOSE OR AVOID

CHOOSE

Breakfast cereals
Oats
All Bran
Oatibix
Sugar-free muesli (without lots of raisins)

Breads
Oatcakes (sugar-free)
100% wholegrain rye bread
Pumpernickel-style breads
(sonnenbrot, volkenbrot)
100% wholemeal bread

Main meal carbs
Quinoa
Beans or lentils
Squash, swede or carrot
100% wholewheat pasta
Brown basmati rice or low-GL rice
Boiled potatoes

AVOID

Breakfast cereals
Cornflakes
Sugared, processed cereals

Breads
Croissants
Muffins
Bagels
Waffles and pancakes
Biscuits (but low-sugar oat biscuits are OK)
White and refined breads, unless 100% wholemeal

Main meal carbs
White rice
Refined pasta
French fries
Baked potato (or have a half serving only)
Sweet potato (or have a half serving only)

Get to know the foods that have essential fats

You need essential fats and phospholipids, which are vital for your brain, so this means eating:

- Unfried, preservative-free oily fish (salmon, sardines, mackerel, herrings, kippers) three times a week; tuna twice a month.

- Seven free-range or organic, or omega-3-enriched eggs, which are rich in phospholipids and vitamin E, every week.

- A small handful, or a heaped tablespoon, of raw nuts or seeds (ideally make up the Essential Seed Mix on page 357) a day.

The following chart shows you which foods contain the best brain fats. (Read more about brain fats in Chapter 10.)

BEST SOURCES OF BRAIN FATS

Omega-3	EPA and DHA	Arachidonic acid
Flax seeds (linseed)	Salmon	Lean, free-grazed or
Hemp	Mackerel	organic meat
Pumpkin	Herring	Dairy produce
Walnut	Sardines	Free-range eggs
	Anchovies	Squid
Omega-6	Tuna (fresh)	
Corn or maize	Omega-3 eggs	
Safflower	Marine algae	
Sunflower		
Sesame	**GLA**	
Hemp	Evening primrose oil	
Pumpkin	Borage oil	
Walnuts	Blackcurrant oil	

The chart below shows you the quantity of omega-3 in various types of fish; you can see that fresh salmon has the highest amount of these beneficial fats.

OMEGA-3 CONTENT OF FISH

Fish	Omega-3: g per 100g
Fresh salmon	2.70
Fresh mackerel	1.93
Canned sardines	1.57
Canned/smoked salmon	1.54
Fresh tuna	1.50
Herring	1.31
Trout	1.15
Canned tuna	0.37

Avoid the wrong fats and deep-fried food

The wrong kind of fats – called trans fats, or hydrogenated fats – are found in fried or processed food. These are bad news for your brain, so avoid all the following:

- Deep-fried food, including fried fish and meat, as well as all damaged and processed fats, including trans fats. If you sauté a food, or steam-fry food (see page 371), use a small amount of coconut butter or oil, olive oil or organic butter. These fats are much less prone to oxidation than polyunsaturated oils such as sunflower oil.

- Avoid fried eggs, choosing boiled or poached instead. However, eggs may be cooked slowly – scrambled – over a low temperature in a small amount of suitable fat, such as virgin coconut oil or extra-virgin olive oil.

- Avoid high-fat junk food and processed foods. These include most pizzas, confectionery, biscuits, cakes and some crisps (try Nairns Oat Bakes instead).

- No margarine. Have pure butter, or nut butters instead.

Get plenty of antioxidants

Make sure your diet includes plenty of fresh fruit and vegetables for their antioxidants (see Chapter 12 for more details).

- There is no limit on how many vegetables you can eat. Have a serving of a dark green vegetable every day: spinach, greens, broccoli, kale, peas, Brussels sprouts, green cabbage and asparagus or avocado. But most days, make this a serving of cruciferous vegetables – cabbage, kale, cauliflower, broccoli and Brussels sprouts. Make a super-green serving by blending a handful of spinach leaves, watercress, parsley and basil with a tablespoon of extra-virgin olive oil, and a squeeze of lemon juice.

- Have something red, orange or yellow every day – carrots, tomatoes, red or yellow peppers, sweet potato, butternut squash, beetroot. (Or sometimes have something blue instead, such as blueberries.)

- Eat onions, spring onions or shallots. Have a red onion, which is high in quercetin (a pigment that reduces allergic reactions), and/or some garlic most days.

- Fruit is also good, although some fruits, such as grapes, mangos, dates, raisins and bananas, are high in fast-releasing sugars and are best limited. Have no more than half a banana a day or a quarter of a mango, or ten grapes or raisins a day. The best low-GL choices are apples, pears, peaches, cherries and plums. Whenever you can, choose fresh, organic produce and have two servings a day.

- Have a serving of berries every day (blueberries, strawberries or raspberries), preferably fresh or use frozen out of season. These have the highest antioxidant content. Also good are pomegranates, acai and goji berries.

- Fruits are best chewed, not drunk.

- Herbs and spices are also good sources of nutrients and antioxidants. So have lots of garlic, turmeric, cayenne pepper, black pepper, mustard, dill, rosemary, herbal blends, cinnamon and ginger. Add a sprinkling of nutmeg to occasional dishes.

- Avoid adding salt to your foods – instead use Solo sea salt.

Drink eight glasses of water a day

Your body needs more water than you think. By the time you are thirsty you are already dehydrated. So develop the habit of drinking. Have a glass of water when you wake up, for example, and one before each meal and snack. You can drink this water as herbal teas – try red bush (rooibos) tea and Yogi teas – or green tea (see Drinks on page 354) and diluted fruit juice, although we recommend no more than one or two glasses of fruit juice (preferably apple or orange, not grape) diluted 50:50 with water a day.

Stay away from diet colas and other drinks sweetened with aspartame (usually listed as NutraSweet on packaging). Many are high in phosphates and, usually, caffeine. These are junk drinks.

Food allergies in the DIY diet

In Chapter 14 we explored the subject of food allergies and explained the kinds of symptoms and the tests that determine them. If you have had a hidden food allergy test, and you tested positive, you'll need to adjust your diet accordingly. The most

continues ▶

common allergy-provoking foods are wheat and milk. Many of
the recipes in this book and the guidelines we give you are
compatible with a wheat-free and dairy-free diet. At its simplest
you can replace wheat cereal or bread with oat cereal and
oatcakes; eat rice, quinoa and buckwheat pasta instead of wheat
pasta, and rice or soya milk instead of cow's milk. Cook with
coconut butter or extra-virgin olive oil instead of butter or
sunflower oil, and use olive oil or tahini (sesame spread) instead
of butter on wholegrain toast.

The when and how of eating

As we've said before, the most important meal of the day is breakfast. If you eat the right breakfast, containing low-GL carbs such
as oatmeal porridge or a wholegrain low-GL bread or oatcakes,
this literally keeps your blood sugar in check for the day, making
you less hungry for sugar and stimulants. Studies show that this
improves your concentration and keeps your blood sugar more
stable for up to ten hours.[2] Remember to eat some protein with
carbohydrate; for example, seeds with your oatmeal. This further
stabilises your blood sugar levels.

Have two main meals (lunch and dinner), a mid-morning
snack and a mid-afternoon snack. Eating little and often in this
way keeps your blood sugar level even. If you are supplementing
tryptophan or 5-HTP or tyrosine, take these with a carbohydrate
snack, such as a piece of fruit or fruit juice.

Leave at least three hours between dinner and bedtime. If you
don't sleep well, have more carbohydrate and little or no protein
for dinner and during the evening. If you do this, make sure your
lunch is higher in protein to balance this out. If you have a serving
of lentils or beans with your dinner this helps even out your blood
sugar rise when you eat breakfast the next day, so it helps you feel
fuller, more satisfied and less tired the next day. Helping your

blood sugar to remain level in this way will increase your energy and reduce your craving for sugar and drugs; it will also help you get a good night's sleep.

Slow down and chew your food thoroughly – until the food is liquid – before swallowing. This will normally take at least 20 chews. Chewing properly helps to draw the nutrients out. This is why your mouth has teeth whereas your stomach doesn't.

Relax when you eat. Every now and then stop for a minute and enjoy your food, the surroundings and good company. Take a moment to be grateful. Eating the right foods is one of the most important things you are likely to do today. Most of all enjoy what you eat.

Your action list

1. If you have any allergens, avoid them in your diet.

2. Eat breakfast every day.

3. Have two snacks of protein and carbs each day.

4. Avoid caffeinated and sugary drinks, or those made with artificial sweeteners.

5. Eat low-GL meals to keep your blood sugar even.

6. Eat carbohydrate foods with protein foods.

7. Eat foods that contain the healthy fats: oily fish, eggs, nuts and seeds.

8. Avoid the bad fats and deep-fried foods.

9. Get plenty of antioxidants by eating fresh fruit and vegetables.

10. Drink eight glasses of water a day.

29.

THE SUPPLEMENTS

In Parts 2 and 3 we explained the importance of a whole host of supplemental nutrients: amino acids, vitamins, minerals, essential fats, phospholipids and a few other specific nutrients. These recommendations are based both on substantial published research and our experience with thousands of people who have successfully given up addictive substances and alleviated their abstinence symptoms.

Eating healthy foods and supplementing your diet with the optimal level of nutrients, which are almost invariably higher than the basic RDAs (the recommended daily amounts to prevent scurvy and other chronic deficiency diseases), makes all the difference. You can achieve the RDA levels of nutrients from diet alone, and our assumption is that you will be achieving these levels by following the How to Quit Diet explained in the previous chapter. However, you cannot achieve optimum nutrition through food alone.

The optimal amount of these nutrients you need to recover your brain's chemical balance, and to help correct reward deficiency, is greater than the amount that you need on an ongoing basis to maintain your health at the highest level. To determine which combination of nutrients are most important for you, refer to the chapter in Part 3 that applies to your specific addiction. At the end of this chapter you will find details on the specific prescriptions for each addiction on easy-to-read charts, and full instructions on how to take them.

Are nutrients safe?

Once again we would like to emphasise that the levels of nutrients we are promoting are completely safe, based on substantial published research and our extensive experience. Very rarely, minor side effects (such as nausea) will be reported in people who have taken too many pills with too little food. This is probably because you need some digestive juices to break the pills down. These types of symptoms are minor – they go away immediately on cutting back, and pale into insignificance alongside the scale of reduction most people experience in their abstinence symptoms.

In the next chapter, which is aimed at those with serious addictions, we talk about intravenous (IV) nutrient therapy, which bypasses the digestive tract. This method is most helpful for those whose digestive tract is damaged or where their digestive processes are shut down (such as those with a chronic alcohol problem).

Nutrients for recovery and maintenance

In this chapter, we show you the optimal intakes of key nutrients for *recovery*, which for many people means the first four to twelve weeks, and for *maintenance*. How long you need to be on the recovery level of nutrients depends largely on how quickly your abstinence symptoms recede. The disappearance of these symptoms is one of the most useful indicators that, for example, you are no longer in a state of reward deficiency. If you are giving up a substance with the guidance of a nutritional therapist, doctor or health-care practitioner, they may wish to run appropriate tests to find out if you are ready for maintenance supplementation. If you are not, see the box below, Chart Your Progress, to find out when you are ready to go from recovery supplementation to maintenance supplementation.

Chart your progress

How do you know when it's time to switch to maintenance mode? The best guide is your score on the Scale of Abstinence Symptoms Severity. Have a look at the questionnaire you completed on page 26. Now pick the five symptoms you'd most like to eliminate. Write these down, together with the scores you had for each of them on your start date. Keep this list of symptoms and your beginning total score. After four weeks, and then weekly, add up your total score for these five symptoms again. Once your total score for these five of your worst abstinence symptoms is two-thirds (66 per cent) less than your starting score, you can switch to maintenance supplements. For example, if your total score for these five symptoms was 30 when you started and is now nine, it is time to stop taking the extra supplements recommended.

1 _____

2 _____

3 _____

4 _____

5 _____

continues ▶

Beginning total score:

Calculate two-thirds (66 per cent):

Score after 4 weeks:

Score after 5 weeks:

Score after 6 weeks:

Score after 7 weeks:

Score after 8 weeks:

Score after 9 weeks:

Score after 10 weeks:

Score after 11 weeks:

Score after 12 weeks:

Start with the basics

Assuming you eat a diet similar to the How to Quit Diet, it is still beneficial to supplement optimal levels of vitamins, minerals, amino acids and essential fats.

Aren't supplements just 'making expensive urine'?

No doubt you've heard that taking supplements is unnecessary. Consider this recent study, however, conducted by Dr Gladys Block at the University of California. She investigated the health status of three groups of people: those who took no supplements, those who took a daily multivitamin based on the RDA, and those who took many supplements, more akin to what we are recommending.

The study was partly motivated by the concern that taking large amounts of supplemental nutrients might lead to adverse effects from overdosing, but the results showed startling health benefits and disease-risk reductions the more supplements were taken, with no apparent downside.

The risk of diabetes was 73 per cent less and the risk of coronary heart disease was 52 per cent less in the multiple-supplement takers compared to those who didn't take any supplements. On self-assessment, the multiple-supplement takers were 74 per cent more likely to rate their health as 'good' or 'excellent'.

Where homocysteine levels fit in

One of the best overall indicators of health is your homocysteine level, as we discussed in Chapter 9, and the ideal level is below 7. The lower your homocysteine, the lower your risk of heart disease, strokes, Alzheimer's disease, depression, chronic pain, certain cancers, osteoporosis, pregnancy complications, liver disease and addiction, and the lower your risk of premature death from all causes.

In the study mentioned above, four times as many people not taking supplements (45 per cent) had elevated homocysteine levels (averaging 9.6) compared to the multiple-supplement takers (11 per cent – averaging an optimal 6.1). Single-supplement takers were three times more likely (37 per cent) to have raised homocysteine levels. Multiple-supplement takers also had significantly higher HDL ('good' cholesterol), lower triglycerides, a better HDL–cholesterol ratio and lower blood pressure – all reliable indicators of a reduced risk of cardiovascular disease.

There was no indication of a risk of overdosing or negative side effects from taking multiple supplements. So, far from wasting your money 'making expensive urine', this study strongly suggests that popping a handful of supplements a day is likely to add years to your life and life to your years.

The role of supplements in optimal health

The above findings are completely consistent with the emerging science helping to define what 'optimum nutrition' really means. More people are realising that intelligently supplementing your healthy diet (as defined above) is necessary if you want to achieve optimal health. The ideal level of basic nutrients we recommend is based on estimates of optimum daily amounts (ODA), explained on the website www.patrickholford.com/supplements.

The four basic supplements: our Basic Supplement Pack

Everybody can benefit from the following four basic supplements, taken twice a day, every day. We take these every day despite having no addictions or abstinence symptoms. You will, however, need specific amino acids as well, depending on your abstinence symptoms and on the substance you are quitting (more on this later). These are:

1. An optimum nutrition multivitamin and mineral

2. Additional vitamin C, ideally with berry extracts (bioflavonoids)

3. Essential omega-3 and 6 fats (ideally providing GLA, DHA, DPA and EPA)

4. Phospholipid complex (ideally providing phosphatidyl choline, serine, DMAE, TMG and either glutamine or pyroglutamate)

Multivitamin–mineral

The starting point of any supplement programme is a high-potency multivitamin and multimineral. This should provide the following nutrients:

Multivitamin A good multivitamin should contain at least 2,250mcg (7,500iu) of vitamin A (women of child-bearing age should not exceed 10,000iu daily), 15mcg (600iu) of vitamin D, 100iu of mixed natural vitamin E, 250mg of vitamin C, and 25mg each of vitamins B_1, B_2, B_3, B_5 and B_6, 10mcg of vitamin B_{12}, 200mcg of folic acid and 50mcg of biotin.

Multimineral This should provide at least 200mg of calcium, 150mg of magnesium, 10mg of zinc, 2.5mg of manganese, 20mcg of chromium and 25mcg of selenium.

Multivitamin and mineral You simply can't fit all of the above vitamins and minerals into one tablet. So we recommend two or more tablets a day of a good combined multivitamin and mineral formula to meet these levels. The bulkiest nutrients are vitamin C, calcium and magnesium. These are often insufficiently supplied in multivitamin and mineral formulas. Vitamin C, in particular, is best taken separately simply because you'll never get at least 1,000mg into a multi tablet.

Vitamin C supplement

The ideal vitamin C supplement should provide around 1,000–2,000mg, as a daily amount. It is often taken in two tablets (10,000 daily or more with heroin recovery). Some formulas also provide other key immune-boosting nutrients such as zinc, bioflavonoids or anthocyanidins in the form of black elderberry and bilberry.

CAUTION When taking very high-dose vitamin C, always make sure that you are well nourished with both magnesium and vitamin B_6 (these are included in the Basic Supplements).

Essential fatty acids

The best way to take the essential fats you need is to remove the guesswork from the equation and have your blood tested (see Appendix 5 on tests on the website www.how2quit.co.uk), and then supplement as appropriate. If that's not possible, the ideal essential-fat supplement should provide the most potent omega-6 fat, GLA, and the most potent omega-3 fats, EPA, DPA and DHA. The easiest way to calculate how much omega-3 to take is to add together the EPA, DPA and DHA quantities shown on your supplement packaging. You will need to take 1,000mg a day, usually in two doses. You then need 100mg omega-6 GLA: this can be from evening primrose, borage or blackcurrant oil.

You may want to increase these dosages if you have had a brain-unfriendly lifestyle (bad diet, drinking and drugs) or are prone to ADHD, depression, suicidal feelings, anxiety, panic attacks, bipolar disorder, irritability, anger, aggressive behaviour, poor concentration or memory loss. In which case you can easily double or triple these amounts to 2,000–3,000mg omega-3 (EPA + DPA + DHA, as above) plus 200–300mg GLA (evening primrose, borage or blackcurrant oil).

Phospholipids

The ideal phospholipid supplement should provide phosphatidyl choline, phosphatidyl serine and DMAE. There are other nutrients and nutrient derivatives that help support brain function, which include glutamine, SAM, NADH, phosphatidyl inositol and pyroglutamate, plus the methylating nutrients, especially TMG, B_6, B_{12} and folic acid.

A cheap source of phospholipids is lecithin, which comes in 1,200mg capsules and in granules (a heaped teaspoon being equivalent to a 1,200mg capsule). This provides almost as much phosphatidyl choline as found in an egg, which provides 2,000mg of lecithin, containing about 200mg of phosphatidyl choline.

Amino acid supplements

You will find the specific amino acids that you will most likely need under the prescription for your particular addictive substance on pages 403–28. However, it is important for you to understand that your amino acid supplements may vary according to your abstinence symptoms and how you feel from day to day.

General guidelines for taking amino acid supplements

- When you are feeling anxious, stressed or tense, take GABA, tryptophan, 5-HTP or taurine.
- When you have low energy or feel apathetic, take tyrosine.
- When you are having difficulty concentrating, or you have memory problems or feel mentally 'fuzzy', take tyrosine.
- When you are feeling hypersensitive to noise, lights, touch or pain, take DL-phenylalanine (this is a combination of D- and L- phenylalanine).
- When you are having trouble sleeping, take tryptophan or 5-HTP, GABA, and/or taurine.
- When you are irritable, take tryptophan or 5-HTP.
- To offset cravings, take glutamine or GABA.
- When you are depressed and apathetic, take tyrosine. When depressed, tense and agitated, take 5-HTP or tryptophan.

This means taking four supplements, twice a day, in addition to your specific amino acids. It is important that you choose supplements that provide the optimal amount of key nutrients. There are many supplements, some of which we've listed in the Resources section (see page 488), that do provide these kinds of levels. Whatever you choose you must check by looking at the level provided in the supplement. For example, the optimal level of zinc in two multis (the daily dose) is 10mg, and of magnesium is 150mg. There is no point taking a multi that provides 1mg of zinc and 10mg of magnesium, yet there are many multis available that provide these insignificant amounts: they cost half the price, but they do not represent value for money. It's important to get the basics right because we'll assume when we recommend additional magnesium for promoting sleep or to help you if you are cutting out alcohol, for example, that you are already supplementing this basic amount from your multivitamin–mineral.

Finding your ideal supplement programme for recovery

Your ideal supplement programme depends on both your primary addiction and the abstinence symptoms you are experiencing at any particular time, as well as four other critical issues:

1. Do you have significant **digestive problems**? (See the questionnaire on page 146.)

2. Is your **homocysteine level** raised, indicating poor methylation? (See the questionnaire on page 154.)

3. Is your **liver's detox capacity** under par? (See the questionnaire on page 233.)

4. Are you currently suffering from **sleeping problems** and are consequently sleep deprived? (See the questionnaire on page 204.)

The goal is to have you digesting and absorbing well, methylating well, detoxifying well and sleeping well. If, when you take the questionnaires, you test positive you will need the additional recommended nutrients until such a time as you test negative, either by a reduction – or disappearance – in your symptoms.

For simplicity, we will call the supplements you need to correct each issue the **Digestion Prescription**, the **Methylation Prescription**, the **Liver-detox Prescription** and the **Sleep Prescription**. 'Prescription', in this sense, is a combination of supplements that you can buy over the counter. It is not a combination of drugs that your doctor must prescribe.

So, if you have none of these problems all you need is the Basic Supplements (multi, plus vitamin C, plus essential fat complex, plus phospholipid complex). If, for example, you are a heavy drinker and consequently score poorly on the digestion questionnaire and the liver detox questionnaire, but you sleep fine and don't have a raised homocysteine level, you'll need the Basic Supplements + Digestion Prescription + Liver-detox Prescription.

Your Digestion Prescription

To check whether you need to support your digestion, complete the questionnaire, How's Your Digestion? on page 146. If you score 5 or more you would benefit from the following supplements.

- Supplement digestive enzymes with each meal.

- Take 4–8g (1–2 rounded teaspoons) of glutamine powder on an empty stomach. (Glutamine powder should not be taken if there is severe liver damage, i.e. cirrhosis or liver failure.)

- Take a probiotic supplement containing *Acidophilus* and *Bifidobacteria*.

- An optional added extra is a shot of aloe vera juice.

Your Methylation Prescription

The amount of extra methylation nutrients you need depends on your homocysteine level. To check whether you need to improve your methylation, go to page 154 and complete the questionnaire Test Your Methyl IQ. If your questionnaire score is below 5 there is no need to supplement extra. If it is raised we recommend at least one homocysteine-lowering formula and, ideally, testing your homocysteine level (see page 153). The chart on page 394 shows you how much of these key nutrients you need based on your homocysteine blood test results. Look for a supplement that provides this kind of level. If your score is 'high' you will need two, if it is 'very high' you will need three, and if it is 'much too high' you will need four, spread throughout the day. You need to take these for three months only, then retest to find your new score. Notice that in the trial on page 387 the supplement takers had an average homocysteine level of 6.1μmol/L, which is ideal. The chances are that your level will be closer to ideal within three months – and you'll be feeling much more 'connected'.

The most powerful and quickest way to restore a normal 'H score', below 7 μmol/L, is to supplement specific homocysteine-lowering nutrients. These include vitamins B_2, B_6, B_{12}, folate, glycine (TMG), zinc and NAC. Here are the guidelines:

KEY NUTRIENTS FOR LOWERING HOMOCYSTEINE LEVELS

Your H score μmol/L	OK 7–9	high 9–14	very high 15–19	much too high more than 20
Folate	250mcg	500mcg	750mcg	1,000mcg
Methyl B_{12}	250mcg	500mcg	750mcg	1,000mcg
B_6	20mg	40mg	60mg	80mg
B_2	10mg	20mg	30mg	40mg
Zinc	5mg	10mg	15mg	20mg
TMG	500mg	1g	1.5g	2g
NAC	250mg	500mg	750mg	1,000mg
Number of homocysteine-lowering supplements, per day	1	2	3	4

Your Liver-detox Prescription

To find out whether you need to detox your liver go to page 233 and complete the liver-detox questionnaire. If your score is 4 or more you are likely to benefit from this Liver-detox Prescription. If it is 7 or more we strongly recommend it.

Our first recommendation is to supplement a combination of digestive enzymes and probiotics. Digestive enzymes digest your food, minimising the chances of whole food proteins getting into the blood. Probiotics are essential beneficial bacteria, which also play a part in the digestive process. You need two strains: *Lactobacillus acidophilus* and *Bifidobacteria*. You can find a probiotic supplement either in capsules or powder form in any health-food store.

Our second recommendation is a teaspoon of glutamine powder last thing at night (glutamine is direct fuel for the gut lining and helps the liver detoxify). This will help maintain the integrity of the gut wall: your first line of defence from toxins. (Glutamine powder should not be taken if there is liver damage.)

Our third recommendation is an all-round antioxidant or liver-support formula (see Resources). Pick a formula that has as many of the key liver support nutrients shown below as possible. The ones in bold are the most important, and are needed in substantial quantities (outlined below), so you may need to take these separately:

Vitamin C

Vitamin E

Coenzyme Q_{10}

Glutathione

N-acetyl cysteine (NAC),* 500mg twice a day

Glycine

Glutamine, ** 1–2 teaspoons (4–8g) a day, on an empty stomach

Calcium-D-glucarate

Milk thistle (silymarin), taking this with phosphatidyl choline helps its utilisation

DIM (broccoli extract)

MSM (a form of sulphur)

Trimethyl glycine (TMG),* 1g twice a day. (If you can get it, 400mg of SAM* twice a day is even better.)

Turmeric (which is high in curcumin) 500mg twice a day. This yellow spice is rarely found in combination formulas.

Bupleurum as found in sho-saiko-to herbal formula (for liver repair, see Appendix 3 on our website www.how2quit.co.uk)

* Although NAC, TMG and SAM may be extremely helpful, these are best given under medical supervision if you have liver damage (see www.how2quit.co.uk for more details on liver regeneration).** Those with advanced liver cirrhosis or a history of a risk of liver failure must not take large amounts of glutamine, unless under the supervision of a medical practitioner. All amino acids contain nitrogen, which the liver has to process. In advanced liver damage this may be compromised.

There is some crossover between the Digestion Prescription and the Liver-detox Prescription. This is because if your gut is healthy there will be fewer toxins for the liver to detoxify. There is no need to double up on digestive enzymes, probiotics and glutamine powder, so the only added extra is a liver detox formula (see Resources), usually taken twice a day for one to four weeks.

NOTE If you have been diagnosed with liver damage or cirrhosis, or have a liver test with a reading in the orange or red (AST above 33, ALT above 32), we do not recommend glutamine or large amounts of other amino acids without the supervision of a health-care practitioner. This is because when the liver is dys-functional, it can create toxic by-products from excess amino acids. As an alternative we recommend IV nutrient therapy targeted to support liver recovery and regeneration (see the next chapter and www.how2quit.co.uk), under medical supervision. Milk thistle, however, is very helpful. Supplement 600mg a day.

Your Sleep Prescription

Are you sleep deficient? Test yourself by completing the questionnaire on excessive daytime sleepiness, on page 204. If your score is 10 or more you would benefit from this Sleep Prescription. As well as following our recommendations in Chapter 13 these supplements can help you get to sleep and stay asleep. We have given four options for the main 'ingredient' in the prescription. This is because we are all different: some people respond best to tryptophan, some to 5-HTP, some to a mixture of both and others to melatonin.

Tryptophan, 1,000 to 3,000mg (1,000mg of tryptophan is available on prescription as Optimax)

or

5-HTP, 100 to 200mg

or

Tryptophan, 500mg (supplements are limited to 220mg, so take 2) with 5-HTP, 100mg

(All the above options work best one hour before bed, taken with a light carbohydrate snack; for example, some fruit or juice. Do not take if you are on antidepressants.)

or

Melatonin, 1–3mg under the tongue. (This is an alternative to tryptophan or 5-HTP.)

Melatonin is available over the counter in some countries. In the EU it is classified as a medicine and available on prescription.

Niacinamide (vitamin B3) or inositol hexanicotinate, 1,000mg (in truth, you can triple this amount if you need to)

Magnesium, 200mg (in the form of magnesium taurate, glycinate or ascorbate)

Vitamin B6, 50mg (ideally 25mg of pyridoxal-5-phosphate – P5P – and 25mg pyridoxine)

Try any or all of the above. If they don't work, and you feel anxious or stressed, try:

GABA, 1,000–2,000mg (classified as a medicine in the EU, but not in the US)

or

Glutamine, 4–8g (1–2 teaspoons taken in water on an empty stomach) and taurine, 500–1,000mg

The most potent herbal sedative is valerian: 600–1,200mg about 1 hour before bedtime. While this will help you get a good night's sleep as you are coming off your addictive substance, it is important to note that it doesn't restore your brain's chemistry so it isn't a replacement for the amino acids recommended above.

Glycine, 500mg under the tongue. If you suffer from panic attacks take 2g under the tongue, repeated every 4 minutes, until relief (usually two to three times, but do not exceed 10g a day).

What's your addiction?

Depending on your addiction there are specific nutrients that help restore brain chemistry the most rapidly. We will tell you generally what works best for your particular addiction, but you will also need to use your own judgement and adjust what you take according to the symptoms you are experiencing. Ensure you read Chapter 7 for more guidance.

Here are all the prescriptions we use:

Stimulant Prescription For people either coming off caffeine, nicotine, cocaine, methamphetamine, Ritalin and other pre-scribed stimulant drugs, or still suffering abstinence symptoms having quit.

Alcohol Prescription For people either coming off alcohol or still suffering abstinence symptoms having quit.

Opiate Prescription For people coming off heroin, methadone or painkillers, or still suffering abstinence symptoms having quit.

Mood Prescription For people coming off antidepressant med-ication or still suffering abstinence symptoms having quit. This is also the best nutrient combination if you are coming off sugar or excessive cannabis use, or you are still suffering abstinence symptoms having quit.

Chill-out Prescription For people coming off tranquillisers, sedatives or sleeping pills, or still suffering abstinence symp-toms having quit. Please note that this is the same as the Sleep Prescription, discussed on page 397, for taking if you have sleep or relaxation issues. As you'll see in the questionnaire, one of the criteria for benefiting from these additional supplements is that you are coming off tranquillisers, sedatives or sleeping pills or still suffering abstinence symptoms having quit them.

Getting your prescriptions together

You will find these prescriptions on pages 403–24.

If, as an example, you were quitting cigarettes, and you weren't sleeping well you'd need to supplement what's recommended in the following:

Basic Supplements + Sleep Prescription
+ Stimulant Prescription

You would continue with these until your abstinence symptoms were substantially reduced and your sleeping was no longer an issue. At this point your maintenance supplements would simply be the Basic Supplements. If, on the other hand, you were over your cigarette withdrawal symptoms, but you still weren't finding it easy to get to sleep or stay asleep, you would continue to take the Basic Supplements and the Sleep Prescription.

If you are using many substances, perhaps to help you recover from your main addictive substance, we recommend you focus in on your main addictive substance – the one you would miss the most. If you are dealing with more than one *addiction* (such as alcohol, cigarettes and cocaine) again we recommend you take the prescription that best addresses the primary addictive substance that you are quitting. (If you are giving up alcohol first, start with the Alcohol Prescription, then if you give up cigarettes two weeks later, switch to the Stimulant Prescription.) (However, if you have multiple addictions you will get the best results using IV nutrient therapy; see Chapter 30.)

The specific additional nutrients in each of these prescriptions are given on pages 403–24. In Resources you will find a list of suppliers with products that provide the levels of supplements you need.

When you have worked out what you need, and obtained your supplements, see when and how to take them below.

When and how to take supplements

Take your supplements three times a day during the *recovery* phase and twice a day during the *maintenance* phase. Generally supplements are best taken with food, so during the *maintenance* phase, if you are on just the Basic Supplements, take the supplements with breakfast and lunch. But, as you have learned, amino acids are often better absorbed either on a relatively empty stomach or, in the case of tyrosine, tryptophan and 5-HTP, with a carbohydrate snack. So, during recovery, when you will be taking more supplements, we recommend you spread them out across the day to be taken at least three times; for example, take on three occasions from the following: breakfast, lunch, a morning or afternoon snack, dinner or during the evening. By spreading the supplements over the day you will get a better and quicker result.

The table on page 425 shows which supplements are best to take when and how. We have found the best way to approach this, and avoid confusion or missed supplements, is in a way similar to a military operation, as described below. It is much better to do it *before* you quit: if you have a serious addiction you might lose the plot during withdrawal! If you've lost the plot already get someone to help you.

1. Get a supplement box or some small plastic bags, so that you can make up your groups of supplements. (These can be bought from most mail-order supplement companies.)

2. Order enough supplements for the first four weeks.

3. Using the chart on page 425 (When to Take Supplements), assign them to one of the following piles: breakfast; morning carb snack; lunch; afternoon carb snack; dinner; one hour before bed.

4. Now, put them into your supplement box or the bags.

Most importantly, don't forget to take them. If it's too complicated you won't do it. So, if need be, condense your supplements into three piles only. (By the way, a nutritional therapist will work this all out for you if you prefer to consult one – see Resources on page 485. He or she will also work out your optimal diet.)

Finding out your specific needs

Since you are unique, the ideal is to have biochemical tests to find out exactly what your nutrient status is, as well as your neurotransmitter balance. In Resources you can find out about clinics and practitioners who can do this for you. The kind of tests they should be running are explained in Appendix 5 (which is on our website www.how2quit.co.uk). In terms of giving up the substance long term and becoming free of symptoms, three of the most important tests you should be given are for essential fats, hidden food allergies and saliva cortisol/DHEA levels for adrenal function.

Your action list

1. Begin with your supplements for recovery and switch to your supplements for maintenance when the total score of your five worst abstinence symptoms is two-thirds of your beginning score.

2. Regardless of your specific addiction, it is important to take the recommended basic supplements (the Basic Supplements): multivitamin/mineral, extra vitamin C, essential fats, and phospholipids; then take the amino acid supplements appropriate for your addiction. Find the prescription appropriate for your addiction from those listed on pages 403–24.

3. Take additional supplements for specific digestion, liver, homocysteine or sleep problems, if you need them.

The following pages contain our **ADDICTION PRESCRIPTIONS** ▶

ADDICTION PRESCRIPTIONS

STIMULANT PRESCRIPTION

These supplements are recommended to support people coming off caffeine, nicotine, cocaine, metamphetamine, Ritalin and other prescribed stimulant drugs or still suffering from abstinence symptoms having quit.

Supplement	Daily amount	Taken as	With/without food	Notes
Tyrosine	2,000mg	1,000mg × 2	Empty stomach or with carbohydrate snack	
NAC (N-acetyl cysteine)	1,500mg	500mg × 3	As above	Optional but recommended for cocaine
Ginseng (American, Korean, Siberian)	1,000mg	500mg × 2	With or without food	Best taken morning and afternoon, not evening. Must be standardised to guarantee potency
B vitamins:				
B₅ (pantothenic acid)	200mg	100mg × 2	With food	Assumes 50mg with Basic Supplement Pack
B₆	40mg	20mg × 2	With food	Assumes 20mg with Basic Supplement Pack
Folic acid	400mcg	200mcg × 2	With food	Assumes 200mcg with Basic Supplement Pack
B₁₂	20mcg	10mcg × 2	With food	Assumes 10mcg with Basic Supplement Pack
Chromium	400mcg	200mcg × 2	With food	
NADH	10mg	5mg × 2	With or without food	

Stimulant prescription: Notes

Tyrosine is the precursor for dopamine, noradrenalin and adrenalin – the neurotransmitters that addictive stimulants mimic. It is therefore the most important amino acid to take if you are coming off stimulants. It's absorbed best on an empty stomach between meals. You can break open a capsule and tip some under your tongue for a quicker effect. If you are struggling with tiredness, overeating and drug craving you could try double this amount. As an excess may be over-stimulating, it is not recommended for someone who is nervous, highly agitated, irritable, suffering from cancer (including melanomas), high blood pressure or with a history of mania, unless under professional supervision. Tyrosine should not be taken by phenyl- ketonurics, or on a continuous basis by those who are pregnant or breastfeeding.

NAC (N-acetyl cysteine) is a precursor of glutathione and helps to raise glutamate levels in the brain. This reduces craving for stimulants and also helps to repair the brain. A maintenance level is 1,000mg a day. More is needed for those with acute stimulant addiction.

Gingseng This is an adaptogen, a class of substances – also including reishi mushrooms, rhodiola and ashwagandha – that help restore adrenal function. Ginseng restores vital energy throughout the entire body, helping to overcome stress. Allergy can occur with the use of ginseng, but this is rare. Menstrual irregularities and breast tenderness have been reported with the use of Asian ginseng. If you experience these symptoms stop taking it.

Siberian ginseng is the safest and healthiest known stimulant, with generally no negative side effects.

How much you need depends both on the total combination of what you are taking, and the potency or concentration of active ingredients in the herb. In other words, there is potent and weak ginseng. You should be looking for ginsengs with a 'standardised' extract that contains at least 4 per cent ginsenosides. Aim for a total of 700–2,000mg of total adaptogens. It's best not to use them for more than three months at a time, then give yourself a one-month break. Many Asian doctors have traditionally recommended a routine of five days on, two days off, during those three months, to ensure continued effectiveness.

B vitamins Most of these B vitamins will be found in high-dose multivitamins, but not in sufficient quantities. If you are also taking a methylation/homocysteine-lowering formula this will also provide extra B_6. However you are unlikely to get enough pantothenic acid (vitamin B_5) and therefore will need to buy a separate supplement of this.

Chromium helps to stabilise blood sugar balance and, in high doses, is a potent antidepressant in those suffering from atypical depression (see page 296). You need 400–600mcg a day for this effect. Most supplements come in 200mcg tablets, so start with two. Chromium is best taken in the morning and during the day, not in the evening. There is no toxicity below 10,000mcg. Best forms are chromium polynicotinate and chromium picolinate.

NADH (or nicotinamide adenine dinucleotide) in reduced form, is a small organic molecule found naturally in every living cell. It is necessary for thousands of biochemical reactions within the body, playing a key role in the energy production of cells, particularly in the brain and central nervous system. It stimulates cellular production of the neurotransmitters dopamine, noradrenalin and serotonin, improving mental clarity, alertness and concentration. The more NADH a cell has available, the more energy it can produce, and the more efficiently it can perform. It also enhances physical performance and energy. We have found it very useful as part of the treatment of chronic fatigue syndrome, depression and ADHD. There are no known cautions. You will need to obtain separate supplements of this, as it is not generally included in multi formulas.

Making it easy

Some formulas for supporting those reducing stimulants combine tyrosine with adaptogens such as ginseng and B vitamins, especially B$_5$ (pantothenic acid). If you find the right one, this 'kills three birds with one stone'. We will call this a 'combination stimulant formula'. Your supplement planner will then be:

EASY PLANNER: STIMULANT PRESCRIPTION

Supplement	Morning	Afternoon	Evening
Combination stimulant formula	2 on waking	2 mid afternoon	
NADH 5mg	1 on waking	1 mid afternoon	
Chromium 200mcg	1 on waking	1 with lunch	

Plus the Basic Supplement Pack (page 388)

ALCOHOL PRESCRIPTION

These supplements are recommended to support people coming off alcohol or still suffering abstinence symptoms, having quit.

Supplement	Daily Amount	Taken as	With/without	Notes
Tryptophan	2,000mg	1,000mg × 2	Away from main meal	
or				
5-HTP	200mg	100mg × 2	(30 minutes before; 2 hours after) with some carbohydrate such as fruit or an oatcake	
or				
Tryptophan with 5-HTP	500mg 150mg	250mg × 2 75mg × 2		
Methyl nutrients (B_6, B_{12}, folic acid, TMG)	× 2		With food	Find the right formula (see below)
or				
SAM	800mg	400mg × 2	On waking, empty stomach	Not OTC in the EU
and				
Methyl nutrients (as above)	× 1		With food	Find the right formula (see below)
Omega-3 EPA/ DHA	2,000mg	1,000mg × 2	With food	You want 1,000mg of EPA + DHA (see page 408)

Supplement	Daily Amount	Taken as	With/without	Notes
GABA	1,000mg	500mg × 2	With or without food	A high dose can cause tingling in fingers or face
or				
Glutamine with taurine	500mg 500mg	250mg × 2 250mg × 2	With water	
or				
Glutamine alone	8,000mg	4,000mg × 2	With water; not a hot drink	
Magnesium	150mg	75mg × 2	Morning and afternoon, can help sleep in the evening. With or without food	Assumes extra 150mg with Basic Supplement Pack
Vitamin C*	2,000mg	1,000mg × 2	With meals	Assumes 2,000mg in Basic Supplement Pack

OTC: over the counter

*Buy vitamin C powder. If detoxifying, put 10–20g in a bottle of one-third juice and one-third water. Drink frequently throughout the day. If you get loose bowels, lower the dose until your bowels settle. Very quickly, once you are free of your initial withdrawal symptoms, you can stop the high-dose powder and you can start taking basic oral supplements: 2–4g a day. Otherwise supplement 3–4g a day, one with each meal. The Basic Supplement Pack provides 2g, so this means having another 1g or 2g a day.

Alcohol prescription: Notes

5-HTP is about ten times more potent than tryptophan. So 100mg of 5-HTP is equivalent to 1,000mg of tryptophan. Tryptophan is only available in supplements up to 220mg. Therefore, if you take four you will be getting 880mg, close to 1g. Tryptophan is also available on prescription as Optimax in 1,000mg capsules. Some people respond better to tryptophan, others to 5-HTP. The ideal is probably to take some of both. There are no dangers associated with either tryptophan or 5-HTP at these levels provided you are not on antidepressant medication. Many antidepressants stop the body being able to break down serotonin. Therefore, giving large amounts of either tryptophan or 5-HTP is not recommended until you are off antidepressants. A doctor may prescribe both, but you should be under the auspices of a health practitioner to do this.

Methyl nutrients are found in combination in homocysteine-modulating formulas. What you are looking for is a formula that provides B6, B12 (preferably methyl B12), folic acid, plus TMG and NAC, which also helps lower homocysteine and raise SAM. The levels you want are shown on page 394. These help your body to make SAM. If you live in a country such as the US, where you can buy SAM, a short-term and more effective solution is to supplement 400–800mg of SAM twice daily, along with one of these methyl-nutrient formulas. If not, take two. These nutrients help your body make SAM. Glutathione, the body and brain's most important antioxidant, is made from three amino acids: glutamine, glycine (found in trimethylglycine or TMG) and cysteine (N-acetyl cysteine). So pick a methyl-nutrient formula that contains N-acetyl cysteine (NAC).

SAM must be taken away from food. Ideally take it first thing in the morning, on waking, with water before you eat anything, and again between lunch and dinner. One of the best forms of SAM is S-adenolsylmethionine tosylate disulfate. You can double this dose, but be aware that too much can make you nauseous. Usually this is short-lived. Some people have also reported irritability, anxiety and insomnia on high doses.

Omega-3 supplements vary greatly in what they contain. You want to select one that has the most EPA + DHA, and relatively more EPA than DHA. It is also worth getting one from a reputable company so that you can be confident it is pure (free from contaminants such as PCBs and mercury). Your goal is to supplement 1,000mg of EPA + DHA a day, probably 600mg of EPA plus 400mg of DHA. Most 1,000mg supplements provide at least 500mg of EPA + DHA, so this means taking two large fish oil capsules. Read the label carefully.

GABA is both an amino acid and a neurotransmitter. It helps you relax and helps rid you of anxiety. If you take too much it can cause tingling in the fingers or face and make you nauseous. So, it is best to increase gradually, starting with 500mg, and not to take more than 2,000mg daily. GABA is classified as a medicine in the UK. It is available from the US for your own personal use. GABA is made from glutamine and works as a relaxing or calming agent similar to taurine. Therefore, the next best thing is to either supplement glutamine on its own, or glutamine plus taurine. Some supplement formulas contain this combination, plus magnesium. In this way you also achieve the desired amount of magnesium. If you choose to take glutamine on its own, it is most economical to take glutamine powder; 1 rounded teaspoon is about 4g. It dissolves in water and tastes fine. Heat destroys glutamine, so don't put it in a hot drink. (Glutamine powder should not be taken if there is liver damage.) Some people respond better to taurine, others to glutamine. For relief of anxiety, GABA is superior to both.

Vitamin C can cause loose bowels as a temporary phenomenon. Some believe the ideal intake, especially if you're in early recovery, fighting a viral infection or under extreme physical or emotional stress, to be the level just below that which gives you loose bowels. If you are detoxing, withdrawing from alcohol or heroin addiction, very large amounts can make a big difference to minimising your withdrawal symptoms. It's not dangerous, so don't be concerned about trying large amounts. Just cut back if you get loose bowels. It's a good idea to be supplementing with extra B$_6$ and magnesium when taking doses at or about 10g daily. This helps prevent calcium oxalate kidney stones induced by high doses of vitamin C.

Making it easy

Some supplements designed to support normal relaxation contain combinations of nutrients (taurine, glutamine, magnesium and 5-HTP), which help you to sleep or chill out. We will call this kind of combination a 'combination chill/sleep formula'. Some methylation formulas also provide N-acetyl cysteine. So, if you pick carefully, you can achieve all these nutrients in more or less the right amounts, by taking three supplements two or three times a day. The chances are you won't need these for long. Your supplement planner will then be:

EASY PLANNER: ALCOHOL PRESCRIPTION

Supplement	Morning	Afternoon	Evening
* Combination chill/sleep formula	1 mid morning	1 mid afternoon	2 in evening or one hour before bed
+ Methyl-nutrient formula	1 with breakfast	1 with lunch	
Omega-3 EPA-rich capsule	1 with breakfast	1 with lunch	
Vitamin C 1,000mg	1 with breakfast	1 with lunch	

Plus the Basic Supplement Pack (page 388)

* If you are already taking these because you have sleeping problems there is no need to double up.

+ If you are already taking these because you have a high homocysteine level there is no need to double up.

OPIATE PRESCRIPTION

These supplements are recommended to support people coming off heroin, methadone or painkillers, or still suffering from abstinence symptoms having quit.

Supplement	Daily Amount	Taken as	With/without	Notes
D-phenylalanine	1,000mg	500mg × 2	Empty stomach	Best for reducing drug craving
GABA	1,000mg	500mg × 2	With or without food	A high dose can make you nauseous
or				
Glutamine	500mg	250mg × 2	With water, not a hot drink	Hot water (heat) destroys glutamine
with taurine	500mg	250mg × 2	on an empty stomach	
or				
Glutamine alone	8,000mg	4,000mg × 2	With water, not a hot drink	
Tryptophan	2,000mg	1,000mg × 2	Away from main meal	
or				
5-HTP	200mg	100mg × 2	Away from main meal with some carbohydrate	
or				
Tryptophan	500mg	250mg × 2	With a carbohydrate snack	
with 5-HTP	150mg	75mg × 2		

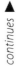

continues

Supplement	Daily Amount	Taken as	With/without	Notes
Niacinamide				
or				
Hexanicotinate	1,500mg	500mg × 3	Any time. With food	Hexanicotinate is a non-blushing niacin
Vitamin C powder*	10g a day or more		Every 1–2 hours throughout the day	
Magnesium	300mg	150mg × 2	Morning and afternoon, can help sleep in the evening. With or without food	Assumes extra 150mg in Basic Supplement Pack
Optional extras:				
NAC (n-acetyl cysteine)	500mg	x 2	Away from main meal (30 minutes before; 2 hours after)	Helps raise enkephalins, improving mood
Turmeric	500mg	x 2	With food (e.g. breakfast and lunch)	Helps enhance detoxification Increases glutathione

Opiate prescription: Notes

D-phenylalanine, as opposed to DL-phenylalanine, specifically raises endorphins (which are much depleted in addicts).

GABA is both an amino acid and a neurotransmitter. It helps you relax. If you take too much it can make you nauseous. So, it is best to increase gradually, starting with 500mg, and not take more than 2,000mg. GABA is classified as a medicine in the UK. It is available from the US for your own personal use. GABA is made from taurine and glutamine. Therefore, the next best thing is to either supplement glutamine on its own, or glutamine plus taurine. Some supplement formulas contain this combination. If you choose to take glutamine on its own, it is most economical to take glutamine powder; 1 rounded teaspoon is about 4g. It dissolves in water and tastes fine. Heat destroys glutamine, so don't put it in a hot drink. (Glutamine powder should not be taken if there is liver damage.) Some people respond better to taurine, others to glutamine. GABA is superior to both.

5-HTP is about ten times more potent than tryptophan. So 100mg of 5-HTP is equivalent to 1,000mg of tryptophan. Tryptophan is only available in supplements, up to 220mg. Therefore, if you take four you will be getting 880mg, close to 1g. Tryptophan is also available on prescription as Optimax in 1,000mg capsules. Some people respond better to tryptophan, others to

5-HTP. The ideal is probably to take some of both. There are no dangers associated with either tryptophan or 5-HTP at these levels provided you are not on antidepressant medication. Many antidepressants stop the body being able to break down serotonin. Therefore, giving large amounts of either tryptophan or 5-HTP is not recommended until you are off antidepressants. A doctor may prescribe both, but you should be under the auspices of a health practitioner to do this.

Niacinamide and **inositol hexanicotinate** are non-blushing forms of niacin (vitamin B₃). There's nothing wrong with niacin, which is cheaper, but it will make you blush, go red, hot and itchy for up to 30 minutes. If you choose to take niacin, take it with meals and make sure you start at a lower dose and can relax, or lie down, when the flushing starts. The more often you take it – for example, twice a day for a week – the less you flush. The flush can leave you feeling deeply relaxed. Some people love it. Others don't.

Vitamin C can cause loose bowels as a temporary phenomenon. Some believe the ideal intake is the level just below that which gives you loose bowels. When you are detoxing very large amounts can make a big difference to minimising withdrawal symptoms. It's not dangerous, so don't be concerned to try large amounts. Just cut back if you get loose bowels, or drink less frequently. It's a good idea to take magnesium and B$_6$ when taking doses above 10g a day (this helps prevent calcium oxalate kidney stones). On the first day of heroin withdrawal increase this dose up to bowel tolerance level, which can be as much as 50 grams.

*Buy vitamin C powder. Put 10–20g in a bottle of one-third juice and one-third water. Drink frequently throughout the day. If you get loose bowels, lower the dose until your bowels settle. High doses are for those coming off heroin/methadone and are only needed for a few days. Very quickly, once you are free of your initial withdrawal symptoms, you can stop the high-dose powder and you can start taking basic oral supplements: 2–4g a day. Otherwise supplement 3–4g a day, one with each meal. The Basic Supplement Pack provides 2g, so this means having another 1g or 2g a day.

Magnesium For short-term use only, intakes of 500mg of magnesium can be very helpful. This level, however, is more than you need on a maintenance programme. Provided you eat greens and seeds most days, supplementing 150–250mg of magnesium a day is sufficient.

Making it easy

Some supplements designed to support normal relaxation contain combinations of nutrients (taurine, glutamine, magnesium and 5-HTP), which help you to sleep or chill out. We will call this kind of combination a 'combination chill/sleep formula'. Some non-blushing niacin formulations contain magnesium. D-phenylalanine comes only as a separate supplement. So, if you pick carefully, you can achieve all these nutrients in more or less the right amounts, by taking three supplements two or three times a day. The chances are you won't need these for long. Your supplement planner will then be:

EASY PLANNER: OPIATE PRESCRIPTION

Supplement	Morning	Afternoon	Evening
*Combination chill/sleep formula	1 mid morning	1 mid afternoon	2 one hour before bed
Niacin 500mg + magnesium	1 with breakfast	1 with lunch	
D-phenylalanine 500mg	1 mid morning	1 mid morning	
Vitamin C powder	throughout the day (until abstinence symptoms abate), then		
Vitamin C 1,000mg	2	2	1

Plus the Basic Supplement Pack (page 388)

*If you are already taking these because you have sleeping problems, there is no need to double up.

MOOD PRESCRIPTION

These supplements are recommended to support people coming off sugar, antidepressants or cannabis or still suffering from abstinence symptoms having quit.

Supplement	Daily Amount	Taken as	With/without food	Notes
Tryptophan	2,000mg	1,000mg × 2	Away from main meal (30 minutes before; 2 hours after) with some carbohydrate such as fruit or oatcake	
or				
5-HTP	200mg	100mg × 2		
or				
Tryptophan with 5-HTP	500mg 150mg	250mg × 2 75mg × 2		
Tyrosine	1,000mg	500mg × 2	Empty stomach or with a carbohydrate snack	
and				
DL-phenylalanine	1,000mg	500mg × 2	Empty stomach	

Supplement	Daily Amount	Taken as	With/without food	Notes
Methyl nutrients (B$_6$, B$_{12}$, folic acid, TMG)	× 2		With food	Find the right formula (see below)
or				
SAM	800mg	400mg × 2	Empty stomach, between meals	Not OTC in the EU
and				
Methyl nutrients (as above)	× 1		With food	Find the right formula (see page 418)
Chromium	400mcg	200mcg × 2	With food	
Omega-3 EPA/DHA	2,000mg	1,000mg × 2	With food	You want 1,000mg of EPA + DHA (see page 419)

OTC: Over the counter

Mood prescription: Notes

5-HTP is about ten times more potent than tryptophan. So 100mg of 5-HTP is equivalent to 1,000mg of tryptophan. Tryptophan is only available in supplements, up to 220mg. Therefore, if you take four you will be getting 880mg, close to 1g. Tryptophan is also available on prescription as Optimax in 1,000mg capsules. Some people respond better to tryptophan, others to 5-HTP. The ideal is probably to take some of both. There are no dangers associated with either tryptophan or 5-HTP at these levels *provided* you are not on antidepressant medication. Many antidepressants stop the body being able to break down serotonin. Therefore, giving large amounts of either tryptophan or 5-HTP is not recommended until you are off antidepressants. A doctor may prescribe both, but you should be under the auspices of a health practitioner to do this.

Tyrosine and **L-phenylalanine** are the amino acid precursors for dopamine, noradrenalin and adrenalin – the motivating neurotransmitters. They are absorbed best on an empty stomach. If your get-up-and-go has got-up-and-gone this can give you a kick-start. If you are struggling with tiredness, overeating and drug craving you could try double this amount. Excess may be over-stimulating. Not recommended for someone who is nervous, highly agitated, irritable, suffering from depression or from cancer (including melanomas), high blood pressure or with

a history of mania, unless under professional supervision. Tyrosine should not be taken by phenylketonurics, or on a continuous basis by those who are pregnant or breastfeeding.

Methyl nutrients are found in combination in homocysteine-modulating formulas. What you are looking for is a formula that provides B_6, B_{12} (preferably methyl B_{12}), folic acid, plus TMG. The levels you want are shown on page 394. These help your body to make SAM. If you live in a country, such as the US, where you can buy SAM, a short-term and more effective solution is to supplement 400mg of SAM, along with one of these methyl nutrient formulas. If not, take two. These nutrients help your body make SAM. Glutathione, the body and brain's most important antioxidant, is made from three amino acids: glutamine, glycine (found in trimethylglycine – TMG). So pick a methyl nutrient formula that contains N-acetyl cysteine (NAC) and cysteine (N-acetyl cysteine). Some formulas designed to support mood already contain most of these, in which case you don't need to supplement extra.

SAM must be taken away from food. Ideally take twice daily on an empty stomach between meals. One of the best forms of SAM is S-adenosylmethionine tosylate disulfate. You can double this dose but be aware that too much can make you nauseous or give you heartburn. This usually goes away within a day or two.

Some people have also reported irritability, anxiety or insomnia on high doses.

Chromium helps to stabilise blood sugar balance and, in high doses, is a potent antidepressant in those suffering from atypical depression (see page 296). You need 400–600mcg a day for this effect. Most supplements come in 200mcg tablets, so start with two. Chromium is best taken in the morning and during the day, not in the evening. There is no toxicity below 10,000mcg. Best forms are chromium polynicotinate and chromium picolinate.

Omega-3 supplements vary greatly in what they contain. You want to select one that has the most EPA + DHA, and relatively more EPA than DHA. It is also worth getting one from a reputable company so that you can be confident it is pure (free from contaminants such as PCBs and mercury). Your goal is to supplement 1,000mg of EPA + DHA a day, probably 600mg of EPA plus 400mg of DHA. Most 1,000mg supplements provide at least 500mg of EPA + DHA, so this means taking two large fish oil capsules. Read the label carefully.

Making it easy

Some supplements designed to support mood contain combinations of 5-HTP, tyrosine, DL-phenylalanine plus methylating B vitamins and TMG. We will call this kind of combination a 'mood nutrient formula'. Your supplement planner will then be:

EASY PLANNER: MOOD PRESCRIPTION

Supplement	Morning	Afternoon
Mood nutrient formula	2 on waking	2 mid afternoon
Chromium 200mcg	1 on waking	1 with lunch
Omega-3 EPA rich capsule	1 with breakfast	1 with lunch

Plus the Basic Supplement Pack (page 388)

CHILL-OUT PRESCRIPTION

These supplements are recommended to support people coming off tranquillisers, sedatives or sleeping pills or still suffering from abstinence symptoms having quit.

Supplement	Daily Amount	Taken as	With/without	Notes
Tryptophan	2,000mg	1,000mg × 2	Away from main meal (30 minutes before; 2 hours after)	
or				
5-HTP	200mg	100mg × 2	with some carbohydrate such as fruit or an oatcake	
or				
Melatonin	3mg	3mg × 1	Taken under the tongue in the evening	
GABA	1,000mg	500mg × 2	With or without food	A high dose can cause tingling in fingers or face and make you nauseous
Glutamine with Taurine	500mg 500mg	250mg × 2 250mg × 2	With water. Empty stomach	
or				
Glutamine alone	8,000mg	4,000mg × 2	With water, not a hot drink, on an empty stomach	Hot water (heat) destroys glutamine

Supplement	Daily Amount	Taken as	With/without	Notes
Niacinamide/ inositol hexanicotinate	1,000mg	500mg × 2	With food	
Magnesium	300mg	150mg × 2	Morning and evening, can help sleep in the evening. With or without food	Assumes an extra 150mg in Basic Supplement Pack. Best forms are taurates, glycinates or ascorbates
Vitamin B$_6$	50mg	25mg × 2	With food	Ideally, half as pyridoxal-5-phosphate (P5P) (see notes, page 423)
Valerian	600mg	300mg × 2	Empty stomach	Take in the evening or one hour before bed

Chill-out prescription: Notes

5-HTP is about ten times more potent than tryptophan. So 100mg of 5-HTP is equivalent to 1,000mg of tryptophan. Tryptophan is only available in supplements, up to 220mg. Therefore, if you take four you will be getting 880mg, close to 1g. Tryptophan is also available on prescription as Optimax in 1,000mg capsules. Some people respond better to tryptophan, others to 5-HTP. The ideal is probably to take some of both. There are no dangers associated with either tryptophan or 5-HTP at these levels provided you are not on antidepressant medication. Many antidepressants stop the body being able to break down serotonin. Therefore, giving large amounts of either tryptophan or 5-HTP is not recommended until you are off antidepressants. A doctor may prescribe both, but you should be under the auspices of a health practitioner to do this.

Melatonin is made from serotonin, which is made from tryptophan so, ideally, it's better to have tryptophan or 5-HTP because it helps you make both serotonin and melatonin. Melatonin is specifically required for sleeping. So, if you are really finding it hard to unwind and go to sleep since quitting your addictive drug, ask your doctor for a prescription of melatonin. In some countries it is available over the counter. Melatonin's side effects include nausea, dizziness and loss of libido and its long-term safety has not been determined. Headache and transient depression have been reported. In people who are depressed, melatonin may worsen symptoms. Melatonin is best taken under medical supervision and is available only by prescription in the UK.

GABA is both an amino acid and a neurotransmitter. It helps you relax. If you take too much it can cause tingling in your fingers or face. So, it is best to increase gradually, starting with 500mg, and not take more than 2,000mg a day. GABA is classified as a medicine in the UK. It is available from the US for your own personal use. GABA is made from glutamine and works similarly to taurine as a relaxing, calming neurotransmitter. Therefore, the next best thing is to either supplement glutamine on its own, or glutamine plus taurine. Some supplement formulas contain this combination. If you choose to take glutamine on its own it is most economical to take glutamine powder; 1 rounded teaspoon is about 4g. It dissolves in water and tastes fine. Heat

destroys glutamine, so don't put it in a hot drink. (Glutamine powder should not be taken if there is liver damage.) Some people respond better to taurine, others to glutamine. GABA is superior to both.

Niacinamide and **inositol hexanicotinate** are non-blushing forms of niacin (vitamin B₃). You can triple the given amount if you need to. There's nothing wrong with niacin, which is cheaper, but it will make you blush, go red, hot and itchy for up to 30 minutes. If you choose to take niacin, take it with meals and make sure you can relax, or lie down, when the flush starts. The more often you take it – for example, twice a day for a week – the less you flush. The flush can leave you feeling deeply relaxed. Some people love it. Others don't.

Magnesium is vital for nerve function and, if you are feeling strung out or on edge, having enough can really help. Pumpkin seeds are one of the best food sources, so snack on these. Ideally, you want to supplement up to 500mg a day. If there's 150mg in your basic multivitamin–mineral supplement, then you are looking to add another 200–400mg. If you have magnesium in the form of magnesium taurate (bound to taurine), ascorbate (bound to vitamin C) or magnesium glycinate (bound to glycine), you get more of these other important nutrients.

Vitamin B₆ (pyridoxine), together with magnesium, helps to convert tryptophan into serotonin and melatonin, tyrosine to dopamine and noradrenalin and glutamine to GABA. There is another form of B₆ called pyridoxal-5-phosphate (P5P) which is especially bio-active. This is possibly twice as effective, so think of 50mg of P5P as equivalent to 100mg of B₆. Ideally you want to achieve a total intake of B₆ between 50mg and 100mg a day. A good multivitamin will provide between 20mg and 50mg. If you are taking a homocysteine-modulating formula, this will probably provide you with enough, together with a multi-vitamin. Otherwise you may need a little more. Ideally, pick a formula that contains some P5P. Some also provide magnesium.

Standardised valerian is one of the most effective and studied herbs for the treatment of anxiety and insomnia, sometimes being referred to as 'nature's Valium'. It has been used as a folk remedy for thousands of years. As a natural relaxant, it is useful for several disorders seen in recovery from addictions, including restlessness, nervousness, insomnia (especially problems with falling asleep), menstrual problems and 'nervous' stomach. It has also been used in conjunction with St John's wort in treating anxiety. A word of caution: valerian can interact with some drugs, including alcohol, certain antihistamines, muscle relaxants, psychotropic drugs and narcotics. At high doses (above 1,600mg a day) over a long period of time, it has been linked to 'hangover' symptoms, and in rare cases withdrawal-like symptoms. It is therefore best to use valerian only under the supervision of a health-care practitioner unless you have come off all drugs. Make sure that the valerian is standardised. This means you have a guaranteed quality of active herb. Hops and passionflower also have sedative effects.

Making it easy

Some supplements designed to support normal relaxation contain combinations of nutrients (taurine, glutamine, magnesium and 5-HTP), which help you to sleep or chill out. We will call this kind of combination a 'combination chill/sleep formula'. Some non-blushing niacin formulations also contain magnesium. Your supplement planner will then be:

EASY PLANNER: CHILL-OUT PRESCRIPTION

Supplement	Morning	Afternoon	Evening
* Combination chill/sleep formula	1 mid morning	1 mid afternoon	2 in the evening or one hour before bed
Niacin 500g*/magnesium	1 with breakfast	1 with lunch	
+ B₆ 25mg	1 with breakfast	1 with lunch	
Valerian 500–800mg			2 in the evening or one hour before bed

Plus the Basic Supplement Pack (page 388)

* If you are already taking these because you have sleeping problems there is no need to double up.

+ If you are already taking extra in your methylation formula because you have a high homocysteine level, there is no need to double up.

WHEN TO TAKE SUPPLEMENTS, HOW TO TAKE THEM AND THEIR CONTRAINDICATIONS

Supplement	When best to take	With what?	Contraindication
VITAMINS AND MINERALS			
B vitamins	Best in the morning or during the day. Never take a single B vitamin without also taking a multivitamin	Ideally with food	None
Vitamin C	Morning and evening	With food	Very high dose causes loose bowels
Chromium	In the morning and during the day, not in the evening	With food	None
Magnesium	Afternoon; before bed if you can't sleep	(Best forms are as taurates, glycinates or ascorbates)	None, but calcium also needed in a support multivitamin–mineral
NADH	Morning and evening	With or without food	None

Supplement	When best to take	With what?	Contraindication
Niacinamide or Inositol hexanicotinate	Best in the morning or during the day	With food	Very high doses (above 3g a day) might stress the liver if you have liver dysfunction. Monitor by testing liver enzymes (AST/ALT)
Niacin	Twice daily when you have time to relax/lie down afterwards for up to 30 minutes because of blushing	With food	
Omega-3 and 6	Morning and evening	With food	None, but don't have omega-6 without omega-3
AMINO ACIDS			
5-HTP/tryptophan	Morning, if you wake up depressed; 1 hour before bed if you can't sleep. Twice a day, on waking and before bed, if you have low mood and insomnia	Away from main meal (30 minutes before; 2 hours after) with some carbohydrate such as fruit or oatcake	Don't take if you are on any antidepressant drugs without professional advice
D-phenylalanine and DL-phenylalanins	Twice daily	With a carbohydrate snack or on an empty stomach	Should not be taken by people with phenylketonuria. Don't take if you have a history of mania, unless under professional supervision

Supplement	When best to take	With what?	Contraindication
GABA	Morning and evening	With or without food	Do not exceed 3g. Makes some people nauseous
Glutamine alone or with taurine	Twice daily. Start with 500mg per day and increase gradually	Empty stomach with water, not a hot drink	Glutamine is not recommended if you have cirrhosis, except under medical supervision
Melatonin	In the evening, not in the day	Take under the tongue	Gives some people headaches. Do not exceed 3mg a day. In people who are depressed, melatonin may worsen symptoms. Best taken under medical supervision and is available only by prescription in the UK
SAM	Between breakfast and lunch and lunch and dinner	Empty stomach	Makes some people nauseous and hyper. Too much can make you nauseous or give you heartburn

Supplement	When best to take	With what?	Contraindication
Tyrosine	Morning and afternoon	Empty stomach or with a carbohydrate snack	Don't take if you have a history of mania, unless under professional supervision. Should not be taken by phenylketonurics. Not suitable for people suffering from cancer (including melanomas), high blood pressure, or on a continuous basis by those who are pregnant or breastfeeding
HERBS			
Adaptogenic herbs (ginseng, American or Korean, or Siberian ginseng)	Morning and afternoon, not evening. After taking for 3 months stop for 1 month During 3 months, have 5 days on 2 days off	With or without food	High doses can cause menstrual abnormalities
Valerian	In the evening, or an hour before bed	Empty stomach	Don't take with sedative drugs, muscle relaxants, antihistamines, psychotropic drugs or narcotics

30.

INTRAVENOUS NUTRIENT THERAPY: THE FAST TRACK FOR CHRONIC ADDICTION

The critical turning point in becoming free from addiction, cravings and abstinence symptoms is recovering normal brain chemistry. The longer you have been abusing alcohol and/or other drugs, and the worse your nutrition has been, the more likely you are to suffer from profound brain chemistry deficiencies and imbalances. As long as this abnormal brain chemistry persists, you are likely to continue to suffer from chronic abstinence symptoms – cravings, depression, anxiety, insomnia, irritability, hypersensitivity and chronic fatigue – and as a direct consequence your chances of relapse are much higher.

To help rapidly reverse these chemical deficiencies, imbalances and chronic abstinence symptoms, the single most effective means is one week of intravenous (IV) nutrient treatment, alongside other nutritional supplements (because some need not, or cannot, be given by IV – such as essential fats and herbs) and the How to Quit Diet.

IV nutrient therapy for chronic late-stage addicts

Often, people who seek IV treatment do so as a last resort. They are not people who are in the early or middle stages of addiction or those who are easy to treat. They may have 'failed' at multiple attempts at recovery in the past and are willing to try this therapy only because they have nothing else to try. They may have lost all hope of being able to give up the substance, let alone live without it. On the other hand they may have been sober or clean from drugs for years, but are miserable because they still suffer from multiple abstinence symptoms. In many cases those who seek IV nutrient therapy are sicker and feel more hopeless than others with addictions and will have a long history of relapse. The sickest, hardest to treat alcoholics are paradoxically the very best candidates for IV treatment, with, in our experience, the highest level of success.

Many people find comfort and serenity following conventional treatment, but it is for those who don't that IV nutrient therapy can be truly a life-saving miracle.

Why is IV so effective?

The intravenous delivery of nutrients direct into the bloodstream assures a more rapid, predictable and reliable delivery of key brain recovery nutrients, achieving therapeutic levels not normally obtainable with oral supplements alone. Also, infusing essential vitamins, minerals, trace minerals, amino acids and nutrient derivatives intravenously often avoids potential negative side effects, such as nausea, that people might experience when taking high doses of certain supplements orally. If you have been eating a poor diet or simply not eating enough, drinking too much alcohol and/or coffee or taking painkillers on a regular basis, there's a good chance that your digestion and absorption of nutrients is messed up. If your digestion is damaged and absorption of nutrients compromised, there can be a vast difference between how much of a nutrient you take by mouth and how much will actually get into the brain. Not only can the same dose be more effective with IV nutrient therapy, but more can be given than can be taken orally.

The benefits

Among the benefits observed with IV nutrient therapy (which should always be accompanied by an optimal diet plus supplementation) are:

- Brain chemistry is rapidly rebalanced. Some people experience rapid relief of symptoms after only two or three days of IV nutrient therapy – in particular, a complete lack of cravings.

- Destructive free radicals, toxins, metabolites and fat-soluble addictants, which invariably build up in the brain and body of an addict, are removed.

- In conjunction with daily healthy meals, the body's nutritional status is restored.

- A healthy brain, as well as gut and liver cell membranes, is restored.

- Immune and liver functions are restored.

- Recovery is accelerated, with many of the common mental, emotional and physical symptoms that are suffered after quitting a substance being reversed. So, accomplishing in six days what would normally take 30, or more.

- For those going through a treatment programme, IV nutrient therapy allows them to take part in the other critically important treatments and counselling more fully, productively and earlier on, and to do so with more clarity, motivation and commitment.

The absence of craving is a particularly pleasant surprise for those receiving IV nutrient therapy. Craving has been part of their lives for so long they don't remember what it feels like not to have it. However, one of the most remarkable benefits to most people is the clarity of thought they possess after just a few days of IV nutrient therapy.

Case study HOWARD

Thirty-year-old university graduate, Howard, said, 'I haven't been able to think and write this clearly since high school, over a decade ago.'

Case study SAM

Sam, who had previously experienced some fairly long periods without alcohol with the help of AA, commented that his thinking was clearer after five days using IV nutrient therapy than it had been after a year of giving up alcohol in the past. 'I feel like I'm starting recovery with my first year behind me,' he said.

There is also a dramatic change in the person's appearance, especially in the eyes. People who come for treatment look very ill, often failing to make eye contact, and are rarely friendly or smiling. But after treatment they suddenly look alive, smile easily, with their eyes alive and bright.

Proof it works

We have 25 years' experience giving IV nutritional therapy as well as several years' experience giving IV nutritional therapy specifically for addiction recovery. For the vast majority of people (85 per cent) this produces a rapid reduction in abstinence symptoms and a much lower relapse rate.

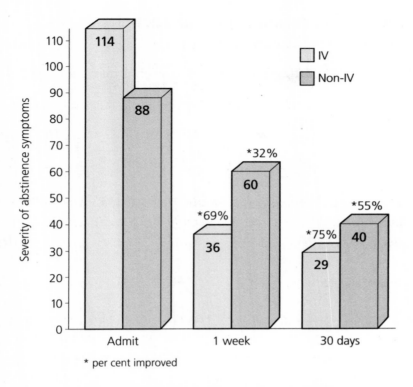

Comparing IV and non-IV nutrient therapy

To understand the effectiveness of IV nutrient therapy, consider the results of a study we did comparing the effects of one group of 16 people receiving diet and oral supplements alone for a month, and another group of 36 people receiving one week of IV nutrient therapy, followed by three weeks of the same diet and oral supplements.

Firstly, both the 16 non-IV and the 36 IV nutrient therapy clients remained drug-free (participants had a mixture of addictions: alcohol, heroin, cannabis, Ecstasy and cocaine).

We then measured each person's symptoms using the Scale of Abstinence Symptoms Severity, both at the start, daily during the week of IV and then weekly for the next three weeks. The charts that follow show a typical before-and-after Scale of Abstinence Symptoms Severity for those who received IV therapy.

SCALE OF ABSTINENCE SYMPTOMS SEVERITY
(BEFORE FIRST IV SESSION)

Name: Malcolm. 30 years old, addicted to alcohol, marijuana and nicotine

	Low level										**High level**
1. Craving/drug or alcohol hunger	(0)	1	2	3	4	5	6	7	8	9	10
2. Craving for sweets/sugar/bread	0	1	2	3	(4)	5	6	7	8	9	10
3. Craving for salt	0	1	(2)	3	4	5	6	7	8	9	10
4. Loss of appetite	(0)	1	2	3	4	5	6	7	8	9	10
5. Overeating/always hungry	0	1	2	3	4	(5)	6	7	8	9	10
6. Bloating or sleepiness after eating	0	1	2	3	(4)	5	6	7	8	9	10
7. Sense of emptiness/incompleteness	0	1	2	(3)	4	5	6	7	8	9	10
8. Feel tense, jittery	0	(1)	2	3	4	5	6	7	8	9	10
9. Anxiety/nervous for no apparent reason	0	1	2	(3)	4	5	6	7	8	9	10
10. Internal shakiness/shaky inside	0	1	2	3	4	5	(6)	7	8	9	10
11. Restlessness	0	1	(2)	3	4	5	6	7	8	9	10
12. Impulsiveness/act before thinking	0	(1)	2	3	4	5	6	7	8	9	10
13. Difficulty concentrating or focusing	0	1	(2)	3	4	5	6	7	8	9	10

continues ▶

14. Fuzzy thinking/head cloudy/
brain fog   0 1 (2) 3 4 5 6 7 8 9 10

15. Memory problems/memory loss   0 1 2 3 (4) 5 6 7 8 9 10

16. Depressions   0 1 2 (3) 4 5 6 7 8 9 10

17. Mood swings   0 1 2 3 (4) 5 6 7 8 9 10

18. Negative self-talk   0 1 2 3 (4) 5 6 7 8 9 10

19. Irritability/impatience/quick
tempered   0 1 2 3 4 5 6 (7) 8 9 10

20. Daytime sleepiness/drowsiness   0 1 2 3 (4) 5 6 7 8 9 10

21. Problems getting to or staying asleep   0 1 2 3 (4) 5 6 7 8 9 10

22. Fatigue/lack of energy/worn out   0 (1) 2 3 4 5 6 7 8 9 10

23. Hypersensitivity to stress   0 (1) 2 3 4 5 6 7 8 9 10

24. Hypersensitivity to sound or noise   0 1 2 (3) 4 5 6 7 8 9 10

25. Hypersensitivity to pain   0 1 2 (3) 4 5 6 7 8 9 10

26. Aches/muscle or joint pain/
headaches   0 1 2 3 4 (5) 6 7 8 9 10

Total Score: 78

SCALE OF ABSTINENCE SYMPTOMS SEVERITY
(AFTER SIXTH IV SESSION)

Name: Malcolm

	Low level									High level	
1. Craving/drug or alcohol hunger	(0)	1	2	3	4	5	6	7	8	9	10
2. Craving for sweets/sugar/bread	(0)	1	2	3	4	5	6	7	8	9	10
3. Craving for salt	(0)	1	2	3	4	5	6	7	8	9	10
4. Loss of appetite	(0)	1	2	3	4	5	6	7	8	9	10
5. Overeating/always hungry	(0)	1	2	3	4	5	6	7	8	9	10
6. Bloating or sleepiness after eating	0	(1)	2	3	4	5	6	7	8	9	10
7. Sense of emptiness/incompleteness	(0)	1	2	3	4	5	6	7	8	9	10
8. Feel tense, jittery	(0)	1	2	3	4	5	6	7	8	9	10
9. Anxiety/nervous for no apparent reason	0	(1)	2	3	4	5	6	7	8	9	10
10. Internal shakiness/shaky inside	(0)	1	2	3	4	5	6	7	8	9	10
11. Restlessness	(0)	1	2	3	4	5	6	7	8	9	10
12. Impulsiveness/act before thinking	(0)	1	2	3	4	5	6	7	8	9	10
13. Difficulty concentrating or focusing	(0)	1	2	3	4	5	6	7	8	9	10

continues ▶

14. Fuzzy thinking/head cloudy/
brain fog   (0) 1 2 3 4 5 6 7 8 9 10

15. Memory problems/memory loss   0 (1) 2 3 4 5 6 7 8 9 10

16. Depressions   (0) 1 2 3 4 5 6 7 8 9 10

17. Mood swings   (0) 1 2 3 4 5 6 7 8 9 10

18. Negative self-talk   0 (1) 2 3 4 5 6 7 8 9 10

19. Irritability/impatience/quick   0 (1) 2 3 4 5 6 7 8 9 10
tempered

20. Daytime sleepiness/drowsiness   0 (1) 2 3 4 5 6 7 8 9 10

21. Problems getting to or staying asleep 0 (1) 2 3 4 5 6 7 8 9 10

22. Fatigue/lack of energy/worn out   (0) 1 2 3 4 5 6 7 8 9 10

23. Hypersensitivity to stress   (0) 1 2 3 4 5 6 7 8 9 10

24. Hypersensitivity to sound or noise   (0) 1 2 3 4 5 6 7 8 9 10

25. Hypersensitivity to pain   (0) 1 2 3 4 5 6 7 8 9 10

26. Aches/muscle or joint pain/
headaches   (0) 1 2 3 4 5 6 7 8 9 10

Total Score: 7

As we saw in the chart on page 433, those receiving the IV nutrient therapy had more severe abstinence symptoms to start with than those receiving the diet and supplement regime (an average score of 114 compared to 88). However, within only one week, those receiving IV nutrients reported 69 per cent less severity of abstinence symptoms – a now lower score of 36, while those on diet and supplements alone, had cut their symptom score by 32 per cent to an average score of 60. Thus, the IV group attained a greater reduction in the severity of symptoms in one week than the non-IV group did in 30 days. At the end of the month those in the IV group had a 75 per cent reduction in abstinence symptom scores, now averaging a score of 29, whereas those on oral supplements plus diet had a 55 per cent reduction, now averaging a score of 40.

Generally, we find that people who reduce their abstinence symptom score to below 30 and keep it there are unlikely to relapse. However, it is important for those who have undergone the treatment to keep up the How to Quit Diet and supplements for as long as it takes to keep their score down, before switching to the maintenance programme.

One year on: how good are the success rates?

We contacted 23 people who had received IV nutrient therapy (along with other treatment approaches) one year after treatment. Of those we contacted 21 were clean and sober at the time of contact – that's 91 per cent. Of these, sixteen had remained clean and sober continuously (70 per cent). We also contacted seven others who have yet to complete a year since the IV treatment. Not one had relapsed. This kind of success rate is unprecedented in the field of addiction.

When evaluated independently most treatment programmes talk about a success rate of about 20 per cent after a year. The best non-nutritional treatment programmes achieve a 30–40 per cent success rate (still clean or dry one year after giving up).

Which treatment centres offer IV treatment?

To date, our work with IV nutrient therapy has mostly taken place in the US, where the treatment is widely available. Unfortunately there are few treatment centres in the UK which offer it (those that do are listed on the website www.how2quit.co.uk/treatmentcentres). However, we hope that this book will inspire more treatment centres to add this invaluable approach to their treatment strategies and offer a training programme for doctors wishing to train in this approach (see the website).

What does IV nutrient therapy involve?

The purpose of IV nutrient therapy is to specifically address your brain's nutrient and neurotransmitter deficiencies and damaged brain cell membranes. So, the first step is a blood test to find out about your deficiencies and imbalances. Then, a specific combination of amino acids, vitamins, minerals and essential fats are given to correct these deficiencies and imbalances.

On the morning of each IV session, the 30 or so ingredients are carefully mixed in the IV solution of normal saline. These are then slowly delivered by means of an intravenous drip, under medical supervision, over a four-hour period. During that four hours most treatment centres arrange other activities, including acupuncture, auricular therapy (see page 270), counselling and educational events, although you can watch television, read a book and move around, albeit in a limited way. You've probably seen the IV drips on stands in hospitals.

Usually, you will be working with a team, including a doctor or psychiatrist, a nurse who administers the IV, a nutritional therapist and a counsellor. IV nutrient therapy is just one piece of addiction treatment and needs to be part of an integrated approach.

We strongly recommend it for anyone in the early stages of recovery from significant addictions because most people have poor digestion and absorption due to damaged digestive tracts. Delivering nutrients straight into the bloodstream, bypassing the gut makes good sense, at least in the first week or two of therapy. It's a much faster, more reliable way of nourishing the body and brain of a person who is in recovery. Usually, IV nutrient therapy lasts for six to ten days, followed by a continuation of the oral supplements.

The IV packs are expensive to prepare, and each IV nutrient therapy costs in the order of £250 to £300. Therefore, a six-day treatment is usually in the order of £1,500, excluding oral supplements.

The other keys to its success

Two additional key ingredients in the success of IV nutrient therapy are already clear: education and ongoing nutritional support. People who have been educated about the nature of their addiction and the importance of nutrition, and who develop a good relapse prevention plan, are less likely to relapse. You need to know the importance of maintaining good nutrition and healthy brain chemistry to understand that what makes you feel like relapsing is probably abstinence symptoms. Knowing what to do when you are feeling down or empty, or craving a substance, is a vital piece of the equation. Therefore, studying this book in detail, as well as the educational package provided by the treatment centre, is a vital part of recovery.

How safe is IV treatment?

IV nutrient therapy is a very safe procedure. Occasionally, a person who has eaten just before they receive IV nutrient therapy may feel nauseous and could even vomit. However, this is easily avoided by having a last pre-treatment meal at least an hour before IV nutrient therapy (make sure it is light, and chew it well). Some people get a mild blush or facial tingling at the start of the IV infusion. This goes away in a few minutes and doesn't need to be treated.

In 25 years' experience giving IV nutrient therapy, both for addiction recovery and other conditions, we have seen one man who reacted allergically. He reacted to glutathione and was treated and recovered quickly. Glutathione sensitivity is very rare, occurring in an estimated one in every 28,000 IV infusions. Other than glutathione hypersensitivity, we have neither seen nor heard of any other serious reaction requiring medical attention, nor has there been any occurrence reported to us from any of the many treatment centres using IV nutrient therapy or from the providers of IV ingredients, over the past 25 years. This kind of safety record, compared to the number of adverse reactions attributed to prescribed medication, is remarkable (over 10,000 deaths per annum are attributed in the UK to prescribed medication).

To minimise this already minimal risk during IV nutrient therapy, nutrients are introduced very slowly in the first ten minutes, because most severe anaphylactic allergic reactions occur in this time – and can then be treated accordingly.

Conventional medical vs IV nutritional detox

Some treatment centres use IV nutrient therapy as a ten-day detox process, dramatically reducing symptoms of acute withdrawal. Others start the IV nutrient therapy after a medical detox. (Keep in mind that even if you have quit an addictive substance months or even years ago, but you still suffer from abstinence symptoms, you can still benefit greatly from IV nutrient therapy – see Bob's story on page 444.)

Conventional medical detox

During conventional medical detoxification from alcohol or benzodiazepines, for example, a prescription drug is given to ease the severity of withdrawal symptoms. The dose is gradually reduced as the symptoms subside. For example, Librium or Valium are often used to detox someone withdrawing from alcohol because these drugs calm the brain and allow the body to adjust to the absence of alcohol gradually. During this process the patient can still experience severe discomfort with tremors, nausea, vomiting and occasionally seizures.

However, conventional medical detox takes longer than the IV treatment because the addicted person has to also withdraw from the substitute drug and his or her brain chemistry is not being restored to normal.

Detoxing with IV nutrient therapy and oral supplements

Starting IV nutrient therapy immediately, as part of the initial detox, tremendously improves your chances of success. In addition, IV nutrient therapy and oral supplements can often be used instead of prescription medication, making early detox faster because, once detoxed, there is then no need to withdraw the substituted medications gradually. Patients treated with IV nutrients often report that their withdrawal symptoms are mild enough that they do not feel the need for any medications to help them through withdrawal (in particular those tough early days). Also, those who are on psychiatric drugs when they first enter treatment can more easily be tapered off using IV therapy.

The one important exception to the above approach is with alcoholics thought to be at high risk of life-threatening withdrawal seizures or delirium tremens (commonly known as the DTs). Here, we strongly advise that these individuals first be treated with the traditional acute medical detox protocol using medications, before IV therapy is introduced. However, immediately following traditional detox, IV therapy is remarkably effective. (There are reports of some centers using IV therapy in place of traditional medical detox and although this approach may one day become the treatment of choice for high-risk alcoholics, much more research needs to be done in this area).

The first couple of days of IV nutrient therapy detoxification may be a little uncomfortable, but nothing like that which addicts have experienced with other types of detox.

Case study **ERIC**

Eric told his counsellor when he came for an IV nutritional detox that he had never made it more than three days in a detox programme and he had tried numerous other methods. People who knew him jokingly called this Eric's three-day syndrome. He said if he was still there on day four it would mean something was working. The first couple of days he was mildly uncomfortable, had trouble sleeping, and was a bit irritable. But it was far from intolerable and for the first time he was not thinking of leaving. By day three he was feeling good, sleeping, and was very hopeful that, finally, he had found a way past his three-day syndrome. On day four he told his counsellor that his three-day syndrome was now 'history'. He had not only made it through the detoxification period but was already experiencing clarity of thought, which is usually not present with conventional treatment, even at the end of a 28-day programme. Following the IV nutrient therapy he went on to further treatment, which had never been possible before because he had never made it through detox.

Eric's symptoms even during the first couple of days were far less severe than other forms of detox. No matter how effective a treatment programme is in helping a person adjust to giving up and developing the skills for living without alcohol or drugs, it can't help a person who finds withdrawal so painful that he or she leaves before ever getting the toxic substance out of the body. Treatment programme recovery rates seldom include the people who leave before they complete the detox; the treatment centres count only those who stay around – but IV nutrient therapies succeed in keeping them around.

IV treatment will end long-term abstinence symptoms

Many people who have succeeded in giving up for months or years following traditional treatment, struggle with symptoms of impaired brain chemistry that never go away. These symptoms are relieved with IV nutrient therapy. So, it can improve your quality of life even if you quit some time ago but still feel s**t.

Case study **BOB**

Bob had 12 years without touching alcohol. He still attended AA regularly and thought that his life was as good as it was going to get. He was grateful for AA and the years of abstinence it had given him. He helped others stop drinking and stay away from alcohol through AA, but he was never really comfortable. He was stress-sensitive and sometimes quite irritable, and he had diffi-culty concentrating. Mainly he had a sense of internal discomfort that he could not describe but which never went away. He was not even close to drinking but he did want to feel better. He met someone who had received IV treatment and he couldn't believe this person could be feeling so good so early in recovery. He began to wonder if it would work for him, even though he hadn't had a drink in 12 years. So he decided to try it. He immediately found relief from the ongoing discomfort that had been with him for so long. Two years later he is still an enthusiastic sup-porter of the treatment and tells anyone who will listen about a way to feel better, even if they are no longer using drugs.

Getting the most out of IV nutrient therapy

Poor nutrition or the use of nicotine or prescription drugs or even severe stress can reduce the beneficial effects of IV nutrient therapy. However, if you are addicted to either benzodiazepines or psychoactive prescription drugs, especially if you are on more than one of these drugs, we recommend you consult your doctor with the aim of tapering them off before starting IV treatment, otherwise it is likely to be less effective. We also highly recommend that following IV treatment you continue taking supplements of essential fats, antioxidants, methylating B vitamins, amino acids and other key nutrients daily, and continue to follow our How to Quit Diet. This will help you maintain the balanced brain chemistry that has been restored by the IV nutrient therapy.

You will have to make many changes to stay off whatever you have given up, but these changes are very difficult when you are craving, depressed, nervous, irritable, feeling confused and unable to concentrate. After IV treatment and oral supplements, you will be better able to do the other work of recovery because your craving will have gone, your mind will be clear, and you will feel so much better. Even people who have had extended periods of being clean and sober in the past often say they feel better than they have ever felt in their lives.

IV treatment is part of recovery – not the whole thing

Sometimes patients feel so good after IV nutrient therapy that they are overconfident about their ability to stay off the substance. They have no desire to drink or use, so they believe they never will. But addiction is much more than brain chemistry. It affects all areas of life. In recovery you must also learn new patterns of behaviour and thinking. You may have to change your priorities; you will have to integrate regular exercise, perhaps change your friends and may need to address your spiritual needs. You will definitely have to change the way you eat. This doesn't happen automatically simply because your brain's chemistry is now in better balance.

SUMMARY

▶ IV nutrient treatment involves a four-hour intravenous drip, given daily for six to ten days. The drip is a combination of up to 30 nutrients, the kind and dose dependent on your nutrient and neurotransmitter imbalances.

▶ IV nutrient treatment rapidly reduces abstinence symptoms by two-thirds, making you feel dramatically better within one or two days, if not immediately. This tremendously increases your chances of staying clean or sober.

▶ IV nutrient treatment must be done in conjunction with an optimum nutrition diet and oral supplements, and followed up with an ongoing healthy diet and supplement programme.

31.

THE FOUR LIFESTYLE ESSENTIALS

As well as improving your diet and taking the right supplements, there are four lifestyle essentials that are key to reducing your addictive tendencies. These are:

1. Getting enough good-quality sleep.

2. Taking regular exercise to raise endorphins.

3. Generating vital energy.

4. Getting the past out of your future – emotional healing.

Getting essential sleep

Without enough sleep everything is worse, as we explained in Chapter 13: more tiredness, depression, anxiety and hence more desire for addictive substances.

Following these guidelines will help you sleep:

- Exercise regularly, but not after 7pm.

- Listen to alpha-wave-inducing music (see Resources) while in bed. This really works.

- Avoid caffeine after breakfast.

- Don't have a lot of sugar in the evening but do have more carbs and less animal protein with your evening meal. For example, have a vegetarian dinner of a tomato-based pasta sauce with vegetables.

- Avoid alcohol and nicotine, which, along with caffeine, are the most common causes of sleep problems.

- Leave at least three hours between eating and sleeping.

- Remove the TV, phone and computer from your bedroom. Your bedroom is for sleeping; it's not your office or TV room.

- Have a warm bath or shower before bedtime.

- If something is really bugging you, or you remember something and can't get it out of your mind, write it down to deal with tomorrow.

- If you are still struggling with sleep, take our Sleep Prescription (see page 397).

Find new pleasure in life by raising endorphins

When you raise your endorphin level you increase your feelings of pleasure and even euphoria. There is a variety of ways to do that, as we explained in Chapter 16. The most important, perhaps, is exercise – it really does make a big difference. Make a commitment to making exercise a part of your daily routine.

- If you are totally unfit, start by walking round the block, then build up to a leisurely walk for 15–20 minutes.

- If you are under 50, build up over time to a slow jog, first around the block, or a track, slowly increasing the distance and speed. For maximum benefit, build up to a full jog that lasts between 30 and 45 minutes, four to six days a week.

- If you are older – between 50 and 75 – briskly walk for 30 minutes five or six days a week (this will lower your risk of premature death by 70 per cent).

- Get a bike and cycle to close destinations, or round your local park.

- Join an aerobics class or learn to dance. There are many different options these days.

- Go swimming at the local pool.

- Go on a trekking/walking holiday.

If you do any of these for five days a week, you will start to feel fabulous, and look good too. Most important of all is to do something you enjoy, even though it might require some willpower to get started. The more you enjoy an exercise, the more likely you are to stick with it.

Other essential parts of a healthy lifestyle that also raise your endorphin level include:

Laughing There is nothing quite like a good belly laugh to raise endorphins and give you a surge of pleasurable feelings. Laughter should be a part of your daily life, no matter how grave you feel your circumstances might be.

Playing Having fun is as important to your well-being as working. It is as vital as other forms of nourishment. Play may take the form of socialising with friends, joining a group of friends in a game of football or in an evening of stimulating conversation. What is fun for you? Whatever it is, get a big dose of it every day.

Enjoying nature, music, art and water There are things to enjoy all around you. The important thing is to add colour to your life. When life is dull and drab the unhealthy things that you have associated with pleasure in the past will call to you. Turn a deaf ear to them by using endorphin-raising activities, which offer greater pleasure than the unhealthy activities you have given up.

Generate vital energy

As we saw in Chapter 4 all drugs deplete vital energy – what the Chinese and Japanese call chi or ki, and which we further explain in Chapter 17. Take up some form of exercise or practice that helps you generate your own vital energy. Here are a few possibilities:

• Yoga

• Psychocalisthenics (see Resources)

• T'ai chi, qigong or aikido

• Meditation

We also recommend that you try acupuncture and/or auricular therapy.

Get the past out of the future – emotional healing

Ultimately, the only person who can change you is you. It is best to get some help if you feel that you've become stuck in a rut and keep repeating negative emotional patterns, or if you always feel angry or sad, or you can't move on from things that happened in the past. Read Chapter 18 to find out more. Make a commitment with yourself to get some help. Here are some things you could try:

• Use the 12 Steps of Alcoholics Anonymous or a relevant fellowship.

• Practise the wisdom of the serenity prayer (*God grant me the serenity to accept the things I cannot change, courage to change the things I can and the wisdom to know the difference*).

- Find a good counsellor (if he or she is also interested in nutrition, even better – more on this in the next chapter).

- Check out the Hoffman Process; an intensive one-week residential course aimed at healing the addictive nature of our personality and getting back in touch with our bigger self or soul. (See Resources for contact details.)

In the next chapter we show you how to find the help you need and how to help yourself.

32.

WHAT YOU CAN DO FOR YOURSELF

During the process of recovery, you will begin to realise that as time passes without an addiction you have the freedom to choose. You are free to change your own behaviour, because mood-altering substances are no longer making your choices. With the freedom to choose comes responsibility. You are free to make responsible choices.

But you will find many things standing in the way of responsible behaviour. Habits developed while using will continue to plague you, but you can exercise your right to make your own choices and break patterns of behaviour that need to change. It takes effort and courage to change, and you may make some mistakes along the way, but that's how you learn. Mistakes are not failure; they are just mistakes.

Although we find comfort in the familiarity of old ways of thinking, feeling and behaving, we don't have to do things a certain way just because that's the way we have always done them. Change is a process; it doesn't happen suddenly and it's often difficult. Take one day at a time and be satisfied, as long as you are making progress. Here are some things that you can do.

Getting a little help from your friends

The world will not change just because you have given up and are on the recovery road. But you can still ask for what you need, and it's OK to ask others for their support. Support can come from many sources – there are many people willing to help if you are willing to tell them what you need. Don't assume that they will know without being told how they can give you support.

Social friends

A successful recovery involves developing new and more mean-ingful social networks. That means finding resources and making contacts that will enable you to meet new people who can offer more than just company to drink with, eat with, or get high with. Especially in the case of drug and alcohol use, it is important to develop new friends, because it can be hazardous to your health to hang around with the ones you got high with.

The people you associated with while using are tied to your addiction-related lifestyle. It is not that they are bad; you just have one central thing in common with them. If you choose to spend more of your time hanging around people you got high with, their expectations for you can become stressful or even impossible to ignore.

A mutual-help group such as Alcoholics Anonymous (AA), Smokers Anonymous (SA), or Overeaters Anonymous (OA), is a valuable source for establishing a helpful support network. You will find people there who not only understand your struggles but who will offer friendship, support, acceptance and encourage-ment. These groups usually offer fun activities without the substance you have given up. Don't forget how important it is to learn to have fun with people who do not centre having a good time on mood-altering chemicals. New friends, new activities, new social contacts are all part of recovery.

You will also want the support of friends you already have. Ask these friends for the kinds of help you need. A good friend will want to help but usually will not know what to do or say. For example, suppose you are recovering from a sugar addiction and want to go to a party, but you know there will be a big dessert table there. Confide in your close friend about your new way of eating and discuss the possibility of having healthy food options instead.

No doubt you will have friends who will be relieved that you are making the changes you are because they care about your health. These people will be delighted to offer the right kind of help. They will want to share in your plans and progress and be a strong, central component of your recovery programme.

Using a 'helping person'

This is a responsible adult who does not have a problem with alcohol, drugs or nicotine (whatever the case may be for you) and who is willing to assist in your recovery plans. You will need to have regular contact with him or her – preferably daily. This helping person is someone you can talk to about how your recovery is going and whether or not you are having difficulties. They will be someone who cares about you and wants you to stick with your recovery plans; someone who can point out to you if your thinking starts to change and you begin to move into 'relapse' ways of thinking. With your permission they can communicate with your counsellor (if you have one) to let him or her know if you are having a problem.

Your helping person can be a neighbour or a friend, but not someone you live with or even a relative that you are close to. The reason for this is that in the course of daily living people sometimes get into spats. You do not want those situations to affect your helping-person relationship. The helping person does not need to be a close friend; it can be someone you respect and who you think would be willing to help. It is best if this is someone that you can see on a regular basis or who would be willing to contact you regularly.

Sponsors

AA uses a system of sponsors to help new members, and this may be appropriate for you. The principles of AA are simple, but at first can be misunderstood. So, a practice has developed whereby members with a great deal of experience with the AA programme make themselves available to newer members as a sponsor. A sponsor's responsibility is to provide support during recovery, answer questions, discuss the various aspects of the programme, assist the new members in identifying meetings that would meet their particular needs, and direct them to appropriate literature and resources that they might need to understand the programme fully.

AA sponsors are not therapists or counsellors, nor are they responsible for telling other members how to work their programmes. All members are responsible for interpreting the principles for themselves and developing their own programmes based on those principles. The sponsor is merely a sounding board, a supportive friend and a knowledgeable resource.

Start a group

If you would like to have others to work more closely with you as you seriously attempt to learn more about what it takes to overcome an addiction and live a healthier life, you could form a group. This could be a group of people who want to study and discuss the information in this book and support one another in putting into practice what you are learning – it doesn't matter what addictions people have in the group. You may well know other people who are using this book as a guide. Ask them to join you to create a study group to discuss, personalise and implement what you are learning.

Or perhaps you would like to form a relapse-prevention group. This is a group of people who get together periodically to help each other develop relapse-prevention plans and stick with them. For materials to use for a relapse-prevention group go to www. miller-associates.org.

Self-protective behaviour

When all is said and done, you are responsible for protecting yourself from anything that threatens your ongoing abstinence. Reducing stress in your life and changing whatever you can that triggers abstinence-based symptoms is of prime importance. You are responsible for doing what is necessary to keep high levels of stress from sabotaging what you are trying to accomplish.

Some stress in life is necessary. It keeps you functioning. Without some stress you would not take care of yourself, go to work, or do anything for your family. But too much stress is harmful. Each of us has a level of stress at which we function most effectively. Your best stress level is high enough to keep you productive, yet low enough not to hurt you or the people around you. Finding the level of stress that is useful without being destructive is important to your recovery. You can relapse because of too little stress (no constructive concern about your addiction) or because of too much stress (which produces excessive worry and anxiety – and the stress hormones cortisol and adrenalin).

One of the most agonising abstinence symptoms is stress sensitivity. Most recovering people have a low stress tolerance and overreact to stress. As we have discussed before, this can create problems and sabotage efforts to stay clean (see Chapter 4). There are also actions you can take to reduce stress and increase serenity and peace of mind.

To protect yourself from unnecessary stress you must first identify your own stress triggers, those situations that might bring an overreaction from you. Then learn to change those situations, avoid them, change your reactions, or learn to interrupt them before they get out of control.

Self-protective behaviour means taking charge of potentially stressful situations, whether an isolated event or ongoing situations in your life. You may change some of your activities, eliminate some unnecessary activities or replace competitive ones with cooperative ones. On the other hand, it may be that competitive activities relieve stress for you. If so, you may want to add them. The point is to take charge of your own life – make choices that will strengthen your recovery rather than jeopardising it.

Self-protective behaviour means learning to set limits and asking other people to respect them. Only you can judge what is in your best interest and in the interest of the healthy lifestyle you are learning to live. And it is up to you to let others know what you choose to do and what you choose not to do. It is your life and your health. Make choices that you can *live* with.

Softening your environment

Hypersensitivity to noise (as well as to other sensory stimulation) is a common and most distressing abstinence symptom. When your filtering system does not work well, you cannot filter out unwanted noises. This can cause you to feel overloaded, overwhelmed and bombarded by your environment. But you can learn to soften your environment and separate yourself periodically from unpleasant noises and sensations.

You can use earplugs to sleep. In addition, a 'white-noise' machine might be helpful. These wonderful little gadgets emit a soft, masking sound like a waterfall, an ocean or similar sound that covers up the sounds that you hear as clanging, banging noises. An electric fan may work because it emits white noise of its own. Some people leave a fan on to give them constant white noise. Many of us are truly fans of fans.

There are also things that can be done where you live to quieten the environment. Double-paned glass doors or windows and carpeting on the floor – or even carpeting on the wall – can deaden sound and allow some protection from unwanted sound intrusions. Also, learn to lower the noise levels in your environment. Tone down the music and turn off the television once in a while. The environment can be softened with music, overstuffed furniture, simple, pleasant-to-the-eye decor and harmonious colours.

You can learn to separate yourself periodically from the constant stimuli you live with. You can put a 'Do Not Disturb' sign on the door to your bedroom or study. You can make time for quiet activities like browsing the libraries or museums. Or you can seek the quiet places in the great outdoors. In these ways you can temporarily eliminate noisy, chaotic activities.

Living creatively

If our creativity is blocked, we feel powerless and impotent. To live creatively is to give expression to our inner selves; to give us laughter, love, forgiveness and healing. Creativity might be expressed through cooking, gardening, caring for children, caring for the elderly, writing, playing, making love, decorating, painting, dancing, writing in a diary or journal, teaching, counselling, repairing, designing and many other activities.

If you fail to experience life's meaningful pleasures, however, this will create a void that will often be filled with destructive 'pleasures' that offer no hope and no joy. We need to sharpen our senses rather than deaden them. We need to wake up and see what is already around us. Someone has said that boredom comes from lack of involvement – so get involved.

But living creatively and joyfully does not mean being happy all the time. Struggle is a normal and usually necessary part of creativity – just as labour is a normal part of giving birth. To live joyfully is to experience a fullness of life, and that means to be open to suffering as well as to pleasure. Pain is woven into life's pleasures and comforts, and is even essential to them. When we turn away from struggle, we turn away from progress, and a deeper pain grows. To escape from normal pain and struggle is to escape from life. That is what mood-altering substances do for you. Freedom from addiction allows you to experience the whole tapestry of living.

So, find new ways to allow the creativity in you to be expressed. What could you do that would light up your life? What are you free to do now that you weren't able to do when you were limited by addiction? Now you can get involved.

Spiritual wellness

When we live in harmony with what we believe and value we create spiritual wellness, but where there is a lack of harmony between our values and our behaviour, we experience shame and guilt. Spiritual balance means that we are in harmony with ourselves, with our values, with others and with God (whatever that may mean to us).

Spirituality is not religion

Spirituality and religion are not the same thing. Religion is a set of beliefs about the spiritual and the practices based on those beliefs. Religion certainly is a means by which some people connect to the spiritual, but we may experience a spiritual awakening without being affiliated with a specific religion or religious denomination. A spiritual awakening is a personal experience that opens the door to creative and purposeful living.

Step 11 of the 12 Steps of Alcoholics Anonymous is helpful in giving guidance for achieving spiritual balance: *We sought through prayer and meditation to improve our conscious contact with God, as we understood him, praying only for knowledge of His will for us and the power to carry that out.* Just as we don't have to have any special concept of God to do this, neither do we have to use any certain definition of prayer or meditation. As we find harmony between what we believe and what we do, we are freed from the burden of guilt and shame to find spiritual fulfilment.

A wholesome, harmonious life does not mean that we never do things we regret or feel bad about. It means that we don't need to become discouraged by our inability to be perfect. We accept our humanness and strive for progress. We seek to eliminate activities that cause us to go to extremes at the expense of other important parts of life. We give up the need for immediate gratification in order to achieve a lifestyle that is more fulfilling and meaningful.

The last step of the 12 Steps of Alcoholics Anonymous is also useful to those recovering from any type of addiction. It says: *Having had a spiritual awakening as the result of these steps, we tried to carry this message [of hope] to others and to practise these principles in all our affairs.* A spiritual awakening occurs as we go beyond the struggle of controlling our addiction and, having found meaning beyond ourselves, we discover the joys of living. We experience enriching pleasures that take us beyond just 'not using'. We actively participate in life rather than passively hoping life will offer us something good along the way.

We can experience a spiritual awakening as we learn that spirituality is not separate from our daily lives but encompasses life and brings new meaning to all our affairs. Although spirituality must be defined by each of us for ourselves alone, it is interesting to note that the word is derived from *spiritus*, which means 'breath' and 'an animating or vital principle held to give life'. Our spiritual awakening allows this animating force to be breathed into all areas of our existence.

33.

WHEN AND HOW TO FIND HELP

The How to Quit Action Plan described in this part as well as the details given in Part 3 for your specific addiction provide the guidance you need for healing your brain and body naturally. The diet, supplements and other recommendations we offer for reducing or eliminating your abstinence symptoms are essential for your full recovery. However, some of you will need more; for example, in Part 3, when we talked about your own addiction we explained those conditions where you would need to get medically detoxed. You may not need medical detox, but you may still benefit from other kinds of help.

Addiction treatment centres

For those of you who have a serious addiction to drugs such as alcohol, heroin or cocaine, we strongly recommend that you seek the professional help available at an addiction treatment centre, either on an inpatient or outpatient basis.

Counselling

There are times when you need to tackle emotional or psychological issues that diet and supplements will not fix. We talked about this in Chapter 18. In this case a professional counsellor is the best kind of help for you. The counselling you might have if you get help from an addiction treatment centre is not usually what you need for addressing these issues. For one thing, you will probably not be ready to deal with painful issues from your past when you are learning how to get off and stay off drugs or alcohol. When you are ready, we recommend that you see a professional counsellor who understands addiction.

If you started drinking or using drugs early in life, you may have skipped some developmental stages of growth. During your teens and early twenties you become emotionally and socially mature. However, if you are drinking alcohol and taking drugs during that time, that developmental process may not occur or it may be slowed down. At whatever point in life you decide to give up drug or alcohol use as a way of coping with life, counselling can help you learn to manage your emotions and develop the insights and self-awareness that you may have missed by addictive living.

How a counsellor might help

A counsellor can help you resolve any shame you feel that might affect your recovery. Addiction is often accompanied by shame for a number of reasons. First, you may feel shame because of a condition that existed before your addiction (such as ADHD) and which increased your vulnerability to using mood-altering substances. Second, you may have done things while drinking or using drugs that you would not do when sober and which are very shameful to you now. Third, you may have a history of repeated relapse that you and other people interpret as being weak-willed or lacking strength of character. (Actually, the fact that you have kept trying despite what has been perceived as failure shows how strong your will and character are.) And fourth, there is the stigma that accompanies addiction. Most societies view addiction as a shameful condition. Even though we live in a culture that encourages drinking, overeating, pill popping and other excesses, when a person becomes addicted to alcohol, pills or sugar, they are looked upon as morally lacking, self-centred, pleasure-obsessed individuals. Learning to accept yourself as a person of worth despite the burden of shame that you or society have placed upon you can be a positive outcome of counselling. A counsellor can help you replace misperceptions you may have about yourself, the world or your addiction with accurate perceptions that facilitate behaviour change.

Helping you to live your life without addiction

In recovery you may need to learn or relearn certain life skills. If you want to change behaviour, a counsellor can help. You have developed many skills that have helped you survive addiction. These same skills can be modified to help you live your life without addiction.

If you can find a counsellor trained in Reality Therapy (see Resources) or Choice Therapy, we highly recommend it. (One of the authors of this book, David Miller, is a Reality Therapist.) This is a therapy that works well for people in recovery from addiction. It is a very simple approach to helping you change your behaviour. It asks you some direct questions to help you evaluate what you are doing and to help you make plans to change what you are doing if you really want to change. The questions are:

1. What are you doing now?

2. Is that working for you?

3. If not, what are you going to do instead?

The idea is to work out what is not working in your life and not just eliminate that but to replace it with better behaviour. With Reality Therapy you take small, manageable steps that lead you where you want to go. This is not a therapy for helping you quit if you haven't already. It is a therapy for helping you make other changes in your life that will help you to *stay* clean and sober. See Resources for some useful contacts to help you find a suitable therapist.

Coaching

Unlike counselling, 'coaching' (taken from sports coaching) refers to a partnership between a coach and their client to help them to succeed. Coaching is now being used extensively by people with attention deficit hyperactivity disorder, and it helps them with organisational skills, time management, to improve concentration and to build up confidence, for example. We recommend ADHD-type coaching, along with nutritional therapy, for people recovering from addiction. In the first place, many of you who have had problems with addiction may also have attention deficit hyperactivity disorder, treated or untreated. Second, many of the symptoms of ADHD are experienced by people who are recovering from addiction. Third and most important, many of the skills that people with ADHD need to develop are lacking in those with addictions. So let's talk about the benefits of coaching.

Coaching to enhance performance

The purpose of any coaching is to find your strengths and to build on them to enhance performance. The purpose of ADHD coaching is to enable you to do this by helping you (1) set goals; (2) devise a plan for reaching them; (3) set priorities; (4) make decisions; and (5) keep on track. The coach offers guidance and support while giving responsibility to you. The first phase in the coaching process is setting the agenda: that is, identifying your long-term goals. And remember, this is *your* agenda, not the coach's. The second phase is making short-term goals that will meet your day-to-day needs and lead to the achievement of your long-term goals. During the second phase it is important to check regularly to determine if the long-term goals are still applicable.

How it will benefit you

The value of coaching for you will be having someone available to guide you when you find it difficult to sort things out and prioritise tasks. Someone trained to do so can help you keep on track by continually holding up your goals and identifying whether what you are doing will achieve them. The coach can help you keep moving when you feel blocked by the obstacles you meet as you face the problems that have been created by your addiction. The coach can also help you identify what support you might need to organise to increase your chances for success; determine what you want or need to accomplish between coaching sessions; and decide what tasks will help you accomplish those things.

When you and the coach determine which skills you are lacking that are preventing you from achieving your goals, you will make plans for developing those skills or change your goals according to the skills you already have. The greatest value of having a coach is having someone to provide regular reminders of where you want to go and what you need to do to get there.

Two are more powerful than one

Coaching differs from counselling in that the power lies not in the coach or yourself, but in the relationship you have together (the coaching alliance). You are a full partner in the alliance. Your coach's goal is always to facilitate your agenda. By asking powerful and direct questions, reminding you of your agenda, and keeping you focused, your coach will allow you to plan your own course and to take the necessary steps to keep you on it. The alliance provides a safe environment for you to practise developing life skills.

Mutual-help groups

A mutual-help group is a valuable help resource. (These are frequently called self-help groups, but this is a misnomer, as these are not DIY– do it yourself – groups, but people helping each other.) You will find that these people will not only understand your struggles but also your need for deeper and more meaningful relationships. They will offer you friendship, support, acceptance and encouragement. Mutual-help groups provide fun activities without alcohol or other drugs. Don't forget how important it is to learn to have fun (with people who do not centre their good times on mood-altering chemicals).

In recovery you need the support of others, especially of people who are going through the same circumstances as yourself. For those who have problems relating to the principles or practices of AA or other 12-step groups there are other support groups available. Most groups – whether 12-step or others – encourage a new way of life based on honesty and reaching out to others. They offer a way and a means for making the right changes at the right time. They are based on members sharing their experiences and what has worked for them. These groups are places where you can meet people with whom you can feel safe and comfortable in new and healthy ways, as you attempt to understand the nature of addiction and the best way to stay clean or sober by learning from the experiences of those in the same boat.

Alcoholics Anonymous and other 12-step programmes

The most well-known support group is Alcoholics Anonymous (AA), founded in the 1930s by people who had tried many other methods of abstaining from alcohol but who had failed. They found that the mutual support gave them a tool that enabled them to do what had previously been unattainable. AA has endured over the years, and these principles apply to other 12-step pro-grammes such as Narcotics Anonymous, Overeaters Anonymous and Cocaine Anonymous.

Twelve-step groups are especially helpful for individuals who prefer a spiritually based group. The steps of AA, and others, are spiritual principles. In AA you are encouraged to accept the help of a higher power, although that power can be defined as you choose. It can even be the power of the group itself.

AA offers the recovering person many things that professional treatment cannot offer. It offers a readily available environment that is conducive to ongoing recovery and staying sober. AA is available 24 hours a day in every major city around the world. You are never farther away from a meeting than the telephone. In large metropolitan areas meetings are held at all times of the day and night. You can always have the phone number of someone who will help you avoid that one drinking or drug episode.

AA doesn't cost anything except time, energy and a motiva-tion to quit. You need a place to go to meet other people who are interested in having fun and socialising without drugs or alcohol. Many recovering people begin the social rebuilding process through friends and acquaintances they find at meetings.

Rational Recovery

Rational Recovery is an alternative support programme for various addictions utilised primarily by people who are uncom-fortable with the spiritual nature of Alcoholics Anonymous and other similar groups. As the name implies, Rational Recovery is based on the concepts of rational thinking. It was started by Jack Trimpey using the principles of rational–emotive therapy devel-oped by the American psychologist, Albert Ellis. In Rational Recovery, you learn to be more aware of your emotions and where they come from. You learn to recognise that emotions are not forced upon you by others or by outside situations. They are your own response to situations, and you can learn to take control of how you respond. Rational Recovery suggests five criteria to evaluate an idea to determine whether it is logical:

1. If I believe this thought to be true, will it help me remain sober (or clean, etc.), safe and alive?

2. Is this thought *objectively* true, and upon what evidence am I forming this opinion?

3. Is this thought producing feelings I want to have?

4. Is this thought helping me reach a chosen goal?

5. Is this thought likely to minimise conflict with others?

Rational Recovery helps you identify irrational ideas and beliefs that perpetuate addictive behaviour and then provides the means to change your emotions and behaviour.[3]

Your action list

In addition to the nutritional programme discussed here in Part 4, there are numerous other things you can do to strengthen and support your recovery.

1. If you have a serious addiction such as to alcohol, heroin or cocaine, we recommend that you get help from an addiction treatment centre.

2. You may also get help through counselling, coaching, or a mutual-help group such as AA or Rational Recovery.

REFERENCES

Part 1

1 Action on Smoking and Health, *Ash: Facts at a Glance* (2007) http://newash.org.uk/files/documents/ASH_93.pdf
2 NHS Information Centre: Statistics on Drug Misuse (2007)
3 The British Coffee Association Information Service, www.britishcoffeeassociation.org
4 United Kingdom Tea Council, www.tea.co.uk
5 S.V. Heatherley, et al., 'Caffeine consumption among a sample of UK adults', *The British Feeding and Drinking Group Annual Conference, Birmingham* (2006). See http://caffeine.psy.bris.ac.uk/results.htm
6 The Parliamentary Office of Science and Technology, *Cannabis Update* (March 1998)
7 NHS Information Centre: Statistics on Drug Misuse (2007)
8 ibid.
9 US Substance Abuse and Mental Health Services Administration statement
10 E. Costello, et al., '10-year research update review: The epidemiology of child and adolescent psychiatric disorders. II: development epidemiology', *Journal of the American Academy of Child and Adolescent Psychiatry*, Vol. 42(10) (2003), pp. 1203–11
11 Prescriber, www.escriber.com (5 August 2005)
12 NHS Information Centre: Statistics on Drug Misuse (2007)
13 T. Tarter, et al., 'Psychological factors associated with the risk of alcoholism', *Alcoholism: Clinical and Experimental Research*, Vol. 12(5) (1988)
14 T. Audhya, 'Advances in measurement of platelet catecholamines at sub-picamole level for diagnosis of depression and anxiety', *Clinical Chemistry*, Vol. 51(6) Supplement E-128 (2005)
15 K.A. Smith, et al., 'Relapse of depression after rapid depletion of tryptophan', *Lancet*, Vol. 349(9056) (1997) pp. 915–19
16 K. Beridge, 'Pleasures of the Brain', *Brain Cognition*, Vol. 52(1) (June 2003), pp. 106–28
17 T. Robinson and K. Beridge, 'The psychology and neurobiology of addiction', *Addiction*, Vol. 95, Supplement 2 (2000), pp. 91–227
18 K. Blum, et al., 'Reward deficiency syndrome (RDS): A biogenic model for the diagnosis and treatment of impulsive, addictive and compulsive behaviours', *Journal of Psychoactive Drugs*, Vol. 32 (2000), pp. 1–100
19 N. Volkow, 'The Science of Addiction', *Science World* (December 2006), pp. 16–17
20 K. Blum, et al., 'Reward deficiency syndrome (RDS): A biogenic model for the diagnosis and treatment of impulsive, addictive and compulsive behaviours', *Journal of Psychoactive Drugs*, 32 (2000)
21 J.P. Connor, et al., 'D(2) dopamine receptor (DRD2) polymorphism is associated with severity of alcohol dependence', *European Psychiatry*, Vol. 17(1) (March 2002) pp. 17–23. E.P. Noble, 'Addiction and its reward process through polymorphisms of the D2 dopamine receptor gene: A review', *European Psychiatry*, Vol. 15(2) (March 2000), pp. 79–89
22 D. Ball, 'Addiction science and its genetics', *Addiction*, Vol. 103(3) (March 2008), pp. 360–7

23 B. Molina, et al., 'Children with attention deficit hyperactivity disorder at risk for alcohol problems', *Alcoholism: Clinical and Experimental Research* (April 2007). B. Molina, et al., 'Alcoholism: Clinical and experimental research', *Journal of Abnormal Psychology* (August 2003). M. Johann, et al., 'National Institute on Alcohol Abuse and Alcoholism (NIAAA)', News Release, Vol. 27 (October 2003), pp. 1527–34. 'Substance abuse and learning disabilities: Peas in a pod or apples and oranges?' The White Paper, CASA the National Center for Learning Disabilities, the National Institute on Drug Abuse and the Ira Harris Foundation sponsored Conference (February 1999)

24 P. Shaw, et al., 'Polymorphisms of the dopamine D4 receptor, clinical outcome, and cortical structure in attention-deficit/hyperactivity disorder', *Archives of General Psychiatry*, Vol. 64 (2007), pp. 921–31

25 E. Noble, 'The gene that rewards alcoholism', *Scientific American, Science and Medicine* (March/April 1996), pp. 52–61

26 N.D. Volkow, et al., 'Prediction of reinforcing responses to psychostimulants in humans by brain dopamine D2 receptor levels', *American Journal of Psychiatry*, Vol. 156(9), pp. 1440–3

27 J.P. Connor, et al., 'D(2) dopamine receptor (DRD2) polymorphism is associated with severity of alcohol dependence', *European Psychiatry*, Vol. 17(1) (March 2002), pp. 17–23

28 B.M. D'Onofrio, et al., 'Causal inferences regarding prenatal alcohol exposure and childhood externalizing problems', *Archives of General Psychiatry*, Vol. 64(11) (2007), pp. 1296–304

29 D. Miller, et al., *Overload: Attention Deficit Disorder and the Addictive Brain*, Kansas City, Andrews and McMeel (1996)

30 Li Ting-Kai, et al., 'Isolation of II-alcohol dehydrogenase of human liver: Is it a determinant of alcoholism?', *Proceedings of the National Academy of Science*, Vol. 74(10) (1977), pp. 4378–81

31 A. Kampov-Polevoy, et al., 'Evidence of preference for a high-concentration sucrose solution in alcoholic men', *American Journal of Psychiatry*, Vol. 154(2) (1997), pp. 269–70

32 K Gilliland, et al., 'Ad lib caffeine consumption, symptoms of caffeinism, and academic performance', *American Journal of Psychiatry*, Vol. 138(4) (1981), pp. 512–14

33 L. Hindmarch, et al., 'The effects of black tea and other beverages on aspects of cognition and psychomotor performance', *Psychopharmacology*, Vol. 139 (1998), pp. 230–8. L. Hindmarch, et al., 'A naturalistic investigation of the effects of day-long consumption of tea, coffee and water on alertness, sleep onset and sleep quality', *Psychopharmacology*, Vol. 149 (2000), pp. 203–16

34 L.R. Juneja, et al., 'L-Theanine, a unique amino acid of green tea and its relaxation effects in humans', *Trends in Food Science and Technology*, Vol. OR10 (1999), pp. 199–204. A.C. Nobre, et al., 'Modulation of brain activity by theanine', a report to Unilever by the Department of Experimental Psychology, University of Oxford, 2003

35 Based on analytical testing by Unilever Research: www.lipton.com.au/ltheanine/news/teaandtheanine.html

36 D. Benton, et al., 'The effects of nutrients on mood', *Public Health Nutrition*, Vol. 2(3A) (September 1999), pp. 403–9

37 Dr Tapan Audhya had discovered that the level of serotonin found in platelets (which are tiny disc-like bodies in the blood) correlates very well with the level of serotonin in the brain. T. Audhya, 'Advances in measurement of platelet catecholamines at sub-picomole level for diagnosis of depression and anxiety', *Clinical Chemistry*, Vol. 51(6) supplement, E-128 (2005), pp. E-128. Next, he investigated whether people with depression do actually have abnormal levels of platelet serotonin by measuring platelet levels in normal and depressed volunteers. The difference was striking. In 73 per cent of depressed patients, serotonin levels were barely a fifth of those in the normal subjects (unpublished data).

38 R. Persaud, ed., *The Mind: A User's Guide,* Royal College of Psychiatrists (2007)
39 R. A. Hansen, et al., 'Efficacy and safety of second-generation antidepressants in the treatment of major depressive disorder', *Annals of Internal Medicine,* Vol. 143(6) (2005), pp. 415–26 Review
40 B.D. Healey, et al., 'Efficacy of anti-depressants in adults', *British Medical Journal,* Vol. 330 (2005), pp. 396–404
41 L. Watkins, 'Conference report at annual meeting of the American Psychosomatic Society in Denver' (4 March 2006)
42 G.A. Fava, et al., 'Effects of gradual discontinuation of selective serotonin reuptake inhibitors in panic disorder with agoraphobia', *International Journal of Neuropsychopharmacology,* Vol. 10 (2007), pp. 835–8
43 National Institute of Clinical Evidence, Insomnia – newer hypnotic drugs (No.77) – see www.nice.org.uk/page.aspx?o=ta077
44 See www.netdoctor.co.uk/medicines/100002841.html
45 O. Morgan, et al., 'Association between availability of heroin and methadone and fatal poisoning in England and Wales 1993–2004', *International Journal of Epidemiology,* Vol. 35(6) (2006), pp. 1579–85
46 See www.ppa.org.uk
47 J. Luty, et al., 'Is methadone too dangerous for opiate addiction?', *British Medical Journal,* Vol. 331(7529) (2005), pp. 1352–3

Part 2

1 R. Brown, et al., 'Neurodynamics of relapse prevention: A neuronutrient approach to outpatient DUI offenders', *Journal of Psychoactive Drugs,* Vol. 22(2) (April/June 1990), pp. 173–87
2 B.J. Sahley and K.M. Birkner, *Heal with Amino Acids and Nutrients,* Pain & Stress Publications (2001)
3 S. Ehrenpreis, *Degradation of Endogenous Opioids: Its Relevance in Human Pathology and Therapy,* Raven (1983)
4 L.E. Banderet, et al., 'Treatment with tyrosine, a neurotransmitter precursor, reduces environmental stress in humans', *US Army Research Institute of Environmental Medicine Brain Research Bull,* Vol. 22(4) (April 1989), pp. 759–62
5 E. Braverman, et al., *The Healing Nutrients Within,* Keats Publishing Inc. (1997)
6 K.A. Smith, et al., 'Relapse of depression after rapid depletion of tryptophan', *Lancet,* Vol. 349 (1997), pp. 915–19
7 B.J. Sahley and K.M. Birkner, *Heal with Amino Acids and Nutrients,* Pain & Stress Publications (2001)
8 W. Poldinger, et al., 'A functional-dimensional approach to depression: Serotonin deficiency as a target syndrome in a comparison of 5-hydroxytryptophan and fluvoxamine', *Psychopathology,* Vol. 24(2) (1991), pp. 53–81
9 E.H. Turner, et al., 'Serotonin a la carte: Supplementation with the serotonin precursor 5-hydroxytryptophan', *Journal of Pharmacology Therapy,* 109(3) (March 2006), pp. 325–38
10 E. Braverman, et al., *The Healing Nutrients Within,* Keats Publishing Inc. (1997)
11 Rogers, et al., 'Amino acid supplementation and voluntary alcohol consumption by rats', *Journal of Biological Chemistry,* Vol. 220(1) (1956), pp. 321–3. J.B. Trunnell and J.I. Wheeler, 'Preliminary report on experiments with orally administered glutamine in the treatment of alcoholics', American Chemical Society, Houston, Texas (December 1956)
12 P. Furst, et al., 'Glutamine dipeptides in clinical nutrition', *Nutrition,* Vol. 13(7/8) (1997), pp. 731–7
13 Ackerson and Resnick, 'The effects of l-glutamine, n-acetyl-d-glucosamine, gamma-linoleic acid and gamma oryzanol on intestinal permeability', *Townsend Letter for Doctors* (January 1993), pp. 20–3

14 B. Sahley, *GABA: The Anxiety Amino Acid*, Pain & Stress Publications (1998)

15 A. Abdou, et al., 'Relaxation and immunity enhancement effects of gamma-aminobutyric acid (GABA) administration in humans', *Biofactors*, Vol. 26(3) (2006), pp. 201–8

16 A. Barbeau, et al., *Taurine*, Raven Press (1975)

17 C.A. Lowry, et al., 'Identification of an immune-responsive mesolimbocortical serotonergic system: Potential role in regulation of emotional behavior', *Neuroscience*, Vol. 146(2) (2007), pp. 756–72

18 Y. Tsuda, et al., 'Clinical effectiveness of probiotics therapy (BIO-THREE) in patients with ulcerative colitis refractory to conventional therapy', *Scandinavian Journal of Gastroenterology*, Vol. 42(11) (2007), pp. 1306–11

19 B.R. Goldin, 'Health benefits of probiotics', *British Journal of Nutrition*, Vol. 80(4) (1998), pp. S203–7

20 H. Tiemeier, et al., 'Vitamin B12, folate, and homocysteine in depression: The Rotterdam Study', *American Journal of Psychiatry*, Vol. 159(12) (2002), pp. 2099–101. I. Bjelland, et al., 'Vitamin B12, homocysteine, and the MTHFR 677C->T polymorphism in anxiety and depression: The Hordaland Homocysteine Study', *Archives of General Psychiatry*, Vol. 60(6) (2003), pp. 618–26. T. Bottiglieri, et al., 'Homocysteine, folate, methylation, and monoamine metabolism in depression', *Journal of Neurology, Neurosurgery & Psychiatry*, Vol. 69(2) (2000), pp. 228–32

21 S. Gilbody, et al., 'Is low folate a risk factor for depression? A meta-analysis and exploration of heterogeneity', *Journal of Epidemiology and Community Health*, Vol. 61 (2007), pp. 631–7

22 H. Refsum, et al., 'The Hordaland Homocysteine Study: A community-based study of homocysteine, its determinants, and associations with disease 1', *Journal of Nutrition*, Vol. 136 (2006), pp. 1731S–40S

23 P.R. Jacques, et al., 'Determinants of plasma total homocysteine concentration in the Framingham offspring cohort', *American Journal of Clinical Nutrition*, Vol. 73 (2001), pp. 613–21

24 C. Blasco, et al., 'Prevalence and mechanisms of hyperhomocysteinemia in chronic alcoholics', *Alcoholism: Clinical and Experimental Research*, Vol. 29(6) (2005), pp. 1044–8

25 C. Halsted, 'Lifestyle effects on homocysteine and an alcohol paradox', *American Journal of Clinical Nutrition*, Vol. 73(3) (2001), pp. 501–2

26 S. Bleich, et al., 'Moderate alcohol consumption and the risk of cardiovascular disease', *American Journal of Clinical Nutrition*, Vol. 75(5) (2002), pp. 948

27 E. Giovannucci, et al., 'Alcohol, low methionine-low folate diets, and risk of colon cancer in men', *Journal of the National Cancer Institute*, Vol. 87(4) (V), pp. 265–73

28 P. Verhoef, et al., 'Contribution of caffeine to the homocysteine-raising effect of coffee: A randomized controlled trial in humans', *American Journal of Clinical Nutrition*, Vol. 76(6) (2002), pp. 1244–8

29 M.J. Grubben, et al., 'Unfiltered coffee increases plasma homocysteine concentrations in healthy volunteers: A randomized trial', *American Journal of Clinical Nutrition*, Vol. 71(2) (2000), pp. 480–4

30 'Only doses of 647 to 1032 mcg of B_{12} were associated with 80 per cent to 90 per cent of the estimated maximum reduction in the plasma methylmalonic acid concentration. [That's how you measure B_{12} sufficiency.] The lowest dose of oral B_{12} required to normalise mild B_{12} deficiency is more than 200 times greater than the basic RDA (Recommended Daily Amount) of 3mcg.' J.P. Simone and M. Eussen, 'Oral cyanocobalamin supplementation in older people with vitamin B12 deficiency', *Archives of Internal Medicine*, Vol. 165 (2005) pp. 1167–72

31 M. Malinow, *Nutrition Revues*, Vol. 56 (October 1998), pp. 294–9

32 K. Koyama, et al., 'Nephrology, dialysis, transplantation: Official publication of the European Dialysis and Transplant Association', Vol. 17 (2002), pp. 916–22

33 E. Menzano, et al., *Institute of Medicine, Food and Nutrition Board: Dietary Reference intakes for Vitamin A, Vitamin K, Arsenic, Boron, Chromium, Copper, Iodine, Iron, Manganese, Molybdenum, Nickel, Silicon, Vanadium and Zinc*, National Academy Press, (2001). P.L. Carlen, 'Zinc deficiency and corticosteroids in the pathogenesis of alcoholic brain dysfunction: A review', *Clinical and Experimental Research*, Vol. 18 (1994), pp. 895–901. S. Navarro, et al., 'Role of zinc in the process of pancreatic fibrosis in chronic alcoholic pancreatitis', *Pancreas*, Vol. 9(2) (1994), pp. 270–4

34 D.O. McGregor, et al., 'Betaine supplementation decreases post-methionine hyperhomocysteinemia in chronic renal failure', *Kidney International*, Vol. 61(3) (2002), pp. 1040–6

35 K. Brahmajee, et al., 'Potential clinical and economic effects of homocyst(e)ine lowering', *Archives of Internal Medicine*, Vol. 160 (2000), pp. 3406–12

36 A.J. Barak, et al., 'Chronic ethanol consumption increases homocysteine accumulation in hepatocytes', *Alcohol*, Vol. 25(2) (2001), pp. 77–81

37 T.A. Mori, et al., 'Dietary fish as a major component of a weight-loss diet: Effect on serum lipids, glucose, and insulin metabolism in overweight hypertensive subjects', *American Journal of Clinical Nutrition*, Vol. 70 (1999), pp. 817–25

38 L.J. Stevens, et al., 'Essential fatty acid metabolism in boys with attention-deficit hyperactivity disorder', *American Journal of Clinical Nutrition*, Vol. 62 (1995), pp. 761–8

39 Ibid.

40 L. Buydens-Branchey , et al., 'Polyunsaturated fatty acid status and aggression in cocaine addicts', *Drug & Alcohol Dependence*, Vol. 71(3) (2003), pp. 319–23. L. Buydens-Branchey, et al., 'Polyunsaturated fatty acid status and relapse vulnerability in cocaine addicts', Psychiatry Research, Vol. 120(1) (2003), pp. 29–35

41 A. Richardson, et al., 'The Oxford–Durham study: A randomized, controlled trial of dietary supplementation with fatty acids in children with developmental coordination disorder', *Pediatrics*, Vol. 115 (2005), pp. 1360–6; also see N. Sinn, et al., 'Effect of supplementation with polyunsaturated fatty acids and micronutrients on learning and behavior problems associated with child ADHD', *Journal of Developmental and Behavioral Pediatrics*, 28 (2007), pp. 82–91

42 J. Sontrop, et al., 'Omega-3 polyunsaturated fatty acids and depression: A review of the evidence and a methodological critique', *Preventive Medicine*, Vol. 42(1) (2006), pp. 4–13

43 L. Buydens-Branchey, et al., 'N-3 polyunsaturated fatty acids decrease anxiety feelings in a population of substance abusers', *Journal of Clinical Psychopharmacology*, Vol. 26(6) (2006), pp. 661–5

44 C. Iribarren, et al., 'Dietary intake of n-3, n-6 fatty acids and fish: Relationship with hostility in young adults – the CARDIA study', *European Journal of Clinical Nutrition*, Vol. 58(1) (2004), pp. 24–31

45 J.R. Hibbeln, et al., 'Omega-3 fatty acid deficiencies in neurodevelopment, aggression, and autonomic dysregulation: Opportunities for intervention', *International Review of Psychiatry*, Vol. 18(2) (2006), pp. 107–18

46 M.E. Sublette, et al., 'Omega-3 polyunsaturated essential fatty acid status as a predictor of future suicide risk', *American Journal of Psychiatry*, Vol. 163(6) (2006), pp. 1100–02

47 A. Tanskanen, et al., 'Fish consumption, depression, and suicidality in a general population', *Archives of General Psychiatry*, Vol. 58(5) (2001), pp. 512–13

48 M. Timonen, et al., 'Fish consumption and depression: The Northern Finland 1966 birth cohort study', *Journal of Affective Disorders*, Vol. 82(3) (2004), pp. 447–52

49 M. Raeder, et al., 'Associations between cod liver oil use and symptoms of depression: The Hordaland Health Study, *Journal of Affective Disorders*, Vol. 101(1–3) (2007), pp. 245–9

50 J.R. Hibbeln, et al., 'Essential fats predict metabolites of serotonin and dopamine in cerebrospinal fluid among healthy control subjects, and early- and late-onset alcoholics', *Biological Psychiatry*, Vol. 44(4) (1998), pp. 235–42

51 C.B. Gesch, et al., 'Influence of supplementary vitamins, minerals and essential fatty acids on the antisocial behaviour of young adult prisoners. Randomised, placebo-controlled trial', *British Journal of Psychiatry*, Vol. 181 (2002), pp. 22–8

52 B. Hallahan, et al., 'Omega-3 fatty acid supplementation in patients with recurrent self-harm: Single-centre double-blind randomised controlled trial', *British Journal of Psychiatry*, 190 (Feb 2007) pp. 118–22

53 S. Conklin, PhD., 'Cardiovascular Behavioral Medicine Program, University of Pittsburgh, at the American Psychosomatic Society's Annual Meeting', Budapest, Hungary, March 2007

54 C. Wang, et al., 'N-3 fatty acids from fish or fish-oil supplements, but not -linolenic acid, benefit cardiovascular disease outcomes in primary and secondary-prevention studies: A systematic review', *American Journal of Clinical Nutrition*, Vol. 84(1) (2006), pp. 5–17

55 D. Mozaffarian, et al., 'Dietary fish and n-3 fatty acid intake and cardiac electrocardiographic parameters in humans', *Journal of the American College of Cardiology*, Vol. 48(3) (2006), pp. 478–84. J.N. Dinet, et al., 'Omega-3 fatty acids and cardiovascular disease: Fishing for a natural treatment', *British Medical Journal*, Vol. 328(7430) (2004), pp. 30–5

56 H. Jensen, 'Choline in the diets of the US population: NHANES, 2003–2004', *Experimental Biology* (2007)

57 S.H. Zeisel, 'Choline: Needed for normal development of memory', *Journal of the American College of Nutrition*, Vol. 19(5 Supplement) (October 2000), pp. 528S–531S. S.H. Zeisel, et al., 'Perinatal choline influences brain structure and function', *Nutrition Revues*, Vol. 64(4) (April 2006), pp. 97–203

58 D. Wu, et al., 'Alcohol, oxidative stress, and free radical damage', *National Institute on Alcohol Abuse and Alcoholism Publication* (2004)

59 J. Grant, et al., 'N-acetyl cysteine, a glutamate-modulating agent, in the treatment of pathological gambling: A pilot study', *Biological Psychiatry*, Vol. 5:62(6) (September 2007), pp. 652–7

60 K. Stinson, et al., 'Barriers to treatment seeking in primary insomnia in the United Kingdom: A cross-sectional perspective', *Sleep*, Vol. 29 (April 2007), pp. 1643–6

61 D. Conroy, et al., 'Perception of sleep in recovering alcohol-dependent patients with insomnia: Relationship with future drinking', *Alcoholism: Clinical Experimental Research*, Vol. 30(12) (2006), pp. 1992–9

62 X. Liu, MD, PhD, 'Sleep deprivation can lead to smoking, drinking [Smoking & drinking can also lead to sleep deprivation – a two way street]', Research abstract of study conducted by the University of Pittsburgh at SLEEP, 2007, the 21st Annual Meeting of the Associated Professional Sleep Societies (APSS), 15 June 2007

63 V. Coiro, et al., 'Alcoholism abolishes the growth hormone response to sumatriptan administration in man', *Center for Alcohology, University of Parma, Italy, Metabolism Clinical and Experimental* (1995). A. Heinz, et al., 'Blunted growth hormone response is associated with early relapse in alcohol-dependent patients', *Alcoholism, Clinical and Experimental Research*, Vol. 19 (1) (1995), pp. 62–5

64 N.J. Pearson, et al., 'Insomnia, trouble sleeping, and complementary and alternative medicine: Analysis of the 2002 National Health Interview Survey Data', *Archives of Internal Medicine*, Vol. 166 (2006), pp. 1775–82

65 V. Coiro, et al., 'Alcoholism abolishes the growth hormone response to sumatriptan administration in man', *Center for Alcohology, University of Parma, Italy, Metabolism Clinical and Experimental*, (1995). A. Heinz, et al., 'Blunted growth hormone response is associated with early relapse in alcohol-dependent patients', *Alcoholism, Clinical and Experimental Research*, Vol. 19 (1) (1995), pp. 62–5

66 'Common ones include "daytime sedation, motor incoordination, cognitive impairments (anterograde amnesia), and related concerns about increases in the risk of motor vehicle accidents and injuries from falls', *Lancet*, Vol. 364(9449) (27 November 2004)

67 Editorial, 'Treating Insomnia: Use of drugs is rising despite evidence of harm and little meaningful benefit', *British Medical Journal*, 329 (20 November 2004), pp. 1198–9

68 S. Saul, 'Sleep drugs found only mildly effective but wildly popular', *New York Times* (23 October 2007)

69 P. Lemoine, et al., 'Prolonged release melatonin improves sleep quality and morning alertness in insomnia patients aged 55 years and older and has no withdrawal effects', *Journal of Sleep Research*, , Vol. 16(4) (December 2007), pp. 372–80

70 Review M. Sateia, et al., 'Insomnia', *Lancet*, Vol. 364(9449) (27 November 2004), pp. 1959–73

71 B. Sivertsen, et al., 'Cognitive behavioral therapy vs zopiclone for treatment of chronic primary insomnia in older adults: a randomized controlled trial', *Journal of the American Medical Association*, Vol. 295(24) (28 June 2006), pp. 2851–8

72 B. Feingold, 'Dietary management of behaviour and learning disabilities', in S.A. Miller (ed.) *Nutrition and Behavior*, Franklin Institute Press (1981), p. 37

73 C. Hallert, et. al., 'Depression is a common presenting symptom of coeliac disease', *Scandinavian Journal of Gastroenterology* (1982). Corvaglia, et al., *American Journal of Gastroenterology* (1999)

74 See www.gluten-free.org/reichelt.html

75 S. Størsrud, et al., 'Adult coeliac patients do tolerate large amounts of oats', *European Journal of Clinical Nutrition*, Vol. 57 (2003), pp. 163–9. L. Högberg, et al., 'Oats to children with newly diagnosed coeliac disease: A randomised double blind study', *Gut*, 2003, Vol. 54x, pp. 649–54

76 H. Arentz-Hansen, et al., 'The molecular basis for oat intolerance in patients with celiac disease', *PloS Medicine*, see http://medicine.plosjournals.org/perlserv?request=get-document&doi=10.1371/journal.pmed.0010001

77 P.B. Watkins, et al., 'Aminotransferase elevations in healthy adults receiving 4 grams of acetaminophen daily: A randomized controlled trial', *Journal of the American Medical Association*, Vol. 296(1) (5 July 2006), pp. 87–93

78 S. Nelson, et al., 'Mixing large doses of common painkiller and caffeine may increase risk of liver damage', *Chemical Research in Toxicology* (publication of the American Chemical Society) (15 October 2007)

79 N. Roglans, et al., 'Impairment of hepatic Stat-3 activation and reduction of PPARalfa activity in fructose-fed rats', *Hepatology* online (26 February 2007), pp. 778–88. K. Scribner, et al., 'Hepatic steatosis and increased adiposity in mice consuming rapidly vs. slowly absorbed carbohydrate', *Obesity* (Silver Spring), Vol. 15(9) (2007), pp. 2190–9

80 V. Kirimlioglu, et al., 'Effect of fish oil, olive oil, and vitamin E on liver pathology, cell proliferation, and antioxidant defense system in rats subjected to partial hepatectomy', *Transplantation Proceedings*, Vol. 38(2) (March 2006), pp. 564–7

81 H. Kaya, et al., 'The protective effect of N-acetylcysteine against cyclosporine A-induced hepatotoxicity in rats', *Journal of Applied Toxicology* (27 April 2007) [Epub ahead of print]. R. Ruffmann, et al., 'GSH Rescue by N-acetylcysteine', *Klinische Wochenschrift*, Vol. 69 (1991), pp. 857–62. O. Woo, et al., 'Shorter duration of oral n-acetyl cysteine therapy for acute acetaminophen overdose', *Annals of Emergency Medicine*, Vol. 35(4) (April 2000), pp. 363–8. S. Flora, 'Arsenic-induced oxidative stress and its reversibility following combined administration of n-acetyl cysteine and meso 2,3-dimercaptosuccini acid in rats', *Clinical and Experimental Pharmacology and Physiology*, Vol. 26(11) (November 1999), pp. 865–9. A. Makin, et al., '7-year experience of severe acetaminophen-induced hepatotoxicity (1987–1993)', *Gastroenterology*, Vol. 109(6) (December 1995), pp. 1907–11. P. Villa and P. Ghezzi,

'Effect of N-acetyl-L-cysteine on sepsis in mice', *European Journal of Pharmacology: Environmental Toxicology and Pharmacology*, Vol. 292 (1995), pp. 341–4

82 C. Weber, et al., 'Effect of dietary coenzyme Q10 as an antioxidant in human plasma', *Molecular Aspects of Medicine*, 15 (1994), Supplement S97–102

83 M.E. Shils, J.A. Olsen and M. Shike (eds), *Modern Nutrition in Health and Disease*, 8th edn, Lea & Febiger (1994), pp. 432–48; E. Schwedhelm, et al., 'Clinical pharmacokinetics of antioxidants and their impact on systemic oxidative stress', *Clinical Pharmacokinetics*, Vol. 42(5) (2003), pp. 437–59

84 ibid. Van Haaften, et al., 'Effect of vitamin E on glutathione-dependent enzymes', *Drug Metabolism Reviews*, Vol. 35(2–3) (May–August 2003), pp. 215–53

85 E. Schwedhelm, R. Maas, R. Troost, R.H. Boger, 'Clinical pharmacokinetics of antioxidants and their impact on systemic oxidative stress', *Clinical Pharmacokinetics*, Vol. 42(5) (2003), pp. 437–59

86 M. Touvier, et al., 'Dual association of beta-carotene with risk of tobacco-related cancers in a cohort of French women', *Journal of the National Cancer Institute*, Vol. 97(18) (21 September 2005), pp. 1338–44. J. Virtamo, et al., 'Incidence of cancer and mortality following alpha-tocopherol and beta-carotene supplementation: A postintervention follow-up', *Journal of the American Medical Association*, Vol. 290(4) (23 July 2003), pp. 476–85

87 M. Yoshida, et al., 'Dietary indole-3-carbinol promotes endometrial adenocarcinoma development in rats initiated with N-ethyl-N'-nitro-N-nitrosoguanidine, with induction of cytochrome P450s in the liver and consequent modulation of estrogen metabolism', *Carcinogenesis* (Epub 7 July 2004), Vol. 25(11) (November 2004), pp. 2257–64

88 Y.J. Moon, et al., 'Dietary flavonoids: Effects on xenobiotic and carcinogen metabolism', *Toxicology In Vitro*, Vol. 20(2) (March 2006), pp. 187–210. (Epub 11 November 2005), Review. P. Hodek, et al., 'Flavonoids–potent and versatile biologically active compounds interacting with cytochromes P450', *Chemical and Biological Interactions*, 22 January 2002, Vol. 139(1), pp. 1–21

89 C.D. Kay, et al., 'The effect of wild blueberry (*Vaccinium angustifolium*) consumption on postprandial serum antioxidant status in human subjects', *Journal of Agricultural and Food Chemistry*, Vol. 50(26) (18 December 2002), pp. 7731–7

90 C. Morand, et al., 'Plasma metabolites of quercetin and their antioxidant properties', *American Journal of Physiology*, 275 (1 Pt 2) (1998), pp. R212–9. H. de Groot, et al., 'Tissue injury by reactive oxygen species and the protective effects of flavonoids', *Fundamentals of Clinical Pharmacology*, Vol. 12(3) (1998), pp. 249–55

91 V. Cody, et al., *Plant Flavonoids in Biology and Medicine II: Biochemical, Cellular and Medicinal Properties*, Alan R. Liss (1988), pp. 135–8. H. Chow, et al., 'Modulation of human glutathione s-transferases by polyphenon E intervention', *Journal of Cancer Epidemiology Biomarkers & Prevention*, Vol. 16 (2007), pp. 1662–6

92 K. Hruby, et al., 'Chemotherapy of Amanita phalloides poisoning with intravenous silibinin', *Human Toxicology* 2 (1983), pp. 183–95. H.A. Salmi, et al., 'Effect of silymarin on chemical, functional, and morphological alterations of the liver: A double-blind controlled study', *Scandinavian Journal of Gastroenterology*, Vol. 17(4) (1982), pp. 517–21; 'Virchows Archive B – Cell Pathology Including Molecular Pathology', 64 (1993), pp. 259–263; *Gastroenterology* 109, 1995, pp. 1941–9. K. Kropacova, et al., 'Protective and therapeutic effect of silymarin on the development of latent liver damage', *Radiatsionnaia biologiia, radioecologiia*, 38 (1998), pp. 411–15; R. Campos, et al., 'Silybin dihemisuccinate protects against glutathione depletion and lipid peroxidation induced by acetaminophen on rat liver', *Planta Medica*, Vol. 55 (1989) pp. 417–1915

93 R. Rukkumani, et al., 'Comparative effects of curcumin and an analog of curcumin on alcohol and PUFA induced oxidative stress', *Journal of Pharmaceutical Sciences*, Vol. 7(2) (20 August 2004), pp. 274–83

94 V. Purohit, et al., 'Role of S-adenosylmethionine, folate, and betaine in the treatment

of alcoholic liver disease: Summary of a symposium', *American Journal of Clinical Nutrition*, Vol. 86(1) (July 2007), pp. 14–24. C.H. Halsted, et al., 'Metabolic interactions of alcohol and folate', *Journal of Nutrition*, Vol. 132 (Aug 2002), pp. 2367S–2372S

95 D. Lobstein, et al., 'Beta-endorphin and components of depression as powerful discriminators between joggers and sedentary middle-aged men', *Journal of Psychosomatic Research*, Vol. 33(3) (1989), pp. 293–305

96 J. Blumenthal, et al, 'Exercise and pharmacotherapy in the treatment of major depressive disorder', *Psychosomatic Medicine*, Vol. 69(7) (2007), pp. 587–96

97 M. Ussher, 'Exercise interventions for smoking cessation', *The Cochrane Database of Systematic Reviews*, Issue 3 (2007)

98 A University of Missouri-Columbia researcher has found that interacting and petting animals creates a hormonal response in humans that can help fight depression. In the study both pet owners and non-pet owners were asked to play with a live animal for a few minutes at a time. Johnson draws blood prior to and after the interaction and then compares the blood for hormone levels. Preliminary results indicate a significant increase in the levels of serotonin following interaction with the animal.

99 C. Streeter, et al., 'Yoga Asana sessions increase brain GABA levels: A pilot study', *Journal of Alternative and Complementary Medicine*, Vol. 13(4) (May 2007), pp. 419–26

100 A. Kjellgren, et al., 'Wellness through a comprehensive yogic breathing program: A controlled pilot trial', *BMC Complementary and Alternative Medicine*, Vol. 7 (2007), p. 43

101 *The Alcoholism Treatment Quarterly*, Vol. 11(1994), pp. 13–87. P. Grossman, et al., 'Mindfulness-based stress reduction and health benefits: A meta-analysis', *Journal of Psychosomatic Research*, Vol. 57(1) (July 2004), pp. 35–43

102 J. Brookes and T. Scarano, 'Transcendental Meditation in the treatment of post-Vietnam adjustment', *Journal of Counselling and Development*, Vol. 64 (1986), pp. 212–15

103 ibid.

104 ibid.

105 K.R. Eppley, et al., 'Differential effects of relaxation techniques on trait anxiety: A meta-analysis', *Journal of Clinical Psychology*, 45 (1989), pp. 957–74

106 'Acupuncture: New perspectives in chemical dependency treatment', *Journal of Substance Abuse Treatment*, Vol. 10 (1) (1993). Michael Smith, 'Acupuncture and natural healing in drug detoxification', *American Journal of Acupuncture*, Vol. 2(7) (1979), pp. 97–106

107 Jay M. Holder, et al., 'Increasing retention rates among the chemically dependent in residential treatment: Auriculotherapy and subluxation-based chiropractic care', *Molecular Psychiatry*, Vol. 6(1) (2001). Jay M. Holder, 'Beating addiction from bondage to freedom', *Alternative Medicine* (1999). Lisa Ann Williamson, 'The secret to success: Auriculotherapy treatment helps some with addictions', *Staten Island Advance* (18 March 2002). Kenneth Blum, et al., 'Reward deficiency syndrome: A biogenetic model for the diagnosis and treatment of impulsive, addictive, and compulsive behaviors', *Journal of Psychoactive Drugs*, 32, Supplement (November 2000), pp. 55–7

108 R. Schmitt, PhD, T. Capo, H. Frazier, MD, D. Boren, 'Cranial electrotherapy stimulation treatment of cognitive brain dysfunction in chemical dependence', *Journal of Clinical Psychiatry*, Vol. 45 (1984), pp. 60–63

109 S. Klawansky, A. Yeung, C. Berkey, et al., 'Meta-analysis of randomized controlled trials of cranial electrostimulation: Efficacy in treating selected psychological and physiological conditions', *Journal of Nervous Mental Disorders*, Vol. 183(7) (1995), pp. 478–84

Part 3

1 J. Lane, et al., 'Caffeine affects cardiovascular and neuroendocrine activation at work and home', *Psychosomatic Medicine*, Vol. 64(4) (2002), pp. 595–603

2 M. Grubben, et al, 'Unfiltered coffee increases plasma homocysteine concentrations in healthy volunteers: A randomized trial', *American Journal of Clinical Nutrition*, 71 (2000), pp. 480–4

3 P. Verhoef, et al., 'Contribution of caffeine to the homocysteine-raising effect of coffee: A randomized controlled trial in humans', *American Journal of Clinical Nutrition*, Vol. 76(6) (2002), pp. 1244–8

4 E. Salazar-Martinez, et al., 'Coffee consumption and risk for type 2 diabetes mellitus', *Annals of Internal Medicine*, 140 (2004), pp. 1–8

5 G. Kiejzers, et al., 'Caffeine can decrease insulin sensitivity in humans', *Diabetes Care*, 25 (2002), pp. 364–9. F.S. Thong and T.E. Graham, 'Caffeine-induced impairment of glucose tolerance is abolished by beta-adrenergic receptor blockade in humans', *Journal of Applied Physiology*, Vol. 92(6) (June 2002), pp. 2347–52

6 H.H. Chow, et al., 'Modulation of human glutathione s-transferases by polyphenon-e intervention', *Cancer Epidemiology Biomarkers Prevention*, Vol. 16(8) (2007), pp. 1662–6

7 A. Steptoe, 'The effects of tea on psychophysiological stress responsivity and post-stress recovery: A randomised double-blind trial', *Psychopharmacology*, Vol. 190(1) (January 2007), pp. 81–9

8 A. Hartz, et al., 'Randomized controlled trial of Siberian ginseng for chronic fatigue', *Psychological Medicine*, 34 (2004), pp. 51–61

9 J. Cleary, et al., 'Naloxone effects of sugar-motivated behaviour', *Psychopharmacology*, Vol. 176 (1996), pp. 110–14. S.A. Czirr and L.D. Reid, 'Demonstrating morphine's potentiating effects on sucrose-intake', *Brain Research Bulletin*, 17 (1986), pp. 639–42. L. Leventhal, et al., 'Selective actions of central mu and kappa opioid antagonists upon sucrose intake in sham-fed rats', *Brain Research*, 685 (1995), pp. 205–10. A. Moles and S. Cooper, 'Opioid modulation of sucrose intake in CD-1 mice', *Physiology and Behaviour*, Vol. 58 (1995) pp. 791–6

10 C.B. Pert, *The Molecules of Emotion*, Pocket Books, (1999). Dr Candace Pert is one of the chief scientists who discovered the central role endorphins play in addiction.

11 K. Blum, et al., 'Neuronutrient effects on weight loss in carbohydrate bingers: an open clinical trial', *Current Therapeutic Research*, 48 (1990), pp. 217–233

12 J.R. Davidson, et al., 'Effectiveness of chromium in atypical depression: A placebo-controlled trial', *Biological Psychiatry*, Vol. 53(3) (February 2003), pp. 261–4

13 J.E. Prousky, 'Vitamin B-3 for nicotine addiction', *Journal of Orthomolecular Medicine*, Vol. 19(1) (2004), pp. 56–7

14 M. Sateia and P. Nowell, 'Insomnia', *Lancet*, Vol. 364 (9449) (2004), pp. 1959–73

15 M. Holbrook, Editorial, 'Treating insomnia: Use of drugs is rising despite evidence of harm and little meaningful benefit', *British Medical Journal*, 329 (20 November 2004), pp. 1198–9

16 J.E. Prousky, 'Niacinamide's potent role in alleviating anxiety with its benzodiazepine-like properties: A case report', *Journal of Orthomolecular Medicine*, 19 (2004), pp. 104–10. H. Mohler, et al., 'Nicotinamide is a brain constituent with benzodiazepine-like actions', *Nature*, 278 (1979), pp. 563–6. B. Kennedy and B.E. Leonard, 'Similarity between the action of nicotinamide and diazepam on neurotransmitter metabolism in the rat', *Biochemical Society Transactions*, 8 (1980), pp. 59–60

17 C. Bockting, et al., 'Continuation and maintenance use of antidepressants in recurrent depression', *Psychotherapy and Psychosomatics*, 77 (2008), pp.17–26

18 A. Bjørnebekk, thesis: 'On antidepressant effects of running and SSRI: Focus on hippocampus and striatal dopamine pathways', Department of Neuroscience, Karolinska Institutet. Download: http://diss.kib.ki.se/2007/978-91-7357-246-0

19 V. Darbinyan, et al., 'Clinical trial of *Rhodiola rosea* L. extract SHR-5 in the treatment of mild to moderate depression', *Nordic Journal of Psychiatry*, Vol. 61(5) (2007), pp. 343–8

20 R. Vandrey, et al., 'A within-subject comparison of withdrawal symptoms during abstinence from cannabis, tobacco, and both substances', *Drug and Alcohol Dependance*, Vol. 92(1–3) (2008), pp. 48–54

21 S.D. LaRowe, et al., 'Is cocaine desire reduced by N-acetylcysteine?', *American Journal of Psychiatry*, Vol. 164(7) (2007), pp. 1115–7

22 S.N. Ramage, et al., 'Hyperphosphorylated tau and amyloid precursor protein deposition is increased in the brains of young drug abusers', *Neuropathology and Applied Neurobiology*, Vol. 31(4) (June 2005), pp. 439–48

23 A.F. Libby and I. Stone, 'The Hypoascorbemia-Kwashiorkor approach to drug addiction therapy: Pilot study', *Orthomolecular Psychiatry*, Vol. 6(4) (1977), pp. 300–8

Part 4

1 A. Steptoe, et al., 'The effects of tea on psychophysiological stress responsivity and post-stress recovery: A randomised double-blind trial', *Psychopharmacology*, Vol. 190(1) (January 2007), pp. 81–89(9)

2 K. Lindgärde, 'Having the right (whole) grains for breakfast keeps blood sugar in check all day', Swedish Research Council. Findings presented in a dissertation from the Faculty (Anne Nilsson) of Engineering at Lund University (11 September 2007) (www.vr.se)

3 J. Trimpney, *The Small Book*, Dell Publishing (1989)

RECOMMENDED READING

Braly, J. and Holford, P., *Hidden Food Allergies*, Piatkus, 2005
Braly, J. and Holford, P., *The H Factor*, Piatkus, 2003
Braly, J. and Hoggan, R., *Dangerous Grains*, Penguin-Putnam, 2002
Braly, J., *Dr Braly's Food Allergy and Nutrition Revolution*, Keats Publishing, 1992
Braverman, E., *The Edge Effect*, Sterling Publishing Co. Inc., 2004
Glenmullen, J., *Prozac Backlash: Overcoming the Dangers of Prozac, Zoloft, Paxil and Other Antidepressants with Safe, Effective Alternatives*, Simon and Schuster Paperbacks, 2005
Holford, P., with Colson, D. and Heaton, S., *The Alzheimer's Prevention Plan*, Piatkus, 2005
Holford, P., *The Holford Low-GL Diet Made Easy*, Piatkus, 2006
Holford, P., *The Holford Low-GL Diet*, Piatkus, 2005
Holford, P., *New Optimum Nutrition for the Mind*, Piatkus, 2007
Holford, P. and Cass, H., *Natural Highs*, Piatkus, 2001
Holford, P. and McDonald Joyce, F., *The 9-Day Liver Detox Diet*, Piatkus, 2007
Holford, P. and Colson, D., *Optimum Nutrition for Your Child's Mind*, Piatkus, 2006
Levine, J., Gelmini, J., Stevens, D., *The Miracle of Alphamusic*, Alphamusic Publishing Limited, 2008
Mathews Larson, J., *Seven Weeks to Sobriety*, Fawcett Books, 1992
Miller, D. and Blum, K., *Overload: Attention Deficit Disorder and the Addictive Brain*, Miller Associates, 2000
Miller, M. and Miller, D., *Staying Clean and Sober*, Woodland Publishing, 2005

Cookery

Holford, P. and McDonald Joyce, F., *Food Glorious Food*, Piatkus, 2008
Holford, P. and McDonald Joyce, F., *The Holford Low-GL Diet Cookbook*, Piatkus, 2005
Holford, P. and Ridgway, J., *The Optimum Nutrition Cookbook*, Piatkus, 1995

Other Books by the Authors

Patrick Holford
100% Health
500 Top Health and Nutrition Questions Answered
Balancing Hormones Naturally (with Kate Neil)
Beat Stress and Fatigue
Boost Your Immune System (with Jennifer Meek)
Food Glorious Food (with Fiona McDonald Joyce)
Hidden Food Allergies (with Dr James Braly)
Improve Your Digestion
Natural Chill Highs
Natural Energy Highs
Natural Highs (with Dr Hyla Cass)
Optimum Nutrition Before, During and after Pregnancy (with Susannah Lawson)
Optimum Nutrition for the Mind
Optimum Nutrition for Your Child (with Deborah Colson)
Optimum Nutrition for Your Child's Mind (with Deborah Colson)
Optimum Nutrition Made Easy
Say No to Arthritis
Say No to Cancer
Say No to Heart Disease
Six Weeks to Superhealth
Solve Your Skin Problems (with Natalie Savona)
The Alzheimer's Prevention Plan (with Shane Heaton and Deborah Colson)
The Fatburner Diet
The H Factor (with Dr James Braly)
The Holford Diet GL Counter
The Little Book of Optimum Nutrition
The New Optimum Nutrition Bible
The Optimum Nutrition Cookbook (with Judy Ridgway)

David Miller
Learning to Live Again: A Guide for Recovery from Chemical Dependency (with Merlene Miller and Terence Gorski)
Overload: Attention Deficit Disorder and the Addictive Brain (with Kenneth Blum)
Reversing the Weight Gain Spiral (with Merlene Miller)
Reversing the Regression Spiral (with Merlene Miller)
Reversing the Regression Spiral Workbook (with Merlene Miller)
Recovery Education Program (with Merlene Miller)
Staying Clean and Sober, Complementary and Natural Strategies for Healing the Addicted Brain (with Merlene Miller)

Dr James Braly
Dangerous Grains (with Ron Hoggan)
Dr Braly's Food Allergy and Nutrition Revolution
Food Allergy Relief
Hidden Food Allergies (with Patrick Holford)
The H Factor (with Patrick Holford)

Merlene Miller
Counseling for Relapse Prevention (with Terence Gorski)
Family Recovery: Growing Beyond Addiction (with Terence Gorski)
Lowering the Risk (with Terence Gorski)
Mistaken Beliefs About Relapse (with Terence Gorski)
Phases and Warning Signs of Relapse (with Terence Gorski)
Recovery Education Workbook (with Terence Gorski)
Relapse Prevention Learning Modules (with Terence Gorski)
Staying Sober: A Guide for Relapse Prevention (with Terence Gorski)
Understanding Addictive Disease (with Terence Gorski)

RESOURCES

www.how2quit.co.uk

This website, created by the authors of this book, provides information on nutritional therapists and other health-care professionals using the approaches recommended in this book. You will also find the appendicies referred to in this book, which cover a variety of topics. In addition there are articles, a free e-news and other resources to help you stay healthy and free from addiction. There's a simple online questionnaire to score your abstinence symptoms. You can also share your experiences and read about what's worked for others recovering from addictions.

Useful organisations and websites

Help with addictions

Blenheim Project is a charity providing services to people with drug problems in London. It also specialises in helping people with hepatitis C. Visit www. blenheimcdp.org.uk/.

Benzodiazepine withdrawal A useful support website for sufferers of benzodiazepine addiction wishing to withdraw and recover is www.benzo.org.uk. Another useful support website is www.bataid.org.

Brain Bio Centre is a London-based treatment clinic founded by Patrick Holford that puts the optimum nutrition approach into practice for people with mental health problems, including learning difficulties, dyslexia, ADHD, addiction recovery, autism, Alzheimer's, dementia, memory loss, depression, anxiety and schizophrenia. For more information, visit www.brainbiocentre. com, tel.: 020 8332 9600.

Miller Associates Through their website, David and Merlene Miller provide useful information and articles on addiction and ADHD, recommended reading and information on the road to recovery. You can order David and Merlene's other excellent books. Visit www.miller-associates.org.

Drugscope This is a very useful resource on addictive drugs. Visit www. drugscope.org.uk, tel.: 020 7940 7500. (Open 10.00am–1.00pm Mon–Fri.)

CITA offers help to people suffering from tranquilliser, sleeping tablet and antidepressant addiction. It provides a range of literature including *Back to Life*, available either in hard copy from 0151 281 5496 or in electronic format via the Internet at www.backtolife.uk.com/news. This book provides a comprehensive list of all the SSRIs and programmes for the withdrawal of these drugs and includes updated information on benzodiazepine withdrawal and a benzodiazepine withdrawal protocol. Training regarding prescribed drug addictions is available for health professionals. Visit: www.citawithdrawal.org.uk, tel.: 0151 474 9626.

Counselling

British Association for Counselling and Psychotherapy is an umbrella organisation maintaining a list of registered counsellors in your area. Visit www.bacp.co.uk, address: BACP House, 15 St John's Business Park, Lutterworth, Leicestershire, LE17 4HB, tel.: 01455 883300.

The Institute For Reality Therapy UK The idea behind Reality Therapy is that regardless of what has 'happened' to us, what we have done, or how our needs may have been unmet or violated in the past, to be happy and effective we must live and plan in the present. Visit www.realitytherapy.org.uk, address: PO Box 227, Billingshurst, West Sussex, RH14 0YU, tel.: 020 7870 8359.

Cognitive behavioural therapy

To find a cognitive or behavioural psychotherapist by visit www. babcp.com.

The British Psychological Society has a useful website to help you find someone in your area. Visit www.bps.org.uk or /bps/e-services/find-a-psychologist/ psychoindex$.cfm.

Eating disorders

If you have a concern about eating disorders, we recommend you contact BEAT – the organisation dedicated to beating eating disorders. (Formerly known as the Eating Disorders Association.) Visit www.b-eat.co.uk, address: 103 Prince of Wales Road, Norwich, NR1 1DW, tel. adult helpline: 0845 634 1414; youthline: 0845 634 7650.

Nutrition information

Food for the Brain Foundation is a non-profit educational project founded by Patrick Holford, which aims to promote awareness of the link between learning, behaviour, mental health and nutrition; and to educate and provide educational material to children, parents, teachers, schools, the public, the catering industry, health professionals and the government. The website contains useful information on nutrition, addiction and mental-health issues. For more information visit www.foodforthebrain.org.

Institute for Optimum Nutrition (ION) offers a three-year foundation degree course in nutritional therapy that includes training in the optimum nutrition approach to mental health. There is a clinic, a list of nutrition practitioners across the UK, an information service and a quarterly journal: *Optimum Nutrition*. Visit www.ion.ac.uk, address: Avalon House, 72 Lower Mortlake Road, Richmond, TW9 2JY, tel.: 020 8877 9993.

Nutritional therapy and consultations To find a nutritional therapist near you who we recommend, visit www.patrickholford.com and click on 'consultations'. You can have your own personal health and nutrition assessment online using the 100% Health Programme. Visit www.patrickholford.com and go to consultations.

Acupuncture and AcuDetox

The British Acupuncture Council is the UK's main regulatory body for the practice of traditional acupuncture with details of over 2,800 acupuncturists. Most acupuncturists are trained in AcuDetox. Visit www.acupuncture.org.uk, address: 63 Jeddo Road, London, W12 9HQ, tel.: 020 8735 0400, fax: 020 8735 0404, email: info@acupuncture.org.uk.

Society of Auricular Acupuncturists This society has details of over 300 trained Auricular Acupuncture Detoxification Practitioners all over the United Kingdom. Visit www.auricularacupuncture.org.uk, address: Woodpeckers, 19 Wildcroft Drive, Wokingham, Berkshire, RG40 3HY, tel.: 01189 773 433, fax: 01189 775 957, mobile: 07966 205811, email:mail@auricularacupuncture. org.uk. Or visit www.smart-uk.com (provider of auricular acupuncture for health-care professionals working with substance misuse).

National Acupuncture Detox Association (NADA) provides training for health professionals. Visit www.acudetox.com, address: NADA, PO Box 1927, Vancouver WA 98668-1927, e-mail: NADAOffice@Acudetox.com, tel.: (360) 254 0186, fax: (360) 260 8620.

Relaxation and mindfulness

Alpha-wave music Available from Health Products for Life (see page 488) or www.patrickholford.com/CD. The relaxation CDs *Silence of Peace* and *Orange Grove Siesta* by John B. Levine will bring you into an alpha state within four minutes. Very helpful for sleeping problems.

Meditation There are a number of different approaches and courses available. Two that have received good feedback are the one-day Learn to Meditate course offered by Siddha Yoga Meditation Centre, 32 Cubitt Street, London, WC1X 0LR, tel.: 0207 278 0035 and courses offered by the London Buddhist Centre at 51 Roman Road, London E2 0HU tel.: 020 8981 1225. Both groups have regional networks.

Courses and training

Arica Institute, founded by Oscar Ichazo, offers a one-day training session in the Doors of Compensation as part of a series that provide a clearly defined map of the human psyche in order that each of us can discover the basis of our ego process and transcend this process into a higher state of consciousness. Visit www.arica.org/trainings/schedule.cfm for details of trainings worldwide. In the US contact the Arica Institute Inc., address: P.O. Box 645, Kent, CT 06757-0645, USA, tel: 860/927-1006, email info@arica.org.

Hoffman Institute UK The Hoffman Process is an eight-day intensive residential course in which you're shown how to let go of the past, release pent-up stress, self-limiting behaviours and resentments, and start creating the future you desire. Visit www.hoffmaninstitute.co.uk, Box 72, Quay House, River Road, Arundel, West Sussex, BN18 9DF, tel.: 0800 068 7114 or +44 (0) 1903 88 99 90, email info@hoffmaninstitute.co.uk.

Courses are also offered in South Africa, Australia, Singapore and other parts of the world. For details on these and other international centres visit www.hoffmaninstitute.com.

Exercise

Psychocalisthenics is an exercise system that takes less than 20 minutes a day, and develops strength, suppleness and stamina, as well as generating vital energy. The best way to learn it is to do the Psychocalisthenics training. See www. patrickholford.com (seminars) for details on this or call +44 (0) 20 8871 2949. Also available in the book *Master Level Exercise: Psychocalisthenics* and on the Psychocalisthenics CD and DVD. For information, see www. pcals.com.

T'ai chi and qigong The Tai Chi Union For Great Britain provides details of teachers near you, events and news. Visit www.taichiunion.com. Also contact The London School of T'ai Chi Chuan and Traditional Health Resources, visit http://taichi.gn.apc.org/, tel.: 0208 566 1677.

Yoga The British Wheel of Yoga can put you in touch with a yoga school or teacher in your area. Visit www.bwy.org.uk/, tel.: 01529 306851, email office@bwy.org.uk.

Laboratory tests

Food Allergy (IgG ELISA), homocysteine and Livercheck tests are available through YorkTest Laboratories, using a home-test kit where you can take your own pinprick blood sample and return it to the lab for analysis. Visit www.yorktest.com, address: Freepost RLUC-GYTE-SGTU, York YO10 5DQ, tel.: freephone (in UK) 0800 4582052. Also see www.thehfactor.com for details of other labs and what to supplement depending on your results.

Biolab carry out blood tests for essential fats, vitamin and mineral profiles, chemical sensitivity panels, toxic element screens, and more. Only available through doctors. Visit www.biolab.co.uk, address: The Stone House, 9 Weymouth Street, London W1W 6DB, tel.: 020 7636 5959.

Individual Wellbeing Diagnostic Laboratories offers a wide variety of tests available to health-care practioners, including an adrenal stress test measuring cortisol and DHEA. Visit www.individual-wellbeing.co.uk.

Totally Nourish offers a selection of home tests referred to in this book. Visit www.totallynourish.com or call 0800 085 7749.

Product and supplement directory

UK

BioCare offer an extensive range of nutritional and herbal supplements, including daily 'packs'. Their products are stocked by most good health-food shops. Visit www.biocare.co.uk. For ordering, tel.: 0121 433 3727 and for further information contact BioCare Product Advisors on 0121 433 8702.

Solgar available in most health stores. Contact Solgar on 01442 890355 for your nearest supplier or visit www.solgar.com.

Totally Nourish offers a wide range of helth products, including all BioCare products available by mail order. Visit www.totallynourish.com, tel.: 0800 085 7749.

Nutriglow stock a zinc taste test called Lamberts Zincatest, along with many Biocare and Solgar products. Visit www.nutriglow.com.

SAM-e is not currently available in the UK. However, Nature Made (www.naturemade.com) produce a high-quality SAM-e product called SAM-e Complete, which is available in the US.

GABA is also widely available in the US and can be purchased from The Vitamin Shoppe (www.vitaminshoppe.com)

Bupleurum is available from Chinese herbalists (minor bupleurum decoction). The Chinese name is *sxiao chi hu wan*.

South Africa

Bioharmony produces a wide range of products in South Africa and other African countries. For details of your nearest supplier visit www.bioharmony.co.za, tel.: 0860 888 339.

Australia

Solgar supplements are available in Australia. Visit www.solgar.com.au, tel.: (free call) 1800 029 871 for your nearest supplier. Another good brand is **Blackmores**.

New Zealand

BioCare products (see above) are available in New Zealand through Aurora Natural Therapies. Visit www.Aurora.org.nz, address: 12a Battys Road, Springlands, Blenheim 7201, New Zealand.

Singapore

BioCare (see above) and **Solgar** products are available in Singapore through Essential Living. Visit www.essliv.com, tel.: 6276 1380.

UAE

BioCare (see above) supplements are available in Dubai from Nutripharm FZCO, address: Post Box: 71246, Dubai, United Arab Emirates, tel.: +971-4-3410008, fax: +971-4-3410009.

INDEX

Patrick Holford's

100%health

transform your diet, your health, your life!

Let me help you stay 100% healthy and informed

- ☐ **FREE e-News**
- ☐ **100%health Newsletter six times a year**
- ☐ **Instant access to over 100 Special Reports**
- ☐ **Useful information on products, services and courses**
- ☐ **Your questions answered**
- ☐ **Events diary of worldwide seminars and workshops**
- ☐ **Books details on titles available in every country**
- ☐ **Personal referral to the best nutritionists**

These services are available worldwide from
www.patrickholford.com
call **0044 (0)20 8871 2949** for a FREE special report

www.patrickholford.com

---

health products for life

Be all you can be

Health Products for Life is an online shop stocking a wide range of supplements, tests and products recommended by Patrick Holford.

- • Patrick Holford's formulated products by Biocare
- • Skincare by Environ
- • Health tests, including allergy and homocysteine tests, from YorkTest

EASY ORDER

Shop and order online @

www.healthproductsforlife.com

or call FREEPHONE ☏ **0800 085 7749**

Try our No. 1 Bestseller

OPTIMUM NUTRITION PACK

Your essential daily supplements in a handy tear-off strip

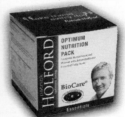

OPTIMUM NUTRITION FORMULA   ESSENTIAL OMEGAS   IMMUNEC®

AM
PM

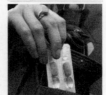